Phlebotomy
A Competency-Based Approach

4e

Kathryn A. Booth, RN-BSN, RMA(AMT), RPT, CPhT, MS
Lillian Mundt, EdD, MLS(ASCP)SH, LMT(NCBMT)

McGraw Hill Education

PHLEBOTOMY: A COMPETENCY-BASED APPROACH, FOURTH EDITION

Published by McGraw-Hill Education, 2 Penn Plaza, New York, NY 10121. Copyright © 2016 by McGraw-Hill Education. All rights reserved. Printed in the United States of America. Previous editions © 2013, 2009, and 2002. No part of this publication may be reproduced or distributed in any form or by any means, or stored in a database or retrieval system, without the prior written consent of McGraw-Hill Education, including, but not limited to, in any network or other electronic storage or transmission, or broadcast for distance learning.

Some ancillaries, including electronic and print components, may not be available to customers outside the United States.

This book is printed on acid-free paper.

1 2 3 4 5 6 7 8 9 0 RMN/RMN 1 0 9 8 7 6 5

ISBN 978-0-07-351384-3
MHID 0-07-351384-9

Senior Vice President, Products & Markets: *Kurt L. Strand*
Vice President, General Manager, Products & Markets: *Marty Lange*
Vice President, Content Design & Delivery: *Kimberly Meriwether David*
Managing Director: *Chad Grall*
Executive Brand Manager: *William R. Lawrensen*
Director, Product Development: *Rose Koos*
Product Developer: *Michelle Gaseor*
Senior Product Developer: *Michelle Flommenhoft*
Market Development Manager: *Kimberly Bauer*
Executive Marketing Manager: *Roxan Kinsey*
Director, Content Design & Delivery: *Linda Avenarius*
Program Manager: *Angela R. FitzPatrick*
Content Project Managers: *April R. Southwood/Christina Nelson*
Senior Buyer: *Michael McCormick*
Design: *Srdjan Savanovic*
Content Licensing Specialists: *Lori Hancock/DeAnna Dausener*
Cover Image: © *tiero, Veer*
Compositor: *Laserwords Private Limited*
Printer: *R. R. Donnelley*

Library of Congress Cataloging-in-Publication Data

Booth, Kathryn A., 1957- , author.
    Phlebotomy: a competency-based approach / Kathryn A. Booth, Lillian Mundt.—Fourth edition.
      p. ; cm.
    Includes bibliographical references and index.
    ISBN 978-0-07-351384-3 (alk. paper)—ISBN 0-07-351384-9 (alk. paper)
    I. Mundt, Lillian A., author. II. Title.
  [DNLM: 1. Phlebotomy—methods. 2. Clinical Laboratory Techniques. 3. Professional Competence. QY 25]
  RB45.15
616.07'561—dc23

                                 2014030354

The Internet addresses listed in the text were accurate at the time of publication. The inclusion of a website does not indicate an endorsement by the authors or McGraw-Hill Education, and McGraw-Hill Education does not guarantee the accuracy of the information presented at these sites.

www.mhhe.com

Dedication

To the users of this program, congratulations on your selection of an essential healthcare career. The skills and abilities learned in this program will provide you a lifetime of employment in a much-needed profession. To my family, all of whom have made this a great year, and especially to TJ and Jennifer for their perseverance and achievement of their goals.

—Kathryn A. Booth

Thank you to my family and friends who were patient and encouraged me while I spent valuable time away from them working on this project.

—Lillian Mundt

About the Authors

Kathryn A. Booth, RN-BSN, RMA(AMT), RPT, CPhT, MS is a registered nurse (RN) with a master's degree in education as well as certifications in phlebotomy, pharmacy tech, and medical assisting. She is an author, educator, and consultant for Total Care Programming, Inc. She has over 30 years of teaching, nursing, and healthcare work experience that spans five states. As an educator, Kathy has been awarded the teacher of the year in three states where she taught various health sciences, including phlebotomy. Kathy serves on the American Medical Technologists registered Phlebotomy Technician Examinations, Qualifications, and Standards Committee. She stays current in the field by practicing her skills in various settings as well as by maintaining and obtaining certifications. In addition, Kathy volunteers at a free healthcare clinic and teaches online. She is a member of advisory boards at two educational institutions. Her larger goal is to develop up-to-date, dynamic healthcare educational materials to assist other educators as well as to promote the healthcare professions. In addition, Kathy enjoys presenting innovative new learning solutions for the changing healthcare and educational landscape to her fellow professionals nationwide.

Lillian A. Mundt, EdD, MLS(ASCP)SH, LMT(NCBMT) is a medical laboratory scientist, massage therapist, curriculum designer, and author. Her background includes a bachelor's degree in medical technology, a master's degree in health professions education, and a doctorate in educational leadership. For over 30 years, she has developed and taught phlebotomy programs, clinical laboratory science programs, and graduate programs at both hospital and university-based institutions. She has authored and developed course materials used in online continuing education programs for colleges and universities, as well as online continuing education companies. In addition, Dr. Mundt has authored several articles for professional journals; a text for Lippincott, Williams, and Wilkins; and a published dissertation. Dr. Mundt has presented at local, state, and national conventions since 1994. Her current focus is on developing educational materials for medical laboratory science and health professions education. She remains current in both her professions by maintaining employment as a Medical Laboratory Scientist (MLS) as well as by developing and teaching courses on a contractual basis.

Brief Contents

Contents

Preface

Competency is within your reach with the new, fourth edition of *Phlebotomy: A Competency-Based Approach.* With *Phlebotomy*'s pedagogy-rich format and plentiful Competency Checks, easily grasp not only essential phlebotomy skills and competencies, but also the critical soft skills needed for a successful transition from classroom to lab. *Phlebotomy* is also now available with McGraw-Hill Education's revolutionary adaptive learning technology, LearnSmart and SmartBook! You can study smarter, spending your valuable time on topics you don't know and less time on the topics you have already mastered. Hit your target with precision using LearnSmart . . . Join the learning revolution and achieve the success you deserve today!

New to the Fourth Edition

Overview

A number of enhancements have been made in the fourth edition to enrich the user's experience with the product.

- More than 20 brand-new Competency Checks are now included near appropriate content to draw attention to the steps of key procedures, encouraging student remediation. From nasopharyngeal swab collection and glucose testing to blood culture collection via butterfly and syringe, these pedagogical features reinforce the text's competency-based approach. Competency Checklists—now moved to the end of each chapter—also make practicing skills and preparing for certification and accreditation easy.
- Learning Outcomes (LOs) have been streamlined to directly correlate with the corresponding section in each chapter. The section headings are numbered to match the numbered LOs. The LOs are summarized in a table at the end of each chapter with links to the related NAACLS Competencies, which are still listed at the beginning of each chapter.
- Based on market feedback, Chapter 8—formerly "Routine Blood Collection"—is now two chapters: Chapter 8, Venipuncture, and Chapter 9, Dermal/Capillary Puncture. These two new chapters clarify both the differences

and similarities between venipuncture and dermal/capillary puncture.

- Per customer feedback, the answer keys for Checkpoint Questions and Chapter Review questions have been removed from the end of the book. Instructors will now have access to these via an Instructor's Manual, available (password-protected) in the Instructor Resources under the Library tab in *Connect*.
- Checkpoint Questions—previously multiple choice—are now short answer to further encourage critical thinking. There are now at least two Checkpoint Questions at the end of each section.
- More than 50 new photographs—taken by the authors—have been added that accurately reflect the realities of today's phlebotomy workplace.
- *Connect* Phlebotomy has been updated to reflect updates in the chapters and feedback from customers.
- *Phlebotomy* is now available with the LearnSmart Advantage, a series of adaptive learning products fueled by LearnSmart and SmartBook.

Chapter Highlights

While content updates have been made to all of the chapters, here are the highlights:

- **Chapter 2:** Now covers bioterrorism preparation as well as the Global Harmonized System and HMIS Labeling System for hazard communication. The text now reflects current OSHA terminology and standards as well.
- **Chapter 3:** New section and table link phlebotomy-specific terminology to the process of deconstructing medical terminology.
- **Chapter 4:** Now includes a learning outcome for each body system to make the content easier to navigate. New tables identify key blood tests per body system, describe the tests, and pair them with specific diseases and disorders to make basic anatomy, physiology, and pathophysiology relevant to the phlebotomist.
- **Chapter 7:** Includes a new learning outcome on phlebotomy equipment by manufacturer as well as a section on transfer devices. New mnemonic

order of draw table and content added to reinforce student retention of this crucial concept.

- **Chapter 8:** New content on venipuncture complications covers iatrogenic anemia and populations at high risk of exsanguination. Chapter now deals solely with venipuncture.
- **Chapter 9:** Capillary/dermal puncture information is now covered in its own chapter.
- **Chapter 11:** Special procedures routinely performed by phlebotomists have been moved to the front of the chapter, before arterial puncture and venous access device information. Section on blood culture preparative cleaning is completely revised.
- **Chapter 13:** Nasal and nasopharyngeal swabs now included, along with other, less-common swabs. Regulatory compliance information has been expanded and updated.
- **Chapter 14:** Information on diversity in healthcare and cultural awareness has been fully revised. Work experience requirements as well as certification, registration, and licensure information have been updated and reinforced with new details.

For a detailed transition guide between the third and fourth editions of *Phlebotomy*, visit the Instructor Resources in *Connect*!

Phlebotomy Preparation in the Digital World: Supplementary Materials for the Instructor and Student

Instructors, McGraw-Hill Education knows how much effort it takes to prepare for a new course. Through focus groups, symposia, reviews, and conversations with instructors like you, we have gathered information about what materials you need in order to facilitate successful courses. We are committed to providing you with high-quality, accurate instructor support. Knowing the importance of flexibility and digital learning, McGraw-Hill Education has created multiple assets to enhance the learning experience no matter what the class format: traditional, online, or hybrid. This product is designed to help instructors and students be successful, with digital solutions proven to drive student success.

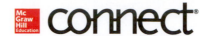

A one-stop spot to present, deliver, and assess digital assets available from McGraw-Hill: McGraw-Hill *Connect* Phlebotomy

McGraw-Hill *Connect*® **Phlebotomy** provides online presentation, assignment, and assessment solutions. It connects your students with the tools and resources they'll need to achieve success. With *Connect* you can deliver assignments, quizzes, and tests online. A robust set of questions and activities, including all of the end-of-section and end-of-chapter questions, additional questions to help your students prepare for certification exams, skills videos, and interactives are presented and aligned with the textbook's learning outcomes. As an instructor, you can edit existing questions and author entirely new problems. *Connect* enables you to track individual student performance—by question, by assignment, or in relation to the class overall—with detailed grade reports. You can integrate grade reports easily with learning management systems (LMSs) such as Blackboard, Desire2Learn, or eCollege—and much more. 24/7 online access to an eBook also comes standard with *Connect*. This media-rich version of the textbook is available through the McGraw-Hill *Connect* platform and allows seamless integration of text, media, and assessments. To learn more, visit http://connect.mheducation.com.

Connect Insight™ is the first and only analytics tool of its kind, which highlights a series of visual data displays—each framed by an intuitive question—to provide at-a-glance information regarding how your class is doing. As an instructor or administrator, you receive an instant, at-a-glance view of student performance matched with student activity. It puts real-time analytics in your hands so you can take action early and keep struggling students from falling behind. It also allows you to be empowered with a more valuable, transparent, and productive connection between you and your students. Available on demand wherever and whenever it's needed, Connect Insight travels from office to classroom!

A single sign-on with Connect and your Blackboard course: McGraw-Hill Education and Blackboard—for a premium user experience

Blackboard®, the web-based course management system, has partnered with McGraw-Hill Education to better allow students and faculty to use online materials and activities to complement face-to-face teaching. Blackboard features exciting social learning and teaching tools that foster active learning opportunities for students. You'll transform your closed-door classroom into communities where students remain connected to their educational experience 24 hours a day. This partnership allows you and your students access to *Connect* and McGraw-Hill *Create*™ right from within your Blackboard course—all with a single sign-on. Not only do you get single sign-on with *Connect* and *Create*, but you also get deep integration of McGraw-Hill Education content and content engines right in Blackboard. Whether you're choosing a book for your course or building *Connect* assignments, all the tools you need are right where you want them—inside Blackboard. Gradebooks are now seamless. When a student completes an integrated *Connect* assignment, the grade for that assignment automatically (and instantly) feeds into your Blackboard grade center. McGraw-Hill and Blackboard can now offer you easy access to industry-leading technology and content, whether your campus hosts it or we do. Be sure to ask your local McGraw-Hill Education representative for details.

Still want single sign-on solutions and using another LMS? See how **McGraw-Hill Campus®** http://mhcampus.mhhe.com/ makes the grade by offering universal sign-on, automatic registration, gradebook synchronization, and open access to a multitude of learning resources—all in one place. MH Campus supports Active Directory, Angel, Blackboard, Canvas, Desire2Learn, eCollege, IMS, LDAP, Moodle, Moodlerooms, Sakai, Shibboleth, WebCT, BrainHoney, Campus Cruiser, and Jenzibar eRacer. Additionally, MH Campus can be easily connected with other authentication authorities and LMSs.

Create a textbook organized the way you teach: McGraw-Hill Create

With **McGraw-Hill Create**, you can easily rearrange chapters, combine material from other content sources, and quickly upload content you have written, such as your course syllabus or teaching notes. Find the content you need in *Create* by searching through thousands of leading McGraw-Hill Education textbooks. Arrange your book to fit your teaching style. *Create* even allows you to personalize your book's appearance by selecting the cover and adding your name, school, and course information. Order a *Create* book and you'll receive a complimentary print review copy in 3 to 5 business days or a complimentary electronic review copy (eComp) via e-mail in minutes. Go to **www.mcgrawhill create.com** today and register to experience how *Create* empowers you to teach *your* students *your* way.

Record and distribute your lectures for multiple viewing: My Lectures—Tegrity

McGraw-Hill Tegrity® records and distributes your class lecture with just a click of a button. Students can view it anytime and anywhere via computer, iPod, or mobile device. It indexes as it records your PowerPoint presentations and anything shown on your computer, so students can use keywords to find exactly what they want to study. Tegrity is available as an integrated feature of **Connect** **Phlebotomy** and as a stand-alone product.

New from McGraw-Hill Education, LearnSmart Advantage is a series of adaptive learning products fueled by **McGraw-Hill LearnSmart®**, the most widely used and intelligent adaptive learning resource proven to improve learning since 2009. Developed to deliver demonstrable results in boosting grades, increasing course retention, and strengthening memory recall, the LearnSmart Advantage series spans the entire learning process from course preparation to providing the first adaptive reading experience found only in **McGraw-Hill SmartBook®**. Distinguishing what students know from what they don't, and honing in on concepts they are most likely to forget, each product in the series helps students study smarter and retain more knowledge. A smarter learning experience for students coupled with valuable reporting tools for instructors, and available in hundreds of course areas, LearnSmart Advantage is advancing learning like no other products in higher education today. Go to **www. LearnSmartAdvantage.com** for more information.

LEARNSMART®

LearnSmart is one of the most effective and successful adaptive learning resources available on the market today and is now available for Phlebotomy. More than 2 million students have answered more than 1.3 billion questions in LearnSmart since 2009, making it the most widely used and intelligent adaptive study tool that's proven to strengthen memory recall, keep students in class, and boost grades. Students using LearnSmart are 13% more likely to pass their classes and 35% less likely to drop out. This revolutionary learning resource is available only from McGraw-Hill Education; join the learning revolution and start using LearnSmart today!

SMARTBOOK®

SmartBook is the first and only adaptive reading experience available today. SmartBook personalizes content for each student in a continuously adapting reading experience. Reading is no longer a passive and linear experience, but an engaging and dynamic one where students are more likely to master and retain important concepts, coming to class better prepared. Valuable reports provide instructors insight as to how students are progressing through textbook content and are useful for shaping in-class time or assessment. As a result of the adaptive reading experience found in SmartBook, students are more likely to retain knowledge, stay in class, and get better grades. This revolutionary technology is available only from McGraw-Hill Education and for hundreds of course areas as part of the LearnSmart Advantage series.

Instructor Resources

You can rely on the following materials to help you and your students work through the material in this book. All of the resources in the following table are available in the Instructor Resources under the Library tab in *Connect*.

Instructor Resources	
Supplement	**Features**
Instructor's Manual	Each chapter has • Learning outcomes and lecture outline • Overview of PowerPoint presentations • Lesson plan • Activities and discussion topics • Answer keys for end-of-chapter and end-of-section questions
PowerPoint Presentations	• Key concepts • Teaching notes • References to learning outcomes
Electronic Test Bank	• EZ Test Online (computerized) • Word version • The exam questions are also available through *Connect* • Questions are tagged with learning outcomes, level of difficulty, level of Bloom's taxonomy, feedback, topic, as well as the accrediting standards of NAACLS, ABHES, and CAAHEP
Tools to Plan Course	• Transition guide, by chapter, from Booth, 3e to Booth, 4e • Correlations by learning outcomes to ABHES, CAAHEP, NAACLS, and more • Sample syllabi • Asset map—a recap of the key instructor resources, as well as information on the content available through *Connect*

Need help? Contact McGraw-Hill Education's Customer Experience Group (CXG). Visit the CXG website at **www.mhhe.com/support**. Browse our FAQs (frequently asked questions) and product documentation and/or contact a CXG representative. CXG is available Sunday through Friday.

Want to learn more about this product? Attend one of our online webinars. To learn more about the webinars, please contact your McGraw-Hill Education sales representative. To find your McGraw-Hill Education representative, go to **www. mhhe.com** and click "Find My Sales Rep."

Best-in-Class Digital Support

Based on feedback from our users, McGraw-Hill Education has developed Digital Success Programs that will provide you and your students the help you need, when you need it.

- Training for instructors: Get ready to drive classroom results with our Digital Success Team—ready to provide in-person, remote, or on-demand training as needed.
- Peer support and training: No one understands your needs like your peers. Get easy access to knowledgeable digital users by joining our Connect Community, or speak directly with one of our digital faculty consultants, who are instructors using McGraw-Hill Education digital products.
- Online training tools: Get immediate anytime, anywhere access to modular tutorials on key features through our Connect Success Academy.

Get started today. Learn more about McGraw-Hill Education's Digital Success Programs by contacting your local sales representative or visit **http://connect.customer.mheducation.com/start/**.

Acknowledgments

Suggestions have been received from faculty and students throughout the country. This is vital feedback that is relied on for product development. Each person who has offered comments and suggestions has our thanks. The efforts of many people are needed to develop and improve a product. Among these people are the reviewers and consultants who point out areas of concern, cite areas of strength, and make recommendations for change. In this regard, the following instructors provided feedback that was enormously helpful in preparing the book and related products.

Manuscript Reviewers

Multiple instructors reviewed the manuscript while it was in development, providing valuable feedback that directly impacted the product.

Pamela Audette, MBA, MT, RMA,
Finlandia University

Tywan Banks, M.Ed., PBT(ASCP),
Columbus State Community College

Belinda Beeman, M.Ed., CMA (AAMA), PBT (ASCP),
Eastern New Mexico University—Roswell and Goodwin College

Laurie Bjerklie, MA, MLS(ASCP),
DeVry University

Rosemarie Brichta, BS, MT(ASCP),
Alverno Clinical Laboratories

Nick Davis, BA, BSED, MA, Ph.D.,
Southern Careers Institute

Vera Davis, MPA, MATD-PHR,
Rasmussen College

Debra Downs, LPN, RMA,
North Georgia Technical College

Cynthia Funnye-Doby, MA.Ed., MLS,
Malcolm X Community College

Denise Garrow-Pruitt, Ed.D.,
Middlesex Community College and Fisher College

Kris Hardy, CMA,
Brevard Community College

Cheryl Harris, AS, MLT, RMA,
Lincoln College of Technology

Cheryl Lippert, MBA, MT(ASCP), CLS(NCA),
Barton Community College

Lynnae Lockett, RN, RMA, CMRS, MSN,
Bryant & Stratton College

David Martinez, MHSA,
Advanced Colleges of America

Tracy Miller, CMA(AAMA), BS,
Eastern Gateway Community College

Adrian Rios, EMT, RMA, NCMA, MA, CPT-1,
Newbridge College

Tammy Rosolik, PBT(ASCP),
Alverno Clinical Laboratories

Andrea Thompson, BS, MLT(ASCP),
Barton Community College

Mary Beth Wall, RN, BSN,
Anderson University

Lisa Wright, CMA (AAMA) MT, SH,
Bristol Community College

Carole Zeglin, MS, BS, MT, RMA,
Westmoreland County Community College

Survey Respondents

Multiple instructors participated in surveys to help guide the early development of the product.

Pamela Audette, MBA, BS, MT(ASCP), RMA,
Finlandia University

Sue Barfield, MT, BA,
York Technical College

Belinda Beeman, M.Ed., CMA(AAMA), PBT(ASCP),
Eastern New Mexico University—Roswell

Cyndi Caviness, CRT, CMA(AAMA), AHI,
Montgomery Community College

Rhonda Davis, ATS, CMA(RMA), RMA(AMT),
Southern State Community College

Colanda Dorsey, AS, CMA,
Columbus Technical College

Debra Downs, LPN, RMA(AMT), AAS,
North Georgia Technical College

Jessica Ennis, BA, CMA(AAMA),
Gwinnett Technical College

Cindy Feldhousen, MSBE, CMA,
Manchester Community College

Suzanne Fielding, CMA(AAMA), BS,
Daytona State College

Tracie Fuqua, BS, CMA(AAMA),
Wallace State Community College

Claudia Guillen, RN, BSN, RMA,
Middlesex Community College

Ariane Hayes, CMA,
Whatcom Community College

Starra Herring, BSAH, BSHA,
 CMA(AAMA), AHI,
Stanly Community College

Dolly Horton, CMA(AAMA), M.Ed.,
*Asheville Buncombe Technical
 Community College*

Judy Hurtt, M.Ed.,
East Central Community College

Nancy Juarez, PBT(ASPT),
Central Arizona Community College

Diana Kendrick, RMA(AMT), RN,
Southern Crescent Technical College

Cheryl Kuck, BS, CMA(AAMA),
James A. Rhodes State College

Constance Lieseke, BS, CMA(AAMA), MLT,
 PBT(ASCP),
Olympic College

Tracy Miller, BS, CMA(AAMA),
Eastern Gate Community College

Brigitte Niedzwiecki, RN, BSN, MSN,
Chippewa Valley Technical College

Leslie Noles, AS, RMA,
Columbus Technical College

Jane O'Grady, M.Ed., RN, CMA, CPC,
Northwestern Connecticut Community College

Stacia Reagan, CMA(AAMA), BA, M.Ed.,
Spokane Community College

Shirley Ripley, CMA(AAMA), RMA, RPT, CPC-A,
Eastern Maine Community College

Cynthia Rutledge, CMA(AAMA),
Chattanooga State Community College

Amy Ryan, CMA,
Augusta Technical College

Lorraine Schoenbeck, MS, CMA(AAMA),
 CAHI(AMT),
Lone Star College—North Harris

Debbie Shaffer, RN,
Southeastern Community College

J. Jennifer Smith, RHIA, RMA, EMT-I,
Neosho County Community College

Elizabeth Sprinkle, BA, CMA(AAMA),
Edgecombe Community College

B. David Sylvia, BBA, AOS, CMA(AAMA),
Erie Community College

Marilyn Turner, RN, CMA(AAMA),
Ogeechee Technical College

Nancy Worsinger, MS, MT(ASCP),
Nash Community College

Lisa Wright, CMA(AAMA), MT(ASCP), SH,
Bristol Community College

Carole Zeglin, MSEd., MT, RMA(AMT),
Westmoreland Community College

Technical Editing/Accuracy Panel

A panel of instructors completed a technical edit and review of the content in the book page proofs to verify its accuracy.

Laurie Bjerklie, MA, MLS(ASCP),
DeVry University

Cynthia Funnye-Doby, MA.Ed., MLS,
Malcolm X Community College

Cheryl A. Harris, AS, MLT(ASCP), RMA,
 AHI(AMT),
Beckfield College

Nancy Kovacs, BSMT, MT(ASCP), NCPT,
Mercy College of Ohio, Toledo

Tammy Rosolik, PBT(ASCP),
Alverno Clinical Labs

Digital Study Tool Development

Special thanks to the instructors who helped with the development of *Connect*, LearnSmart, and SmartBook. These include

Connect Development

Mary E. Free, PBT, CCMA, CET,
Metropolitan Institute of Health and Technology

Stella Nanga-Ndzana, MS-CLS, MT(AMT),
 MLT(ASCP),
Georgia Piedmont Technical College

Kristiana D. Routh, RMA,
Allied Health Consulting Services

Alice L. Spencer, BS MT, MS, CQA(ASQ),
National College

Andrea Thompson, BS, MLT(ASCP),
Barton Community College

Connect Accuracy Checking

Heather Boisot, RN/CEN,
Northeast Technical Institute—Scarborough Campus

Constance Lieseke, BS, CMA(AAMA), MLT,
 PBT (ASCP),
Olympic College

Kathy Smith, MS, PA (ASCP), MT,
Trocaire College

Andrea Stone, MPA, MT(ASCP),
Moraine Valley Community College

Test Bank Development

Justyn Reyes, CPT-1, EMT-P,
*Wagner Training Institute, West Pacific Medical
 Laboratories*

Carole Zeglin, MS, BS, MT, RMA,
Westmoreland County Community College

Test Bank Accuracy Checking

Cyndi Caviness, CRT, CMA(AAMA), AHI,
Montgomery Community College

Shirley Cruzada, Ed.D., MS, MT(AMT),
College of Southern Nevada

Mary Donahee-Rader, BBA, CMA(AAMA),
Schoolcraft College

Kimberly Meshell, CAHI, RTP, RMA, COLT,
 AAS, AMT, ASPT,
Angelina College

Stella Nanga-Ndzana, MS-CLS, MT (AMT),
 MLT (ASCP),
Georgia Piedmont Technical College

Kathleen Tettam, CMA(AAMA), PBT(ASCP),
Dakota County Technical College

Andrea Thompson, BS, MLT (ASCP),
Barton Community College

Mary Beth Wall, RN, BSN,
Anderson University

Carole Zeglin, MS, BS, MT, RMA,
Westmoreland County Community College

LearnSmart/SmartBook Development

Kendra Barker, M.Ed.,
Pinnacle Career Institute

Lynn Egler, BS, RMA, AHI, CPhT,
*Wayne State University School of Medicine, Emergency
 Medicine Research*

Shauna Phillips, CCMA, RMA, CPT, CET,
 CMT, AHI,
Fortis College

Terri Tardiff, AAS,
Mildred Elley College

LearnSmart/SmartBook Accuracy Checking

Laurie Bjerklie, MA, MLS(ASCP),
DeVry University

Connie Lieseke, BS, CMA(AAMA), MLT,
 PBT(ASCP),
Olympic College

Cheryl Lippert, MBA, MT(ASCP),
 CLS(NCA),
Barton Community College

Patricia Raphiel-Brown, MA, BS-CLS, AMT,
Southern University at Shreveport

Kathy Smith, MS, PA(ASCP), MT,
Trocaire College

Kathleen Tettam, CMA(AAMA), PBT(ASCP),
Dakota County Technical College

Acknowledgements from the Authors

We would like to thank the following individuals who helped develop, critique, and shape our textbook and ancillary package.

We thank the extraordinary efforts of a talented group of individuals at McGraw-Hill who made all of this come together. We would especially like to thank our Director of Health Professions, Chad Grall; William Lawrensen, our Executive Brand Manager; Michelle Flomenhoft, our Senior Product Developer; Michelle Gaseor, our Product Developer; Harper Christopher and Roxan Kinsey, our Executive Marketing Managers; Christine Vaughan and April R. Southwood, our Content Project Managers; Mary Conzachi, our Content Production Manager; Christina Nelson, our Media Project Manager; Angela R. FitzPatrick, our Program Manager; Srdjan Savanovic, our Senior Designer; Michael McCormick, our Senior Buyer; Katherine Ward, our Digital Product Analyst; and Lori Hancock and DeAnna Dausener, our Content Licensing Specialists.

We are also deeply indebted to the individuals who helped develop, critique, and shape the text's extensive ancillary package.

Thank you to Adventist Lab Partners, Adventist Health Systems Midwest, for their continued support by providing use of laboratory equipment for the creation of images used in this text. We also want to recognize the valuable input of all those who helped guide our developmental decisions.

Finally, thank you to Roberta Martinak for her expertise and input regarding phlebotomy protocols and best practices.

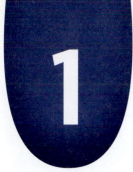

1 Phlebotomy and Healthcare

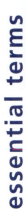
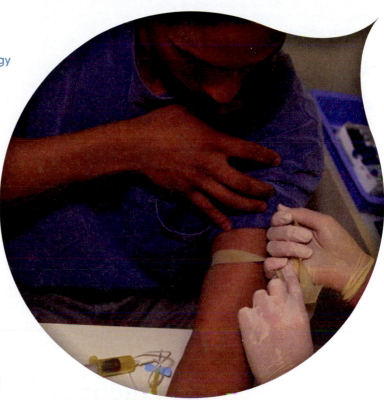

Learning Outcomes

1.1 Summarize the definition and history of phlebotomy.

1.2 Explain the role of the phlebotomist in the various healthcare facilities where he or she may be employed.

1.3 Describe inpatient and outpatient healthcare facilities and their relationship to the practice of phlebotomy.

1.4 Identify the healthcare providers and other members of the healthcare team with which the phlebotomist will interact in inpatient and outpatient facilities.

1.5 Summarize the organization of the medical laboratory.

1.6 Recognize the agencies that regulate hospitals and medical laboratories.

1.7 List the qualities and characteristics of a phlebotomist.

Introduction

The chapter serves as an introduction to the role of the phlebotomist in the delivery of healthcare. It includes information about the phlebotomist's duties in several healthcare settings. In addition, various disciplines within healthcare are briefly defined, as well as specific sections of the medical laboratory. Phlebotomists should also be aware of governmental agencies that regulate how specimens are collected, handled, and tested.

1.1 Phlebotomy

Phlebotomy simply means to cut into a vein. The term comes from *phlebos*, which is Greek for "vein," and *tome*, which means "to cut." Professionals called *phlebotomists* perform this invasive procedure that involves an incision into the skin and blood vessels. At all times during their professional practice, phlebotomists must demonstrate a mastery of the principles and techniques established by the **Clinical and Laboratory Standards Institute (CLSI)**.

The primary role of a **phlebotomist** is to obtain blood specimens for diagnostic testing. These specimens are used to test everything from levels of glucose, proteins, and drugs to blood cell counts, antibodies, and infectious diseases. Blood is obtained either by **venipuncture** (puncturing a vein) or **capillary/dermal puncture** (puncturing the skin). The terms *phlebotomy* and *venipuncture* are often used interchangeably, as are *capillary puncture* and *dermal puncture* (see Table 1-1). Results of laboratory testing are crucial in providing appropriate, quality healthcare. Over 70% of medical decisions are based on laboratory results.

The process of removing blood from the veins may date back as far as 1400 BC; an Egyptian tomb painting shows a leech being applied to the skin of a sick person. Bloodletting was thought to rid the body of impurities and evil spirits or, as in the time of Hippocrates, simply to return the body to a balanced state. Figure 1-1 shows a painting of bloodletting from this era. During the 1800s, anyone claiming medical training could perform bloodletting. Barbers—not unlike those working in salons today—also frequently performed bloodletting procedures.

TABLE 1-1 Two Common Collection Methods

Venipuncture	Insertion of a needle into a vein to allow blood flow into a vacuum tube or syringe	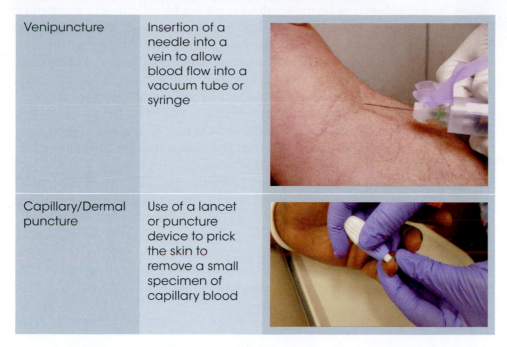
Capillary/Dermal puncture	Use of a lancet or puncture device to prick the skin to remove a small specimen of capillary blood	

In the early 1800s, the popularity of bloodletting created an enormous demand for leeches. Leech farms were established to breed them under controlled conditions. Interestingly, the use of leeches has resurfaced in medicine today (see Figure 1-2). They are prescribed to remove blood that has collected at newly transplanted tissue sites and to decrease the swelling following **microsurgery** (which involves the reconstruction of small tissue structures). Leeches have both anticoagulant and vasodilatation properties. Medicinal leeches may be found in a hospital pharmacy.

Bloodletting also used a process called "venesection," in which the vein was pierced with a sharp object, called a lancet, to drain blood. The lancet, a short, wide, pointed blade, was the most popular medical instrument during the 1800s. Venesection was thought to be an effective procedure for removing unwanted diseases from the body and reducing fever. In fact, the

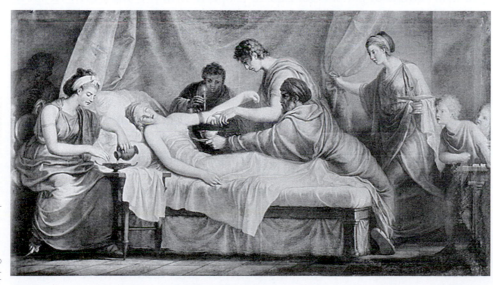

Figure 1-1 Early Romans used bloodletting as a form of healing.

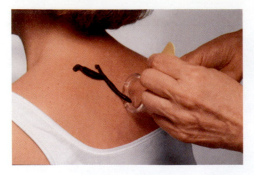

Figure 1-2 Leeches are still used today for localized removal of impurities from the blood.

untimely death of the first U.S. president, George Washington, was believed to be the result of excessive bloodletting in an attempt to treat a throat infection. It is important to note that **aseptic,** or microorganism-free, practices were unknown during that time, so the same lancet was used on several patients without any cleansing.

Another method used for bloodletting was called "cupping." This method produced a vacuum effect by pulling blood to the capillaries under a heated glass cup, which was placed on the patient's back to allow for increased blood flow. Then, a spring-loaded box containing multiple blades pierced the skin to produce bleeding. The procedure typically caused scar tissue.

It was during the 1980s and 1990s that the phlebotomy profession emerged as a result of technology and an expansion of laboratory functions. Initially, only medical laboratory scientists (MLSs, formerly known as medical technologists) and medical laboratory technicians (MLTs) were responsible for collecting blood specimens. However, as technology and the healthcare industry underwent rapid changes, specimen collection was delegated to other groups of trained professionals, including phlebotomists.

> ### ✓ Checkpoint Questions 1.1
>
> 1. Which organization established the principles and techniques that professional phlebotomists must master?
> 2. When did phlebotomy first emerge as a profession?

1.2 Phlebotomist's Role

The phlebotomist is a valuable member of the healthcare team and is responsible for the collection, processing, and transport of blood specimens to the laboratory. This is known as the **pre-examination** (pre-analytical) phase of laboratory testing. Other roles of the phlebotomist may include the removal of blood from donors for blood transfusions and from patients with a condition called polycythemia (overproduction of red blood cells), in which blood must be removed to decrease its viscosity (thickness). Phlebotomists may also give instructions to patients on how to properly collect a urine or fecal specimen, and they are responsible for properly packaging specimens (blood, urine, fecal, cultures, and body fluids). In some settings, the phlebotomist's job also includes accepting incoming specimens, logging specimens into the computer system, and routing specimens to the proper departments for testing and analysis. As a member of the healthcare team, the phlebotomist may assume other responsibilities, such as basic patient care services at inpatient facilities. For example, a phlebotomist also trained as a patient care technician (PCT) may perform additional duties such as delivering meal trays and assisting with the transportation of patients from one department to another.

Several members of the healthcare team are also trained to perform phlebotomy, such as physicians, nurses, medical assistants, paramedics, and patient care technicians. Just as the role of these healthcare team members may include phlebotomy, a phlebotomist may be responsible for performing a variety of other duties, including transporting other specimens—such as arterial blood, urine, sputum, and tissue—to the laboratory for testing. The phlebotomist may also be responsible for performing **point-of-care testing (POCT),** such as blood glucose monitoring. Point-of-care testing is performed at the patient's

TABLE 1-2 Duties and Responsibilities of the Phlebotomist

- Demonstrate professional attire, attitude, and communications.
- Know and follow the facility's policies and procedures.
- Properly identify patients.
- Collect both venous and capillary blood specimens.
- Select the correct specimen container for the specified tests.
- Properly label, handle, and transport specimens following departmental policies.
- Sort specimens received and process specimens for delivery to laboratory departments.
- Perform computer operations and/or update log sheets where required.
- Perform point-of-care testing and quality control checks.
- Observe all safety regulations.

bedside or a work area using portable instruments. POCT can assist the physician in making diagnoses more quickly, which often reduces the length of stay for hospitalized patients. These POCT procedures are explained in the chapter *Waived Testing and Collection of Non-Blood Specimens*. In addition, phlebotomists perform quality control testing and various clinical and clerical duties. Table 1-2 summarizes the essential duties and responsibilities of the phlebotomist.

The phlebotomist must be familiar with the process, equipment, and variables involved in venipuncture and capillary puncture procedures to obtain quality specimens while maintaining patient safety. Nothing is more important in healthcare delivery than patient safety. This means safety not only in the performance of procedures but also in the proper handling of specimens to promote accurate test results, which will influence a patient's diagnosis and treatment. The quality of the specimens sent to the laboratory determines the accuracy of the test results obtained. There is nothing laboratory scientists can do to obtain accurate results on compromised specimens. The phlebotomist is responsible for obtaining the highest-quality specimen possible and ensuring that it is handled properly during transport to the laboratory.

Phlebotomy Training

Entry into phlebotomy training programs usually requires a high school diploma or its equivalent. Training programs are typically offered at hospitals, technical and private schools, and community colleges as well as through continuing education courses. The course can vary from a few weeks to a few months in length, depending on the program.

Various agencies, such as the **National Accrediting Agency for Clinical Laboratory Sciences (NAACLS),** have established standards to which approved programs must adhere. Programmatic approval ensures that students completing the training program are qualified to take a certification examination. In some states, phlebotomists must be both certified and licensed. Certification and licensure are discussed further in the chapter *Practicing Professional Behavior*.

1. Briefly describe the role of the phlebotomist in the delivery of healthcare.
2. What is point-of-care testing?

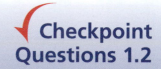

✓ **Checkpoint Questions 1.2**

1.3 Healthcare Facilities

The two main categories of healthcare delivery systems in the United States are inpatient and outpatient services. Phlebotomists are employed in both of these settings as well as in special settings.

Inpatient Facilities

Hospitals, nursing homes, and rehabilitation centers, where patients stay for one night or long term, are examples of inpatient facilities. Phlebotomists employed at inpatient facilities work directly with several members of the healthcare team. Phlebotomists may be part of the medical laboratory staff (see Figure 1-3) or patient care technicians (PCT) with phlebotomy responsibilities. Physicians order specific tests to assist with the evaluation of the patient's condition, and the phlebotomist's role is to collect the blood, properly label the specimen, and transport it to the laboratory.

Outpatient Facilities

Outpatient settings include physician offices, ambulatory care centers, **reference laboratories** (off-site labs), and blood collection centers, where patients visit for a short time and leave the same day. In addition, phlebotomists work for home healthcare agencies, which require them to collect blood in the patient's home. Other special settings include veterinary offices, health maintenance organizations (HMOs), and the American Red Cross, to name a few. The phlebotomist's duties within healthcare facilities vary; however, collecting and processing blood specimens are consistent duties throughout every type of healthcare facility the phlebotomist encounters.

The fastest-growing outpatient settings are ambulatory care centers. These sites are walk-in facilities that patients can go to not only during the day but also after business hours and on weekends, when most physician offices are closed. Lab tests involving chemistry, hematology, urinalysis, serology, coagulation studies, and microbiology are ordered to assist with the diagnosis and treatment of minor conditions, such as sore throat, urinary tract infections, and therapeutic drug monitoring. In addition to blood collection, phlebotomists working in the outpatient setting are responsible for providing instructions to the patient on how to properly collect a urine, fecal, or other specimen. Phlebotomists in these settings may also be responsible for performing other basic patient care duties, such as obtaining vital signs and transporting patients for procedures (such as X-rays).

Physician offices are also considered outpatient facilities. Phlebotomists and medical assistants certified in phlebotomy are usually responsible for collecting and labeling a variety of specimens in the physician office, which are then transported to a reference laboratory for testing. A physician office laboratory may perform only basic lab tests according to the certification it has been granted by the Clinical Laboratory Improvement Amendments (CLIA). Waived tests are the most common and, as defined by CLIA, are "simple laboratory examinations and procedures that have an insignificant risk of erroneous result." These tests are typically performed on small amounts of blood and other specimens

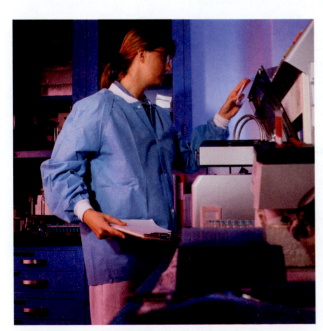

Figure 1-3 An inpatient laboratory is known as a clinical laboratory; personnel perform a wide range of laboratory tests.

such as urine. These tests are discussed in more detail in the chapter *Waived Testing and Collection of Non-Blood Specimens.* (See Figure 1-4.)

Tests such as nasal smears to determine if infection is present and cholesterol level checks are also approved in-office tests. Therefore, depending on the facility of employment, a phlebotomist may be required to perform some of these tests as well as quality control checks on any test he or she performs.

Other outpatient facilities, such as blood banks and the American Red Cross, employ phlebotomists to collect donor blood. The collected blood becomes a unit that might be used for a blood transfusion. Phlebotomists working for agencies are often hired to go into patient homes to collect blood specimens. As healthcare delivery systems change, more care is being provided to patients in nursing homes and in their own residences. Some medical centers provide mobile venipuncture, in which the phlebotomist goes to the patient's home to obtain blood specimens. Additionally, insurance agencies hire phlebotomists to perform in-home phlebotomy as a way of determining a customer's overall health before an insurance policy is written. Other facilities that hire phlebotomists include complementary and alternative medicine (CAM) settings, such as chiropractor offices. Regardless of the work setting, the proper collection, labeling, and handling of all specimens are critical measures for ensuring accurate test results. These steps must be followed correctly to prevent the need for repeating a test unnecessarily or, worse yet, the misdiagnosis or mistreatment of a disorder.

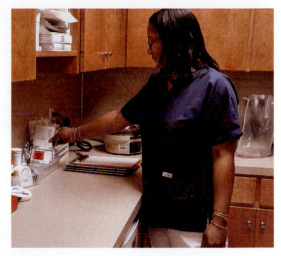

Figure 1-4 A medical assistant or phlebotomist in a physician office laboratory performs "waived" tests, which carry fewer risks to the patient.

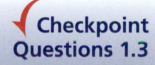

1. Name two types of inpatient facilities.
2. List at least four types of outpatient facilities in which phlebotomists may work.

Checkpoint Questions 1.3

1.4 The Healthcare Team

Whether they are members of the laboratory staff or a nursing unit, phlebotomists must be aware of the healthcare specialties and the professionals found in medical settings. The following pages explain some of the most common healthcare specialties.

- *Anesthesiology* is the management of pain before, during, and after surgery. Anesthesiologists and nurse anesthetists provide this service.

- *Cardiology* is the study, diagnosis, and treatment of conditions pertaining to the heart and circulatory system. The cardiologist is a medical doctor who specializes in disorders of the heart and circulatory system.

- *Diagnostic imaging (radiology)* involves the use of ionizing radiation, X-rays, and specialized procedures such as computed tomography (CT) scans, positron emission tomography (PET), magnetic resonance imaging (MRI), and ultrasound to produce diagnostic images. Radiologic technicians and technologists produce these images, which are then interpreted by radiologists. Radiologists are medical doctors who specialize in diagnosing and treating disease using radiation and imaging processes.

- *Electrocardiography* is the study of the heart's electrical patterns. Nurses, medical assistants, and ECG technicians place electrodes on the skin and record electrical patterns, which are interpreted by cardiologists.
- *Electroencephalography* is the study of electrical activity of the brain. Nurses and EEG technicians place electrodes on the scalp. Neurologists, who are physicians specializing in nervous system disorders, interpret brain activity recordings.
- *Emergency department* doctors and nursing staff specialize in the delivery of acute care for initial treatment of life-threatening or otherwise unplanned medical events. Phlebotomists may need to interact with various healthcare professionals in the emergency department as they respond to trauma assessment and treatment needs.
- *Endocrinology* is the study, diagnosis, and treatment of hormone disorders. Nurses and other healthcare professionals care for patients treated by endocrinologists, who are medical doctors specializing in disorders of the hormone-producing organs and tissues.
- *General medicine (family practice)* is the general care of patients of all ages. Family practice physicians, physician assistants, and nurse practitioners provide this kind of care.
- *Geriatrics* is the diagnosis and treatment of disorders associated with elderly patients. Nurses and other healthcare professionals care for patients treated by gerontologists, who are medical doctors specializing in disorders of the elderly.
- *Internal medicine* is the diagnosis and treatment of disorders related to the internal organs. Physicians who are internists provide this type of care. It is also a common practice area for osteopathic physicians, physician assistants, and nurse practitioners.
- *Neonatology* is the study, diagnosis, and treatment of disorders associated with newborns. Nurses and other healthcare professionals care for these infants, treated by neonatologists, who are medical doctors specializing in disorders of newborns and prematurely born infants.
- *Nephrology* is the study, diagnosis, and treatment of disorders of the kidneys. Physicians specializing in kidney disorders may be nephrologists or urologists.
- *Neurology* is the study, diagnosis, and treatment of disorders of the brain and nervous system. Nurses and other healthcare professionals care for patients treated by neurologists, who are medical doctors specializing in disorders of the brain and nervous system.
- *Nuclear medicine* is the use of injectable radionuclides to diagnose and treat diseases, such as tumors. Medical radiation physicists and physicians specializing in radiotherapy customize treatments for patients based on their disease state and the needs of their particular anatomy.
- *Nutrition and dietetics* is responsible for ensuring that patients receive proper nutritional intervention during and after their hospital stay. Registered dietitians supervise food preparation, develop modified diet plans, and provide special nutrient preparations to patients unable to consume food normally.
- *Obstetrics/gynecology* is the study, diagnosis, and treatment of the female reproductive system. Physicians who are obstetricians and/or gynecologists provide this kind of care.

- *Occupational therapy* enables people to perform meaningful and purposeful activities within the limits of a disability. Occupational therapists and occupational therapy assistants provide this service to people of all ages by using everyday activities as a part of therapy.
- *Oncology* is the study, diagnosis, and treatment of malignant tumors. Nurses and other healthcare professionals care for patients treated by oncologists, who are medical doctors specializing in the study of cancerous tumors.
- *Orthopedics* is the diagnosis and treatment of bone and joint disorders. An orthopedic surgeon provides surgical intervention for these disorders. Physical therapists provide rehabilitation services under the direction of an orthopedic specialist.
- *Pathology* is the study and diagnosis of disease. Pathologists are medical doctors who specialize in this field of medicine. Medical laboratory personnel often work closely with pathologists.
- *Pediatrics* is the diagnosis and treatment of disorders associated with children. Nurses and other healthcare professionals care for children treated by pediatricians, who are medical doctors specializing in disorders of children.
- *Pharmacy* ensures the safe and effective use of therapeutic drugs. Pharmacists and pharmacy technicians dispense physician-prescribed medications and use laboratory results in monitoring appropriate dosages.
- *Physical therapy* is a rehabilitative science that focuses on the development, maintenance, and restoration of maximum movement and functional ability. Physical therapists and physical therapy assistants provide this service to people of all ages, particularly to those whose movement and functionality are threatened by aging, injury, disease, or environmental factors.
- *Psychiatry* is the study and treatment of mental disorders. Nurses and other healthcare professionals care for patients treated by psychiatrists, who are medical doctors specializing in affective, behavioral, cognitive, and perceptual disorders.
- *Respiratory therapy* is the assessment and treatment of breathing disorders. Respiratory therapists, also known as respiratory care practitioners, provide this service through airway management and mechanical ventilation. They work with the laboratory or may perform their own laboratory tests for acid-base balance and blood gas levels.
- *Surgery* uses operative techniques to investigate and treat a pathological condition or to improve bodily function or appearance. General surgeons and surgeons specializing in a specific type of procedure provide this service and are assisted by surgical nurses and surgery technicians.
- *Urology* is the study, diagnosis, and treatment of male and female urinary tract disorders and disorders of the male reproductive system. Physicians specializing in these disorders may be urologists or nephrologists.

These descriptions represent only a sample of the numerous specialties that constitute the medical system. A diverse group of medical specialists cooperate and function as a healthcare team in order to achieve the greatest benefit for the patient (customer). By understanding these different roles and services, the phlebotomist is better prepared to perform a variety of duties for almost any healthcare facility.

Match the following medical specialties with their role in healthcare.

_____ 1. cardiology

_____ 2. pharmacy

_____ 3. physical therapy

_____ 4. psychiatry

_____ 5. respiratory therapy

a. monitoring and adjustment of medication dosages

b. restoration of movement and functional ability

c. diagnosis and treatment of heart conditions

d. assessment and treatment of breathing disorders

e. study and treatment of mental disorders

1.5 The Medical Laboratory

Most hospitals have their own laboratories, which are referred to as "medical" or "clinical" laboratories because they perform a wide range of tests in several specialties.

Each laboratory is organized based on its individual size and complexity. Organizational charts similar to the example in Figure 1-5 are used to show the chain of accountability in the medical laboratory. State licensure laws may dictate the laboratory's structural hierarchy. A hospital laboratory is typically segmented into clinical **pathology** and anatomic pathology. A laboratory director who is an administrative medical laboratory scientist is usually responsible for the overall operation of the clinical portion of the laboratory. A pathologist, on the other hand, is usually responsible for the operation of the anatomic portion of the laboratory. This division of responsibility may vary based on state regulations.

Medical Laboratory Organizational Chart

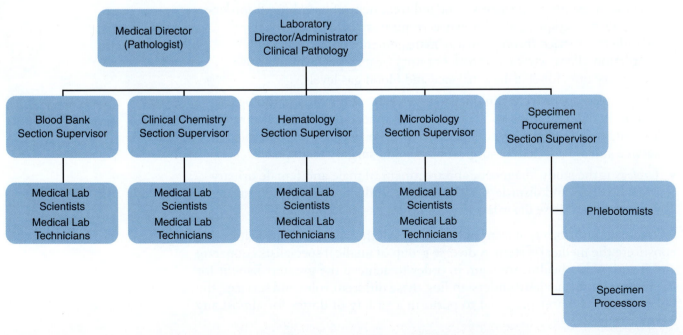

Figure 1-5 Organizational charts similar to this one are used by medical laboratories.

Individual hospital laboratories usually have supervisors who oversee operations for each of the main sections of the laboratory, whereas multihospital organizations may have regional supervisors who travel from site to site, managing operations for their section at each site. Where regional supervisors are used, lead technologists are responsible for the daily functions of laboratory sections. Technicians and scientists perform laboratory tests requested by patients' physicians. Phlebotomists collect and provide the specimens on which these tests are performed.

Medical Laboratory Specialties

Specialty areas of the medical laboratory, along with some of the tests performed in each area, include:

- **Cytology** is the investigation of human cells for the presence of cancer. The most common specimens examined by cytologists are gynecological specimens. (See Figure 1-6.)

- **Histology** is the study of human body tissues and cells. Surgical specimens are sent to histology to be prepared and stained by histologists. (See Figure 1-7.)

- **Clinical chemistry** is the evaluation of the chemical constituents of the human body. Laboratory personnel determine levels of enzymes, glucose, hormones, lipids, proteins, vitamins, iron and other nutrients, therapeutic drugs, drugs of abuse, and trace elements, such as lead. (See Figure 1-8.)

- **Hematology** is the study of blood and blood-forming tissues; it may also include evaluation of hemostasis (coagulation system). Laboratory personnel perform complete blood counts, coagulation tests, bone marrow analysis, body fluid cell counts, and special tests for red blood cell and white blood cell disorders. (See Figure 1-9.)

- **Immunohematology (blood bank)** involves collection and preparation of donor blood for transfusion. Donor phlebotomists screen donors and collect units of blood. Laboratory personnel perform blood group and type analysis and cross-matches, prepare and issue blood products, and conduct transfusion reaction investigations. (See Figure 1-10.)

- **Immunology** and **serology** are the study of the body's resistance to disease and defense against foreign substances. Some of the immunology tests laboratory personnel perform include ANA, Monospot, RPR, and Group A Strep screening. (See Figure 1-11.)

- **Medical microbiology** is the study of medically significant microscopic organisms. In the clinical setting, laboratory personnel perform techniques to identify pathogenic bacteria, fungi, parasites, and viruses. In addition,

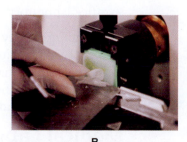

Figure 1-6 Cytology is responsible for examining prepared tissue cells for the presence of cancer.

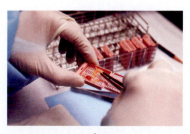
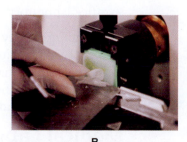
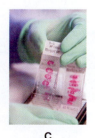

A   B   C

Figure 1-7 Histology is responsible for (A) embedding surgically removed tissues in paraffin, (B) cutting ultrathin slices of the embedded tissue, and (C) affixing them to slides and applying various stains.

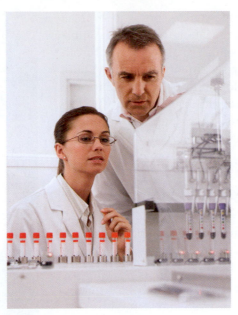

Figure 1-8 The chemistry section of a medical laboratory uses automated analyzers to allow for many tests to be performed in a short amount of time.

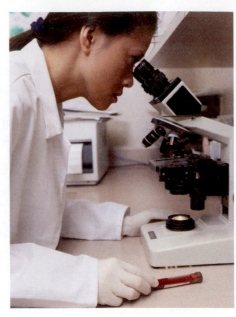

Figure 1-9 This hematology technician is preparing to examine a blood smear.

they identify microorganism resistance or susceptibility to specific antibiotics. (See Figure 1-12.)

- **Molecular diagnostics** is the detection and classification of disease states using molecular and DNA-based testing. Laboratory personnel may perform molecular tests for infectious diseases, such as chlamydia, gonorrhea, and human papillomavirus (HPV); flow cytometry procedures for classification of leukemia and lymphoma; and DNA-based tests, such as gene mutations and tumor cell ploidy analysis. (See Figure 1-13.)

- **Toxicology** is the detection and study of the adverse effects of chemicals on living organisms. Laboratory personnel evaluate blood and body fluids for the presence of trace elements, toxic substances, and drugs. (See Figure 1-14.)

- **Urinalysis** is the examination of urine for physical, chemical, and microscopic characteristics. Laboratory personnel perform routine urinalysis and special confirmatory tests. The urinalysis section may also be responsible for pregnancy testing and testing of other body fluids. Urinalysis may be performed in the general laboratory or a specific department of the laboratory, such as chemistry or hematology. Urinalysis may also be performed in a physician office laboratory. (See Figure 1-15.)

Providing quality healthcare requires a variety of laboratory professionals. These professionals perform analyses of many types to produce the information physicians need to make diagnoses, to form treatment plans, and to monitor outcomes.

Medical Laboratory Personnel

There are various professionals in the medical laboratory with whom the phlebotomist may interact, including the following:

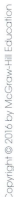

Figure 1-10 The blood bank ensures that blood components are safe for use in transfusion therapy.

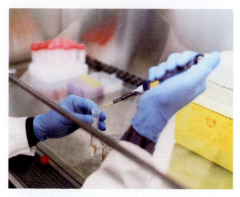

Figure 1-11 Immunology personnel are responsible for detecting the presence of infectious diseases.

- *Medical office staff* greet and assist outpatients needing laboratory services.
- *Medical transcriptionists* prepare pathologist-dictated reports.
- *Medical laboratory assistants (MLAs)* are phlebotomists trained to perform low-complexity testing or assist laboratory staff in other ways.
- *Histologic technicians (HTs)* prepare small sections of surgical specimens for microscopic examination by a pathologist.
- *Histologists (HTLs)* perform more complex functions of the histology laboratory and are responsible for the technical aspects of the histology laboratory as well as new procedure evaluation.
- *Cytologists (CTs)* perform microscopic examination of human cells in order to detect cancer and other diseases. In addition, some laboratories employ professionals with master's degrees or PhDs in specific disciplines, such as microbiology or molecular pathology.

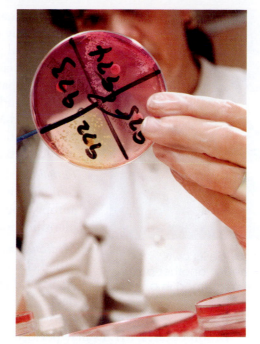

Figure 1-12 Cultures of various specimens are analyzed in the medical microbiology area to identify the causative agent of infections and to determine the appropriate antibiotic to use in combating bacterial infections.

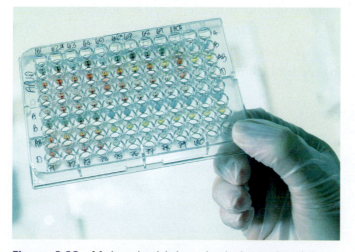

Figure 1-13 Molecular biology techniques involve cellular protein markers or DNA probes to test for various disease conditions.

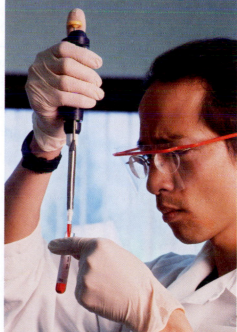

Figure 1-14 Toxicology may be part of the chemistry section and is responsible for drug testing as well as testing for trace elements and environmental toxins.

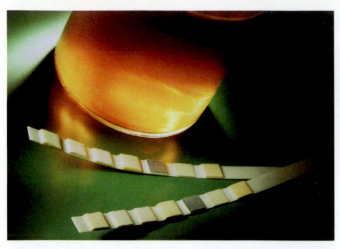

Figure 1-15 Urinalysis testing may be its own laboratory section or be performed in another part of the laboratory; it may also be performed in a physician office laboratory.

- *Pathologists* are medical doctors who specialize in the study of disease, which includes anatomic and clinical pathology. An anatomic pathologist provides diagnoses on surgically removed tissue. A clinical pathologist oversees the interpretation of blood and body fluid test results produced by MLTs and MLSs. Some pathologists also have subspecialties in the various disciplines within the medical laboratory.

- *Pathologists' assistants (PAs)* examine surgically removed tissue samples and collect and examine autopsy specimens. They assist pathologists in the identification of disease states.

- *Medical laboratory technicians (MLTs)*, formerly called clinical laboratory technicians by some agencies, have a minimum of an associate's degree and can perform low-complexity and some moderately complex laboratory testing other than cytology and histology. In some states, MLTs may perform some procedures (those requiring interpretation) under direct supervision of medical laboratory scientists.

- *Medical laboratory scientists (MLSs)*, formerly called medical technologists or clinical laboratory scientists, have a minimum of a bachelor's degree and can perform high-complexity testing other than cytology and histology. They are responsible for the technical aspects of the medical laboratory as well as new procedure evaluation. In addition, some MLSs also have specialties in one or more of the laboratory sections. Some laboratories employ persons with degrees in clinical chemistry or medical microbiology for the position of MLS in specific sections of the medical laboratory.

Medical laboratory technicians and scientists may serve in areas that seem outside the realm of laboratory practice. These areas include laboratory information systems (LIS), marketing and outreach coordination, customer service, and the education of medical laboratory and other medical personnel.

Medical laboratory scientists can also function as the laboratory administrator or laboratory manager. The laboratory manager may have an advanced degree and oversees the day-to-day operations of the laboratory. The laboratory manager works closely with the laboratory's medical director (pathologist) to ensure the quality of laboratory-delivered healthcare.

✓ **Checkpoint Questions 1.5**

Match the following medical laboratory sections to their laboratory testing responsibility.

_____ 1. cytology

_____ 2. hematology

_____ 3. immunohematology

_____ 4. serology

_____ 5. toxicology

a. study the adverse effects of chemicals

b. prepare donor blood for transfusion

c. study the body's resistance to disease

d. detect cancer in gynecological and other specimens

e. study the blood-forming tissues

1.6 Regulatory Agencies

Regulatory agencies routinely visit and inspect laboratories and medical offices to evaluate quality control and quality assurance. Laboratory facilities must have quality assurance programs in place to ensure that tests are effective and accurate. Quality assurance will be discussed in more detail in the chapter *Quality Essentials*.

The 1988 **Clinical Laboratory Improvement Amendments (CLIA '88),** a revision of CLIA '67, were established to ensure that all laboratories receiving federal funds, regardless of size, type, or location, would meet the same standards and be certified by the federal government. This legislation, which became effective in 1992, serves as the main regulatory body for all laboratories, and establishes qualifications for phlebotomists.

Classifications of laboratories are based on the complexity of testing performed and the associated patient risks if the tests are not performed properly. Some laboratories are categorized as "waived" and are not subject to inspections because they perform only simple tests that have minimal associated patient risks, such as dipstick urine testing. Other laboratories are classified as "moderately complex" or "highly complex," and both undergo inspections. Inspections are stricter for higher-complexity laboratories. Personnel qualifications are specified for various levels of test complexity, which are outlined in the CLIA '88 regulations. Failure of any institution to comply with these regulations may result in termination of Medicare and Medicaid reimbursements as well as loss of privilege to perform the procedure.

Hospital laboratories and physician office laboratories are governed by regulations that provide rules and guidelines for quality patient care. **The Joint Commission (TJC)** and the **College of American Pathologists (CAP)** are two accrediting agencies that help ensure a high standard of care for patients. The main accrediting agency for hospitals is TJC. The CAP specifically accredits medical laboratories. The **Department of Health and Human Services (HHS)** oversees the **Centers for Medicare & Medicaid Services (CMS),** formerly the Health Care Financing Administration (HCFA). CMS is the federal agency that established regulations to implement CLIA '88 as well as the **Commission on Office Laboratory Accreditation (COLA)** for accrediting **physician office laboratories (POLs).** Physician offices must keep records for quality control, temperature readings, and equipment maintenance logs.

The Clinical and Laboratory Standards Institute (CLSI), formerly the National Committee for Clinical Laboratory Standards (NCCLS), is a non-profit, private, educational organization that develops and publishes national and international standards for clinical laboratory testing procedures. CLSI standards follow the CLIA '88 mandates and assist medical laboratories in adhering to federal regulations. Clinical laboratories use these standards when developing their procedures and policies. Procedures and policies are documents that outline how specimen collection and laboratory tests are to be performed.

CLSI standards have been categorized into three phases: pre-examination, examination, and post-examination. The terminology for these phases was adopted by CLSI in 2010 due to preferences of the International Organization for Standardization (ISO), the organization with which CLSI aligns its documents. Table 1-3 shows these changes in terminology and explains their meanings.

In addition to the federal government, other agencies oversee various aspects of procedures performed by phlebotomists. The **Centers for Disease Control and Prevention (CDC)** implements public health regulations and reporting requirements for the clinical laboratory and other healthcare providers. The CDC is responsible for categorizing newly developed laboratory tests as waived, moderately complex, or highly complex.

TABLE 1-3 Clinical and Laboratory Standards Institute Alignment of Testing Phase Terminology with the International Organization for Standardization

CLSI Terminology Prior to 2010	CLSI Terminology After Global Harmonization, 2010	Definition of Testing Phase
Pre-analytical	Pre-examination	Every step in the testing process that occurs before the actual performance of a laboratory test, including • ordering and requisitioning of tests. • patient identification. • specimen collection processes, including prioritization. • integrity of the specimen (handling and transport).
Analytical	Examination	Every step in the testing process that occurs during the actual performance of a laboratory test, including • quality assurance of equipment and reagents. • adherence to standards or practices (SOP). • quality control procedures. • test analysis and interpretation. • resolution of result discrepancies.
Post-analytical	Post-examination	Every step in the testing process that occurs after the actual performance of a laboratory test, including • reporting of results. • ensuring proper handling of critical results. • follow-up on reflex testing. • documentation of errors in reporting. • documentation of variances to reporting SOP. • documentation on corrective action. • specimen storage after testing.

The **Occupational Safety and Health Administration (OSHA)** regulates concerns over worker safety for the clinical laboratory. As employees of the clinical laboratory, phlebotomists have the right to a safe working environment and can report concerns regarding unsafe work practices to OSHA without fear of retaliation.

The **Environmental Protection Agency (EPA)** ensures that healthcare providers follow the *Medical Waste Tracking Act (MWTA)*. The MWTA defines medical waste (laboratory specimens and items contaminated by blood or body fluids) and establishes acceptable practices for treatment and disposal of this waste.

The *Department of Transportation (DOT)* establishes requirements for safe packaging and transport of biologically hazardous and other hazardous materials (HAZMATS), such as used or expired laboratory chemicals. The *Nuclear Regulatory Commission (NRC)* regulates handling and disposal of radioactive materials (radionuclides used in therapy). While the medical laboratory minimizes the use of radioactive materials, there are still some tests involving these substances. In addition, there may be times when the blood bank needs to irradiate blood products for transfusion. This may occur when patients need blood in which the white blood cells have been deactivated.

Blood banks undergo additional regulation by the **Food and Drug Administration (FDA)** and the *American Association of Blood Banks (AABB)*. The FDA approves medical and diagnostic equipment, pharmaceuticals, reagents (chemicals used for testing), and diagnostic tests before these can be marketed.

The FDA also regulates content-labeling requirements. Blood and blood products are considered pharmaceuticals. The AABB is an international, not-for-profit association that develops standards and educational programs that focus on blood donor and recipient safety. The AABB also specifically accredits blood banks.

Other organizations that inspect or accredit medical laboratories include state and local agencies and the American Society for Histocompatibility and Immunogenetics (ASHI). Regulatory agencies provide a valuable service to ensure patient safety through regular inspections. The inspection process is designed to assess compliance with regulations and evaluate a laboratory's policies, procedures, and practices. Table 1-4 summarizes regulatory agencies and their relevance to the phlebotomist.

TABLE 1-4 Regulatory Agencies and the Phlebotomist

Agency	Acronym	Relevance to the Phlebotomist
American Association of Blood Banks	AABB	Accredits blood banks and develops standards for blood donor, blood product, and blood recipient safety
American Society for Histocompatibility and Immunogenetics	ASHI	Inspects and accredits laboratories that perform histocompatibility testing
Centers for Disease Control and Prevention	CDC	Categorizes newly developed laboratory tests
Centers for Medicare & Medicaid Services	CMS	The agency that established regulations to implement CLIA '88
Clinical and Laboratory Standards Institute	CLSI	Sets standards for clinical laboratory testing procedures
College of American Pathologists	CAP	Accredits hospital and reference laboratories
Commission on Office Laboratory Accreditation	COLA	Accredits physician office laboratories
Department of Health and Human Services	HHS	Oversees the operations of the CMS
Department of Transportation	DOT	Sets requirements for safe packaging and transport of HAZMATS
Environmental Protection Agency	EPA	Ensures correct disposal of medical waste
Food and Drug Administration	FDA	Approves medical equipment, pharmaceuticals, reagents, and diagnostic tests before use—laboratory-issued pharmaceuticals include blood products
National Accrediting Agency for Clinical Laboratory Sciences	NAACLS	Approves phlebotomy training programs
Nuclear Regulatory Commission	NRC	Regulates handling and disposal of radioactive materials
Occupational Safety and Health Administration	OSHA	Regulates practices to ensure worker safety in the workplace
The Joint Commission	TJC (formerly JCAHO)	Accredits healthcare facilities to ensure high standards of patient care

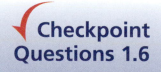

Checkpoint Questions 1.6

1. Which regulatory agency is *most* concerned with the quality of laboratory tests performed in physician offices?
2. What is the purpose of CLIA '88?

1.7 Qualities of a Phlebotomist

A practicing phlebotomist must be professional and display professionalism at all times. A phlebotomist's public image, along with excellent communication and customer service skills, is a necessary quality of this occupation.

Professionalism

Most people do not like having their blood drawn because of the potential discomfort, so **professionalism** and good interpersonal skills are critical attributes. Professionalism includes a sincere interest in providing healthcare, a standard of excellence, training, accountability, and pride in your work. Having a well-groomed and professional appearance demonstrates to others a sense of pride in yourself, your workplace, and your overall profession.

Becoming certified or licensed as a phlebotomist can also send an important message to the patient, and, in turn, the patient will have more confidence in your abilities. Professionalism is covered in more detail in the chapter *Practicing Professional Behavior.*

Critical Thinking

Providing Customer Service

Your patients are your customers, so they should be satisfied with your service. Customer service involves providing customer satisfaction through professionalism, positive communication, and an attitude that promotes resolution of problems.

Example scenario: You are working alone in a busy laboratory because two other phlebotomists have called in sick. The laboratory waiting area is crowded. You expect another phlebotomist to arrive in about 20 minutes. Consider what you would do to promote positive customer service.

Public Image

First impressions are key. Your appearance is the first statement you send to those around you. Phlebotomists are expected to be clean, well groomed, and appropriately dressed for the work setting (this includes closed-toe and closed-heel shoes and socks; no high heels). Basic details such as using good posture, being well rested, and having fresh breath, no unpleasant body odor, clean hair that does not cover the face (tied back if hair is long), minimal to no facial hair, no facial or tongue piercings, and no visible tattoos are mandatory. Lack of good personal hygiene or proper dress can give a negative impression to an already anxious patient.

Many institutions require that phlebotomists wear a lab jacket and specified shoes in order to meet Occupational Safety and Health Administration (OSHA) guidelines. Compliance with the dress code established by your facility is important for establishing a professional public image. Depending on the setting, the phlebotomist may be the only laboratory contact person a patient encounters, so a positive public image is important not only for the credibility of the individual but also for the laboratory department and institution.

Customer Service and Communication

The healthcare industry is service oriented. This means that, as a healthcare professional, you want your customers (patients) to be pleased with both the services you provide and the manner in which you deliver them. This is customer service. Positive communication is a key to customer service.

The process of communication occurs in a loop (see Figure 1-16). The *communication loop* involves four basic elements: (1) the sender, (2) the message, (3) the receiver, and (4) feedback. The sender is the one who begins the communication process by encoding a message to be sent. The message is the thought, idea, or information. The receiver is the person who decodes the meaning of the message. Feedback is the receiver's acknowledgment of and response to the message. If clarification is needed, a role reversal occurs. The receiver now becomes the sender and encodes a message to be sent. Filters or barriers—pain, fear, visitors, or the television—may be present and can interfere with a receiver decoding a message. For the communication loop to occur, the sender and receiver will alternate roles.

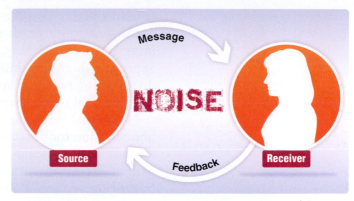

Figure 1-16 The process of communication involves an exchange of message and feedback. Noise (barriers to communication) can interfere with the communication process.

The ability to communicate and provide customer service is crucial for the phlebotomist. Communication can be verbal or nonverbal. *Verbal* refers to the use of language or words to express ideas. The phlebotomist must be able to communicate using nonmedical terms, so that patients can understand what is being said to them. For example, using the term *venipuncture* with a patient instead of simply telling the patient that you will be "drawing some blood" can create a block in communication. The phlebotomist must be capable of explaining procedures to patients of various ages in order to gain their confidence and cooperation.

Never give false reassurance to patients by making statements such as "You won't even feel it" because most patients feel some level of discomfort during phlebotomy procedures. Avoid using slang, or "street" talk, because different words have different meanings to different individuals. Address patients by name, avoiding inappropriate terms such as "honey" or "sweetie." Excessive talking is also to be avoided because it tends to be annoying to patients wanting and needing rest. Speak in a calm and clear voice with a tone appropriate to the patient's needs. For example, you may need to use a louder volume for a patient who is hard of hearing.

Patients receive not only the spoken message but also the nonverbal cues the phlebotomist sends (see Table 1-5). Nonverbal communication begins with attire and includes overall mannerisms and behaviors. Maintaining eye contact during patient interactions is a positive nonverbal response that assists with establishing trust. During the initial greeting, displaying a smile, maintaining erect body posture with relaxed arms, and avoiding the

TABLE 1-5 Nonverbal Communication: Positive versus Negative Gestures

Positive	Negative
• Good body posture	• Drooping shoulders with head held low
• Eye contact	• Looking down or away from patient
• Neat, well-groomed appearance	• Dingy, wrinkled lab coat; too much jewelry
• Respecting personal space	• Immediately approaching patient's space before greeting and explaining procedures

patient's personal space are usually well-received gestures. Personal space is the proximity or distance between individuals a person prefers when interacting with others. Many people feel uncomfortable when strangers approach them and immediately enter their personal space. Appropriate distance for personal space or proximity varies based on gender, culture, and personal preference.

Nonverbal behavior is also the use of communication devices such as cell phones, blue tooth technology, and social media. Using these while on the job not only causes a distraction from job duties but is also rude to your patient. Remember, the patient is your customer who can choose to seek healthcare services at another facility. Many facilities have policies restricting the use of cell phones due to possible electromagnetic interference with medical devices.

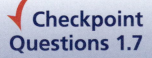

Patient Education & Communication

Using Proper Communication

The phlebotomist may be required to obtain blood from patients who are unable to communicate as a result of a stroke or other medical condition. Regardless of the patient's inability to communicate, the phlebotomist is expected to provide the same greetings, introductions, and explanations as he or she would for any patient.

The mere fact that a patient cannot respond does not necessarily mean that he or she cannot hear! Do not talk in the presence of unconscious patients as if they cannot hear you.

To provide positive communication and customer service when approaching any patient, the phlebotomist should properly introduce him- or herself, state the purpose of the visit, and request that the patient state his or her full name and date of birth. The patient should respond verbally to the request and if he or she is unable to do so another means of identification should be used. Once an initial greeting is established, it is acceptable and necessary to move closer to the patient's bedside or chair, depending on the workplace setting. In addition to professionalism and positive communication, customer service requires common courtesy. As mentioned earlier, when patients are having blood drawn, they may be anxious and not in the best of moods. They may be concerned about the test results or just frightened. You can help their experience by being sympathetic to their situation. Observe their behavior, listen to their concerns, and address any situation promptly and effectively. You should approach any problem with flexibility and the obligation to find a resolution.

✓ Checkpoint Questions 1.7

1. Name four examples of positive nonverbal communication.
2. What is customer service?

Chapter Summary

Learning Outcome	Key Concepts/Examples	Related NAACLS Competency
1.1 Summarize the definition and history of phlebotomy. Pages 2–4.	Phlebotomy means cutting into a vein. It is an invasive procedure performed by phlebotomists; it has evolved from the use of leeches for blood collection to modern-day certified phlebotomists.	1.00
1.2 Explain the role of the phlebotomist in the various healthcare facilities where he or she may be employed. Pages 4–5.	Phlebotomists are responsible for the collection, processing, and transportation of blood specimens, as well as other duties required by their place of employment.	1.1
1.3 Describe inpatient and outpatient healthcare facilities and their relationship to the practice of phlebotomy. Pages 6–7.	Phlebotomists can be employed at hospitals, rehabilitation centers, nursing homes, clinics, physician offices, ambulatory care centers, blood banks, reference laboratories, and insurance companies.	1.2
1.4 Identify the healthcare providers and other members of the healthcare team with which the phlebotomist will interact in inpatient and outpatient facilities. Pages 7–10.	Phlebotomists interact with healthcare professionals from many medical specialties including nurses, physicians, radiologic technologists, respiratory therapists, physical therapists, and surgical technicians.	1.1
1.5 Summarize the organization of the medical laboratory. Pages 10–14.	Medical laboratories are organized based on the needs of the facility in which they serve. Phlebotomists interact with medical laboratory personnel from many laboratory specialties, including clinical chemistry, cytology, hematology, histology, immunohematology, immunology, medical microbiology, molecular diagnostics, and urinalysis.	1.3, 1.4, 1.5
1.6 Recognize the agencies that regulate hospitals and medical laboratories. Pages 15–17.	The regulating agencies for the practice of phlebotomy include CLSI, TJC, HCFA, HHS, CDC, and OSHA.	1.00
1.7 List the qualities and characteristics of a phlebotomist. Pages 18–20.	Proper professionalism, public image, communication, and customer service are necessary traits of a phlebotomist.	9.00, 9.3, 9.6

Chapter Review

A: Labeling

Label the elements of this communication loop. Write the name of each element on the lines provided.

1. [LO 1.7] _____

2. [LO 1.7] _____

3. [LO 1.7] _____

4. [LO 1.7] _____

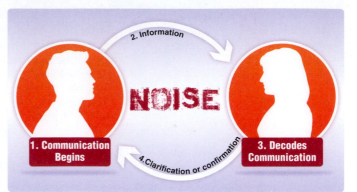

B: Matching

Match each organization with its role in regulating medical laboratories.

_____5. [LO 1.6] sets standards for laboratory testing

_____6. [LO 1.6] is responsible for minimizing work-related injuries

_____7. [LO 1.6] regulates content labeling of blood products

_____8. [LO 1.6] regulates the internal handling of medical waste

_____9. [LO 1.6] monitors and reports diseases

___10. [LO 1.6] sets standards for phlebotomy training programs

a. AABB
b. CAP
c. CDC
d. CLSI
e. EPA
f. FDA
g. NAACLS
h. OSHA

C: Fill in the Blank

Write in the word(s) to complete the statement or answer the question.

11. [LO 1.2] The healthcare professional who has the greatest control over pre-examination variables during blood collection is the _____.

12. [LO 1.5] The medical doctor who works in the laboratory is the _____.

13. [LO 1.7] Becoming _____ or licensed as a phlebotomist sends a positive message to patients.

14. [LO 1.3] What term is used to describe tests that are performed at a patient's bedside?
_____.

List two negative verbal and nonverbal types of communication that should be avoided.

Verbal

15. [LO 1.7] _____

16. [LO 1.7] _____

Nonverbal

17. [LO 1.7] _____

18. [LO 1.7] _____

D: Sequencing

Number the following laboratory personnel in the order of hierarchy in a laboratory's organizational chart from 1 (highest management function) to 5 (lowest management function).

19. [LO 1.5] _____ administrator

20. [LO 1.5] _____ technician

21. [LO 1.5] _____ scientist

22. [LO 1.5] _____ phlebotomist

23. [LO 1.5] _____ section supervisor

E: Case Studies/Critical Thinking

24. [LO 1.7] A patient is having blood work done during her lunch hour. She has waited 25 minutes before being called back for her blood to be drawn. How can you implement customer service in this situation?

25. [LO 1.7] A phlebotomist has been asked to obtain a blood specimen from a hospitalized patient. The phlebotomist enters the patient's room and gives the appropriate greeting but discovers that the patient speaks only Spanish, a language the phlebotomist is unfamiliar with. Should the phlebotomist proceed with the blood collection? What are the phlebotomist's next steps? Explain your answer.

26. [LO 1.7] While explaining the purpose of a visit to a patient, a phlebotomist notices five visitors entering the room. The patient greets the visitors pleasantly and one of the visitors asks the phlebotomist what blood tests have been ordered. How should the phlebotomist handle this situation and why?

27. [LO 1.7] The phlebotomist is scheduled to obtain a blood specimen from a patient in a patient's home. The phlebotomist enters the home and makes the appropriate greetings. The patient is very agitated and states, "I'm just sick and tired of you people drawing my blood. It's not helping me to get any better, so get out! I refuse to be a pincushion for you medical jerks!" What would be a good response for the phlebotomist to make? How should the phlebotomist handle this situation?

28. [LO 1.7] A phlebotomist employed at the outpatient clinic of a large, acute care hospital begins her shift to find the waiting room full of patients. Two of the scheduled phlebotomists have called in sick and it will be at least 20 minutes before any additional phlebotomists can arrive. The phlebotomist begins to call patients back and listens while each patient voices his or her frustration, saying only what is required to collect the specimen and letting the patients leave. Did the phlebotomist make any error? What could he have done differently?

F: Exam Prep

Choose the best answer for each question.

29. [LO 1.1] The term *phlebotomy* comes from Greek words that mean
   a. "draw blood."
   b. "cut vein."
   c. "drain blood."
   d. "dermal cut."

30. [LO 1.2] The minimum requirements for entry into a phlebotomy training program generally include a
   a. nursing degree or CNA certification.
   b. medical laboratory MLT certification.
   c. high school diploma or equivalent.
   d. medical assisting certification.

31. [LO 1.2] The main duty of a phlebotomist is to

    a. interpret laboratory values.

    b. evaluate blood specimens.

    c. process blood specimens.

    d. collect blood specimens.

32. [LO 1.2] The phlebotomist is mainly responsible for which phase of laboratory testing?

    a. Examination

    b. Pre-examination

    c. Post-examination

    d. Reporting

33. [LO 1.2] Which of the following is NOT a phlebotomist's duty?

    a. Aseptic procedures

    b. Capillary puncture

    c. Surgery assistance

    d. Venipuncture

34. [LO 1.3] Opportunities for phlebotomy employment at outpatient facilities include all of these EXCEPT

    a. physician office.

    b. home healthcare.

    c. insurance companies.

    d. nursing homes.

35. [LO 1.4] The diagnosis and treatment of conditions pertaining to the heart and circulatory system are the functions of which medical specialty?

    a. Anesthesiology

    b. Cardiology

    c. Electrocardiography

    d. Electroencephalography

36. [LO 1.4] The assessment and treatment of breathing disorders are the functions of which medical specialty?

    a. Diagnostic imaging

    b. Endocrinology

    c. Physical therapy

    d. Respiratory care

37. [LO 1.4] Restoration of maximum movement and functional ability is the purpose of

    a. occupational therapy.

    b. orthopedics.

    c. physical therapy.

    d. respiratory therapy.

38. [LO 1.7] Which specialty uses ionizing radiation to produce diagnostic images?

    a. Nuclear medicine

    b. Orthopedics

    c. Pathology

    d. Surgery

39. [LO 1.4] Which specialty recommends treatment plans based on therapeutic drug monitoring results from the laboratory?

    a. Nuclear medicine

    b. Pharmacy

    c. Radiology

    d. Surgery

40. [LO 1.5] Surgically removed body tissues are prepared and stained by

    a. cytologists.

    b. hematologists.

    c. histologists.

    d. tissuologists.

41. [LO 1.4] Prepared body tissues are examined and a diagnosis is made by

    a. cytologists.

    b. histologists.

    c. pathologists.

    d. tissuologists.

42. [LO 1.5] Cross-matching of donated blood with a recipient is the function of

    a. cytology.

    b. histology.

    c. immunohematology.

    d. immunology.

43. [LO 1.5] The study of the body's resistance to disease is the function of

    a. clinical chemistry.

    b. histology.

    c. immunology.

    d. microbiology.

44. [LO 1.6] CLIA classifies laboratories based on

    a. number of employees.

    b. size of the laboratory.

    c. number of tests performed.

    d. complexity of tests performed.

45. [LO 1.6] A college dean who wants to offer a phlebotomy training program would seek approval from which organization that sets standards for phlebotomy training programs?

   a. CAP

   b. CLSI

   c. NAACLS

   d. NCCLS

46. [LO 1.7] Filters or barriers that can interfere with clear communication include all of these EXCEPT

   a. eye contact.

   b. fear and anxiety.

   c. pain or discomfort.

   d. television viewing.

47. [LO 1.7] Customer service would LEAST likely include

   a. common courtesy.

   b. complexity.

   c. flexibility.

   d. professionalism.

48. [LO 1.7] Evaluate which of the following scenarios would BEST contribute to customer satisfaction.

   a. A medical office receptionist tells a patient to "have a seat," without making eye contact.

   b. A phlebotomist fumbles with equipment assembly prior to the blood collection procedure.

   c. A healthcare worker encounters a lost visitor and assists this person to his destination.

   d. A medical assistant is always dressed in the latest fashions and jewelry.

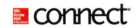

Enhance your learning by completing these exercises and more at connect.mheducation.com.

References

American Association of Blood Banks. (2013). *About AABB*. Retrieved July 23, 2013, from www.aabb.org/about/who/Pages/default.asp

American Association for Respiratory Care. (2011). *American Association for Respiratory Care home page*. Retrieved February 5, 2011, from www.aarc.org

American Dietetic Association. (2010). *Food and nutrition information you can trust*. Retrieved February 5, 2011, from www.eatright.org

American Occupational Therapy Association. (2011). *About occupational therapy*. Retrieved February 5, 2011, from www.aota.org

American Pharmacists' Association. (2011). *About APhA*. Retrieved February 5, 2011, from www.pharmacist.com

American Physical Therapy Association. (2011). *About us*. Retrieved February 5, 2011, from www.apta.org

American Society for Clinical Laboratory Science. (2011). *ASCLS history*. Retrieved February 5, 2011, from www.ascls.org/about-us/ascls-history

American Society for Clinical Pathology. (2011). *ASCP history*. Retrieved February 5, 2011, from www.ascp.org/About-the-ASCP

Clinical and Laboratory Standards Institute. (2010). *CLSI organizational policy on harmonization*. CLSI. Retrieved June 7, 2011, from www.clsi.org/Content/NavigationMenu/Resources/HarmonizedTerminologyDatabase/HarmonizationPolicy0205approved.pdf

National Accrediting Agency for Clinical Laboratory Sciences. (2010). *NAACLS entry-level phlebotomist competencies. Rosemont, IL. NAACLS. Retrieved February 5, 2011, from* www.naacls.org/docs/Guide_Approval-section1b-Phleb.pdf

Pashazadeh, A. M., Aghajani, M., Nabipour, I., & Assadi, M. (2013). An update on mobile phones interference with medical devices. *Radiation Protection Dosimetry* 156(4), 401-406. Retrieved February 15, 2014, from www.academia.edu/3435639/MOBILE_PHONES_INTERFERENCE_WITH_MEDICAL_DEVICES

Stedman's medical dictionary for the health professions and nursing (6th ed.). (2008). Baltimore: Wolters Kluwer Health/Lippincott Williams & Wilkins.

Taber's cyclopedic medical dictionary (21st ed.). (2009). Philadelphia: F.A. Davis.

The Joint Commission. (2013). *Joint Commission history*. Retrieved July 23, 2013, from www.jointcommission.org/assets/1/6/Joint_Commission_History.pdf

Thierer, N., & Breitbard, L. (2007). *Medical terminology essentials*. New York: McGraw-Hill.

Wilson, D. D. (2008), *McGraw-Hill manual of laboratory and diagnostic tests*. New York: McGraw-Hill.

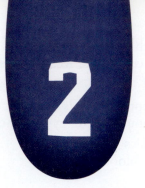

2 Infection Control and Safety

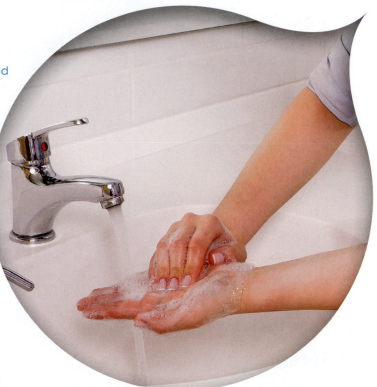

Learning Outcomes

2.1 Identify the elements in the chain of infection and the ways in which disease can be transmitted.

2.2 Demonstrate knowledge of infection control practices and guidelines related to phlebotomy.

2.3 Implement safety practices to reduce the risk of infection from medical biohazards in compliance with state and federal standards and regulations.

2.4 Apply techniques to ensure the physical safety of healthcare workers and patients.

Related NAACLS Competencies

2.00 Demonstrate knowledge of infection control and safety.

2.1 Identify policies and procedures for maintaining laboratory safety.

2.2 Demonstrate accepted practices for infection control, isolation techniques, aseptic techniques, and methods for disease prevention.

2.3 Comply with federal, state, and locally mandated regulations regarding safety practices.

2.4 Describe measures used to ensure patient safety in various patient settings, i.e., Inpatient, outpatient, pediatrics, etc.

Introduction

All healthcare personnel must help to prevent infection and provide for safety. This chapter includes an overview of infection control and emphasizes precautions healthcare workers should take to avoid the spread of infection in clinical settings. In addition, the various hazards that may be present in the clinical setting are presented along with practices for maintaining safety.

2.1 Disease Transmission

Diseases are transmitted in many different ways. For example, they can be passed from person to person through direct contact or can be transmitted through the air. Understanding the elements needed for infections to occur and how diseases are transmitted is the first step in learning to control infections.

Chain of Infection

Most infections can be prevented by hand hygiene and other precautions that break any of the links in the **chain of infection.** The chain of infection contains these six factors (links) that must be present for an infection to occur:

1. An infectious agent
2. A reservoir
3. A portal of exit
4. A mode of transmission
5. A portal of entry
6. A susceptible host

Transmission of an infection can occur at any one of these six links in the chain of infection. Likewise, if the chain is broken at any of the links, an infection will not develop (see Figure 2-1 and Table 2-1).

Drug Resistant Bacteria

Several bacteria have become resistant to antibiotics, making the control of spreading infection difficult. Extra precautions are often taken with patients who are identified as infected with or as reservoirs of these bacteria.

Methicillin-resistant *Staphylococcus aureus* (MRSA), vancomycin-resistant enterococci (VRE), multidrug-resistant *Acinetobacter baumannii* (MDRAB), and *Clostridium difficile* (C-diff) enteritis are examples of infectious agents that are spread by contact transmission. MRSA is a type of bacterium that is resistant to methicillin and other common antibiotics. MRSA and other staphylococci (staph) infections occur most frequently among patients in hospitals, dialysis centers, and nursing homes who have weakened immune systems. MRSA can be transmitted from person to person. Hands are easily contaminated during the process of caregiving or from contact with environmental surfaces,

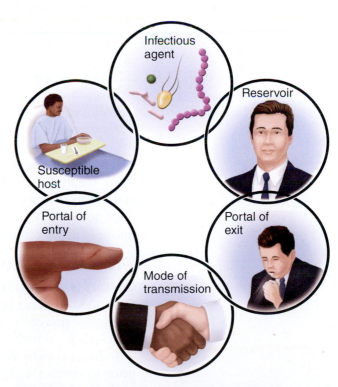

Figure 2.1 If one of the links in the chain of infection is broken, infection can be prevented.

TABLE 2-1 Chain of Infection

Link	Description	How the Phlebotomist Can Break the Links
Infectious agent	Pathogen or disease-producing microorganism	• Perform hand hygiene.
Reservoir	Site where the organism grows and multiplies, such as humans, animals, water, food, or air	• Wear gloves when obtaining and handling any specimens.
Portal of exit	Skin, respiratory tract, gastrointestinal tract, eyes, ears, urinary tract, and reproductive tract	• Dispose of contaminated materials properly.
Mode of transmission	How the pathogen travels; most commonly by contact, droplet, or air, either direct or indirect	• Use required personal protective equipment, including mask, gloves, and eye protection.
Portal of entry	Respiratory system, eyes, ears, urinary tract, reproductive tract, or break in skin	• Perform aseptic technique when required.
Susceptible host	Person at risk for developing an infection from the pathogen, such as one who is immunocompromised; has wounds or drain tubes, poor nutrition, underlying diseases, stress, or lack of sleep; is very young or elderly; or is undergoing invasive procedures	• Follow isolation precautions when required.

such as beds, countertops, and doorknobs. Even though reimbursement is denied for negative results, some hospitals require healthcare workers to swab the nasal passages of newly admitted patients to determine if MRSA is present. This is done to identify potential reservoirs.

Enterococci are bacteria that are normally found in human intestines. These bacteria can cause infections. Sometimes the bacteria are resistant to the antibiotic vancomycin, which is used to treat enterococci infections. VRE are often passed by direct contact from person to person and by people who touch contaminated surfaces. The infection is also spread from the hands of healthcare providers to other people or surfaces.

C-diff is a spore-forming bacterium that can cause diarrhea and can live outside the human body for a very long time. It can spread from person to person and can be found on bed linens, bedrails, and medical equipment. The infection can spread from the hands of healthcare providers to other people or surfaces. Some strains of C-diff have formed resistance to antibiotics such as ciprofloxacin (Cipro) and levofloxacin (Levaquin).

Pseudomonas aeruginosa causes many healthcare-associated infections. Preventing exposure to this bacterium is difficult because it is found on nearly every **fomite** (inanimate object capable of transmitting infectious organisms) from hospital room furniture and bathroom surfaces (such as sinks, faucets, and toilets) to various forms of patient care equipment. Although *Pseudomonas* does not typically cause a rapid, severe infection, its increasing resistance to multiple drugs causes significant health risks.

Modes of Transmission

Contact transmission is the most frequent source of healthcare-associated infections and can occur by either direct or indirect contact. Direct contact requires a physical transfer of pathogens from reservoir to susceptible host (person to person). This transfer can take place by something as simple as a touch.

Indirect contact occurs when a fomite, such as a soiled dressing, is handled prior to contact with a susceptible host (person to contaminated item to person). Indirect contact most often occurs when healthcare employees fail to wash their hands and to change gloves between patients.

Droplet transmission is a form of contact transmission, but the method of transfer is different. This form occurs when droplets from an infected person are propelled short distances (usually up to 3 feet) and enter the susceptible host through the nasal mucosa, the mouth, or the conjunctiva of the eye. Examples of infections spread by droplet transmission are influenza, mumps, and rubella. Droplets are propelled by coughing, sneezing, breathing, and talking. The droplets are not suspended in the air, as they are with airborne transmission. Droplet transmission can also occur with blood or body fluids and during specimen handling.

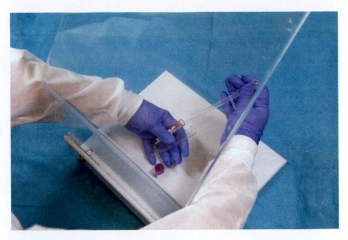

Figure 2-2 A phlebotomist prepares a specimen behind a protective shield.

In **airborne transmission,** small particles carry the pathogens. These particles can be widely dispersed by air currents before being inhaled by a host. Legionnaires' disease, varicella (chickenpox or shingles), and tuberculosis (TB) are examples of infections spread by airborne transmission. Airborne transmission can also occur when **aerosols** are created during the removal of caps from tubes of blood, urine, or other body fluid specimens. Aerosols are tiny, airborne droplets of fluid that are often so small they go unnoticed because you cannot smell or feel them, yet they can carry microorganisms. You should always use appropriate personal protective equipment (PPE), which will be discussed later in this chapter. Use a specimen shield or an approved ventilation hood when opening specimens during processing (see Figure 2-2).

Vehicle-borne transmission occurs when a fomite comes in contact with contaminated items, such as food, linen, or equipment. The fomite becomes a vehicle for spreading disease when it is touched or ingested by a susceptible host. To prevent this mode of transmission, soiled linen and equipment must be cleaned or disposed of properly.

Vector-borne transmission occurs when a living host, such as an animal or insect, comes in contact with a contaminated item, such as food, linen, or equipment. The animal or insect becomes a vector that carries and transmits disease to a susceptible host. A mosquito that carries and spreads the West Nile virus is an example of vector-borne transmission.

1. List the links in the chain of infection.
2. Explain the difference between airborne transmission and droplet transmission.

✓ **Checkpoint Questions 2.1**

2.2 Infection Control

As a healthcare worker, you will come across the concept of infection control on a daily basis. Working safely in any healthcare setting requires careful attention to detail, from routine hand hygiene to more complex infection prevention measures. Protecting the safety of patients, colleagues, and yourself is a key aspect of your career as a phlebotomist.

Standards have been developed by the Centers for Disease Control and Prevention (CDC) to prevent healthcare-associated infections. **Healthcare-associated infections (HAIs),** sometimes called *healthcare-acquired* and

TABLE 2-2 Hand Hygiene Procedures for Phlebotomists

Recommended Practices

- Wash your hands at the beginning of the workday.
- Wash your hands with soap and water whenever they are visibly contaminated with blood or other body fluids.
- If your hands are not visibly contaminated, you can use an alcohol-based hand rub.
- Wash your hands at the end of the workday before leaving the facility.

Indications for Hand Hygiene

- Before putting on and after removing gloves
- Between patient contacts; between different procedures on the same patient
- After touching blood, body fluids, secretions, excretions, or contaminated objects
- After handling specimen containers or tubes
- Before inserting any invasive device
- After contact with the patient's skin
- After contact with wound dressings (bandages)
- After contact with inanimate objects near a patient
- Before eating, applying cosmetics, or manipulating contact lenses
- After restroom visits, eating, combing hair, handling money, and any other time hands get contaminated

Advantages of Alcohol-Based Hand Rubs (Foam or Gel)

- They kill more effectively and more quickly than handwashing with soap and water (only when there is not visible contamination).
- They are less damaging to the skin than soap and water, resulting in less skin irritation.
- They require less time.
- Dispensers can be placed in more accessible areas.

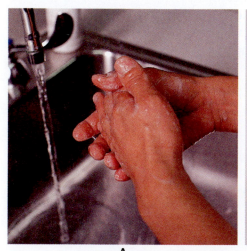 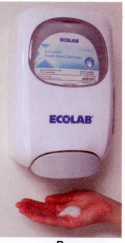

A   B

Figure 2-3 (A) Handwashing. (B) Alcohol-based hand rub.

previously known as *nosocomial infections*, are infections that occur while a patient is hospitalized or is receiving treatment for another condition in any type of healthcare facility. According to the CDC, about 1 in every 20 hospital patients will develop a healthcare-associated infection. Phlebotomists come in contact with many patients and can contribute to these infections if they do not follow infection control standards.

Hand Hygiene

Correct **hand hygiene** is one of the most critical steps in preventing HAIs. Hand hygiene includes both hand washing and the use of alcohol-based hand rubs. Hand washing is the best method of cleaning your hands, but the use of alcohol-based hand rubs is acceptable in many circumstances, such as when you have no visible foliage on your hands (see Table 2-2 and Figure 2-3). Follow the steps in Competency Check 2.1 when performing hand hygiene. Use the competency checklist *Hand Washing* at the end of this chapter to review and practice the procedure.

Hand Hygiene

Competency Check 2-1

Hand Washing

1. Remove all rings and jewelry.

2. Turn on the water and adjust the temperature to warm.

3. Wet your hands liberally with the fingertips pointing down and without leaning your body against the sink area.

4. Apply soap and work up a good lather. Use circular motions while applying friction, being sure to interlace your fingers to clean between them, for 2 minutes at the start of your work day, a minimum of 20 seconds between patients and between procedures on the same patient, and 1 to 2 minutes when your hands are soiled.

5. Rinse each hand, allowing water to run from your wrist toward your fingertips, pointing your fingers downward.

6. Remove contamination from under your fingernails with a tool designed for that purpose, such as an orange stick. If a cleaning tool is not available, scratch the nails of one hand against the palm of the other hand to get the soap worked under the nails.

7. Repeat the preceding steps if your hands are very soiled.

8. Thoroughly wash the wrists.

9. Dry your hands thoroughly by patting them with paper towels and discard the paper towels into a waste receptacle without touching the receptacle.

10. Turn off the water with a clean, dry paper towel, if indicated. Many facilities have sensors that turn the water on automatically when hands are lowered to the faucet. Other facilities have a knee or foot device to turn the water on when depressed and off when released.

11. Clean the area using dry paper towels as needed.

Alcohol-Based Hand Rubs

1. Make sure there is no visible dirt or contamination.

2. Apply 1/2 to 1 teaspoon of alcohol cleanser (either foam or gel) to hands. Check the manufacturer's directions for the proper amount.

3. Rub your hands together vigorously, making sure all surfaces are covered including the fronts and backs of your hands and between your fingers.

4. Continue rubbing until your hands are dry. The drying of the alcohol kills microorganisms.

Respiratory Hygiene and Cough Etiquette

Because of the potential for an outbreak of respiratory illness, especially certain types of flu, the CDC has created the respiratory hygiene and cough etiquette standard. This standard applies to everyone and is added to the standard precautions for healthcare settings. Individuals should cover their cough or sneeze, use the flu salute, and clean their hands frequently. The specifics of the standard are shown in Figure 2-4.

Personal Protective Equipment

The process of blood collection is an invasive procedure. Whenever blood or body fluid from one person comes in contact with another person, there is a major risk of exposure to **bloodborne pathogens,** such as human immunodeficiency virus (HIV), hepatitis C virus (HCV), and hepatitis B virus (HBV).

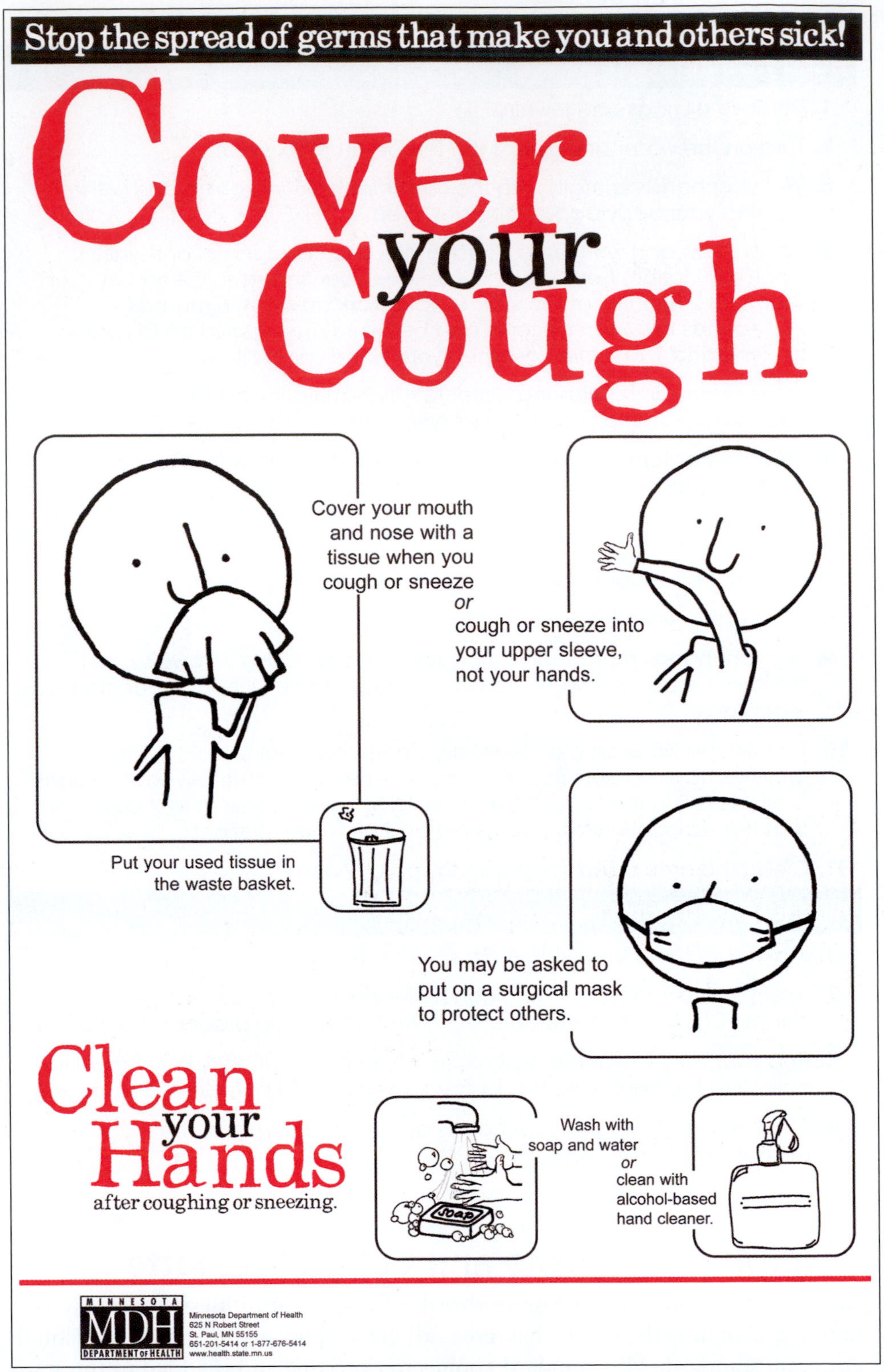

Figure 2-4 Respiratory hygiene and cough etiquette.

The use of **personal protective equipment (PPE)** is mandated by the **Occupational Safety and Health Administration (OSHA)** to minimize exposure to bloodborne pathogens. PPE includes gloves, gowns, masks, and protective eyewear. See Figure 2-5 and Table 2-3 for more information about personal protective equipment and its applications.

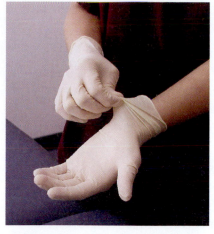 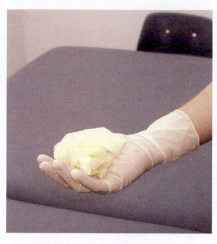 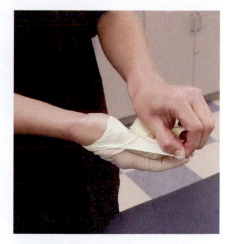

(A) Grasp the outside edge near the wrist. Peel away from the hand, turning the glove inside out. Hold the glove in the opposite gloved hand.

(B) Hold the contaminated glove in the gloved hand while removing the second glove.

(C) Slide the ungloved finger under the wrist of the remaining glove. Peel off from inside, creating a bag for both gloves, and then discard.

Figure 2-5 Removing gloves properly.

TABLE 2-3 Personal Protective Equipment

Type	When Used	Rules for Use
Gloves	For hand contact with blood, mucous membranes, and other potentially infectious materials or when nonintact skin is anticipated; when performing vascular access procedures; or when handling contaminated items or surfaces	• Gloves do not replace handwashing. • Perform hand hygiene before applying and after removing gloves. • When removing gloves, do not touch the outside (contaminated) area of the gloves (see Figure 2-6). • Keep gloved hands away from your face. • Avoid touching or adjusting other PPE. • Remove gloves if they are torn and perform hand hygiene before putting on new gloves. • Limit surfaces and items touched. • Extend gloves over isolation gown cuffs.
Gown	During procedures and patient care activities when contact of clothing/exposed skin with body/body fluids, secretions, or excretions is anticipated	• Always avoid touching the contaminated outside of the gown when removing it.
Mask	During patient care activities likely to generate splashes or sprays of blood, body fluids, secretions, or excretions	• Fully cover your nose and mouth. • Respirator masks, such as N95, N99, or N100, must be used for airborne precautions.
Eye protection	During patient care activities likely to generate splashes or sprays of blood, body fluids, secretions, or excretions	• Goggles should fit snugly over and around the eyes. • Personal glasses are not an acceptable substitute. • You can use a face shield that protects the face, nose, mouth, and eyes. • Face shield should cover your forehead, extend below your chin, and wrap around the side of your face. • Position goggles over the eyes and secure to the head using the earpieces or headband. • Position the face shield over your face and secure it on your brow with the headband.

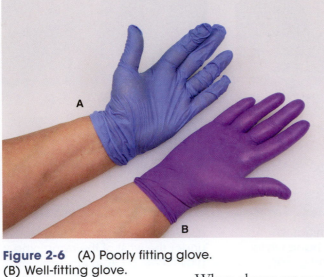

Figure 2-6 (A) Poorly fitting glove. (B) Well-fitting glove.

In general, when using PPE, you should do the following:

- Don (put on) the PPE before contact with the patient, generally before entering the room.
- Apply PPE in correct sequence: gown, mask or respirator, goggles or face shield, then gloves.
- Use PPE carefully to avoid spreading contamination.
- Remove and discard PPE carefully, either at the doorway or immediately outside the patient's room; remove the respirator outside the room.
- Remove PPE in correct sequence: gloves, face shield or goggles, gown, then mask or respirator.
- Immediately perform hand hygiene.

When gloves are required, be sure to wear gloves that fit you properly. Proper fit is important for safety. If your gloves are too small, they may tear. If your gloves are too large, you may drop items or the glove material might interfere with the safe performance of procedures (see Figure 2-6). Follow the steps in Competency Check 2.2 when donning and removing personal protective equipment. Use the competency checklist *Gowning, Gloving, and Masking* at the end of this chapter to review and practice the procedure.

Patient Education & Communication

Using Gloves

When describing the phlebotomy procedure to the patient, explain that you are required to wear gloves to prevent the spread of infection, so he or she will feel more comfortable. Be certain to ask the patient if he or she has had any problems with allergies to gloves or tourniquets. Never expose patients to latex products.

Donning and Removing Personal Protective Equipment

Competency Check 2-2

Gloves
1. Remove gloves by using your dominant hand to grasp the palm of the glove of your nondominant hand.
2. Gently pull the glove off the nondominant hand, turning it inside out and holding it in your dominant hand.
3. Encase the removed glove completely in the dominant hand to prevent the spread of contaminants.
4. Place the thumb or two fingers of the ungloved hand under the cuff of the remaining glove, being careful not to touch the contaminated outside of the glove with your bare hand.
5. Pull the glove over your hand, turning it inside out over the other glove, leaving none of the outside surface exposed.
6. Throw the gloves away in the appropriate waste container.
7. Wash your hands.

Gown
1. Put on a gown with the opening in the back.
2. Secure at the neck and waist.

3. Remove the gown by unfastening the ties.
4. Peel the gown away from the neck and shoulder and do not touch the outside.
5. Turn the contaminated gown outside toward the inside.
6. Fold or roll the gown into a bundle.
7. Discard the contaminated gown.

Mask

1. To put on the mask, place it over the nose, mouth, and chin.
2. Fit the flexible nose piece over the nose bridge.
3. Secure the mask on the head with ties or elastic.
4. Adjust the mask to fit.
5. To remove the mask, untie the bottom, then top tie.
6. Remove the mask from the face without touching the outside.
7. Discard the mask.

Eye Protection

1. To remove goggles or face shield, grasp the ear or headpieces with ungloved hands.
2. Lift them away from the face without touching the outside.
3. Place in designated receptacle for reprocessing or disposal.

Standard Precautions

In the late 1980s, the CDC introduced Universal Precautions to help protect healthcare workers from exposure to bloodborne pathogens. The use of Universal Precautions applied to blood, semen and vaginal secretions, and most body fluids. However, these precautions did *not* apply to feces, nasal secretions, sputum, sweat, tears, urine, or vomitus unless they contained visible blood. This is because the original Universal Precautions were aimed primarily at preventing the transmission of HIV/AIDS, which is not typically transmitted by these means.

In 1996, the CDC expanded its recommendations to include precautions against all types of healthcare-associated infections. At this time, the CDC implemented two levels of precautions: Standard Precautions and Isolation Precautions. The first level is **Standard Precautions,** which are based on the older Universal Precautions. These precautions apply to healthcare employees, combining hand hygiene and personal protective equipment use when working with blood and body fluids, non-intact skin, or mucous membranes. Unlike Universal Precautions, Standard Precautions apply when employees are exposed to *all* body fluids, secretions, and excretions, except sweat, regardless of whether they contain visible blood. The use of Standard Precautions reduces the risk of microorganism transmission from both recognized and unrecognized sources of infection. (See the appendix *Standard Precautions.*)

In addition, the CDC advises that healthcare employees not wear artificial nails because they are more likely to harbor gram-negative and other pathogens, both before and after handwashing, than natural nails. Natural nails should extend no more than one-fourth of an inch beyond the fingertips.

Isolation Precautions

Isolation Precautions, the CDC's second level of precautions, are based on how infectious agents are transmitted. For this reason, they are often called **transmission-based precautions.** The isolation categories include

- Airborne precautions that require special air handling, ventilation, and additional respiratory protection (HEPA or N95 respirators).

- Droplet precautions that require mucous membrane protection (goggles and masks).
- Contact precautions that require gloves and gowns during direct skin-to-skin contact or contact with contaminated linen, equipment, and other fomites.
- Protective environment (PE) precautions that are used for patients who may have a compromised immune system. A healthcare worker could easily transmit disease to these patients. Therefore, healthcare workers should wear gown, gloves, and mask when interacting with patients in PE.

When entering the room of a patient on Isolation Precautions, always wear appropriate PPE. If you are not certain what PPE to wear, consult a licensed practitioner caring for the patient, such as a nurse.

Never take a tray of phlebotomy equipment into an isolation room. Take only the equipment needed for the particular draw. If you need additional equipment, you must remove all PPE before leaving the room, collect the needed supplies, and then don new PPE before reentering the room. Similarly, the only introduced elements to leave the room should be the phlebotomist and the tubes. Any unused equipment or supplies must be left in the room.

A special procedure called **double-bagging** is used to dispose of contaminated waste and equipment from an isolation room. Two biohazard-labeled bags are used for this procedure. One person, wearing appropriate PPE, is in the room and places all items for disposal into the first bag. A second person remains at the doorway, with a second biohazard bag held wide open. The first person carefully places the closed bag into the second bag, making sure not to contaminate the outside of the second bag. The second bag is secured by the person outside the isolation room and can now be safely transported to the disposal area.

You should follow Standard Precautions with every patient when performing phlebotomy. Isolation Precautions are used less often and only with patients who have or are suspected of having specific infections. When Isolation Precautions are mandated for a patient receiving phlebotomy, you will be required to follow the specific guidelines for the type of precautions implemented (see the appendix *Transmission-Based Precautions*).

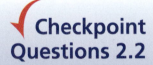

Checkpoint Questions 2.2

1. You have been asked to perform phlebotomy on a patient with an unknown respiratory disease. The patient has not been placed on Isolation Precautions, but as you approach the room, you can hear the patient coughing. What PPE would you use while drawing blood from this patient?
2. Briefly explain the differences between Universal Precautions, Standard Precautions, and Isolation Precautions.

2.3 Medical Biohazards

Biological substances that can threaten human health are called **biohazards.** Medical biohazards include any materials that may be contaminated with infectious agents. They include blood and body fluids, medical waste, and laboratory specimens and cultures. The handling and disposal of biohazardous wastes are regulated both by individual state regulatory committees as well as by OSHA and the CDC at the federal level. As state regulations often exceed federal requirements, be sure you know the applicable laws in your state.

Always wear gloves when handling biohazardous waste and only place them in bags or containers that are red and are clearly labeled as biohazards.

Biohazardous waste containers should be present close to locations where biohazardous waste is generated, such as next to a phlebotomy station.

Bloodborne Pathogens Standard

To help reduce the risk of injury and infection from biohazardous wastes, in 1991 OSHA developed the **Bloodborne Pathogens Standard.** This standard requires that healthcare facilities provide annual employee training on preventing exposure to bloodborne pathogens as well as using the necessary PPE. It applies to all blood products, body fluids, human tissues and cultures, vaccines, and any supplies, instruments, or equipment that have been in contact with any of these items. According to the standard, all potentially biohazardous waste must be discarded in an appropriate manner or processed according to strict guidelines.

To comply with the Bloodborne Pathogens Standard, employers must provide documented training to all employees. Training covers general information about infectious diseases caused by bloodborne pathogens, the use of PPE, Universal Precautions, and devices engineered to prevent exposure. It also includes procedures employees should follow when exposure occurs.

The Bloodborne Pathogens Standard also mandates other requirements. Employers must offer the hepatitis B vaccine (HBV) at no charge to all employees who are reasonably expected to come in contact with blood or **other potentially infectious materials (OPIM).** In addition, each healthcare facility is required to have an occupational **exposure control plan,** which is a protocol to be followed in the event an employee is exposed to blood-borne pathogens.

Needlestick Safety and Prevention Act

One of the most common biohazards in the healthcare setting is the risk of injury or infection from needles. A **needlestick injury** is a percutaneous (through the skin) piercing wound that is caused by the point of a needle. Injuries caused by other sharp instruments or objects, such as lancets, blades, or glass slides, are also included in this category.

Needlestick injuries are preventable with proper education, safety equipment, and the elimination of needles whenever possible. Through the recommendation of the National Institute for Occupational Safety and Health (NIOSH) and OSHA, the Needlestick Safety and Prevention Act was passed in 2001.

The **Needlestick Safety and Prevention Act** mandates the use of safety devices that reduce needlestick injuries in the clinical setting. The introduction of needleless equipment and protected needles has significantly reduced the risk of needlestick injuries. All devices selected for phlebotomy should be equipped with needlestick prevention features, such as one-handed needle covering devices or retractable needles. These devices, called *engineering controls*, will be discussed in more detail in the chapter *Blood Collection Equipment*. To reduce the chance of a needlestick injury, never break off, recap, or reuse needles.

In addition, a sharps container must be used for the proper disposal of needles and other sharps. Immediately after using a needle or other sharp device, engage the safety feature and place it in the sharps container (see Figure 2-7). Empty the sharps container into a designated biohazardous waste container when it becomes three-quarters full.

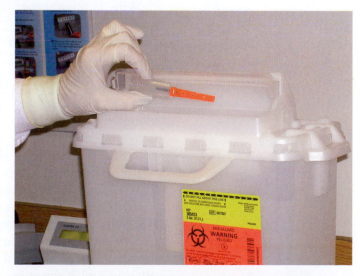

Figure 2-7 A sharps disposal container provides a place to safely dispose of used needles in order to prevent a needlestick injury.

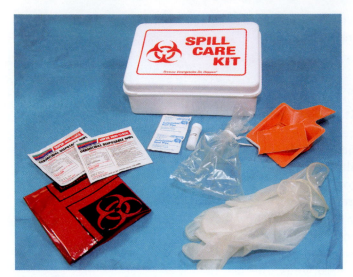

Figure 2-8 A biohazard cleanup kit.

The ultimate objective of the act is to protect both employees and patients from coming in contact with potentially harmful materials, such as contaminated needles and other sharps. Proper disposal of venipuncture equipment greatly decreases the incidence of accidental needlestick injuries and exposure.

Exposure to Hazardous Drugs

Research has shown that long-term exposure to hazardous drugs, such as antiviral and cancer drugs, can cause both acute and chronic illnesses in healthcare workers. In 2004, the National Institute for Occupational Safety and Health (NIOSH) published the NIOSH Alert: Preventing Occupational Exposure to Antineoplastic and Other Hazardous Drugs in Health Care Settings. This Alert is frequently updated and includes a list of hazardous drugs and recommendations for safe handling. Phlebotomists should be aware of the existence of these hazardous drugs, especially when repeatedly drawing blood from patients using them, such as oncology (cancer) patients.

Cleaning Up Biohazardous Spills

No matter how careful healthcare personnel may be, biohazardous spills do occasionally occur. Such spills must be handled carefully and according to federal guidelines. Depending on the type of spill, a biohazard spill cleanup kit may be needed. These kits contain special hazardous waste control products such as disposable dustpans and brushes for cleaning up broken glass that has contained blood or other biohazardous material (see Figure 2-8).

Clean up all biohazardous spills or splatters immediately. Always use appropriate PPE; never allow hazardous substances to come in contact with your skin. If the spill involves broken glass, use the disposable equipment in the spill kit to collect the contaminated glass and to dispose of it in a sharps container.

> **✓ Checkpoint Questions 2.3**
>
> 1. Which agencies regulate the handling and disposal of hazardous wastes?
> 2. What is the ultimate objective of disposing of sharps in a specially made container?

2.4 Safety and Preparedness

Complying with regulations and guidelines not only helps protect patients, personnel, and visitors from potentially contracting infections, but it also keeps everyone safe in other ways. Everyone involved in delivering quality healthcare must be aware of and comply with safety regulations and mandates from all levels of governmental and employer-developed policies.

In hospital laboratories, a designated safety officer is responsible for implementing a laboratory safety program. Injury and illness can occur because of improper handling of equipment during procedures or modification of the steps of the procedures. Each member of the healthcare team is responsible for his or her own safety as well as the safety of patients and other people in the immediate area.

Physical hazards in the healthcare setting are any nonbiological objects that may cause injury or illness to healthcare employees, patients, or visitors.

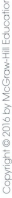

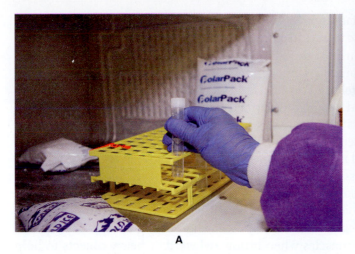 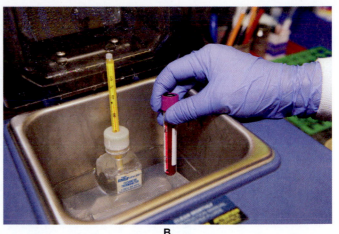

A   B

Figure 2-9 Specimen processing may require (A) cooling or (B) warming samples.

Physical hazards include allergen exposure, chemical hazards, compressed gas cylinders, electrical systems, fire hazards, radiation hazards, temperature hazards, and vacuum systems. In addition, physical hazards can result from using improper ergonomics in the workplace or lack of commonsense practices.

Common Sense and Ergonomics

Commonsense precautions should be applied in almost every environment, but especially in the healthcare setting. Avoid running or rushing, be aware of wet floors, avoid wearing dangling jewelry, and tie back long hair. Dangling jewelry and long hair may be obstacles in performing phlebotomy. More importantly, they can become contaminated and increase the risk of infection transfer, including healthcare-associated infections.

While processing specimens in the laboratory, operate laboratory equipment as recommended by the manufacturer. Again, wearing dangling jewelry and long hair untied may create a hazard when using equipment such as centrifuges. Keeping the workplace clean and organized also helps create a safe work environment.

Phlebotomists may need to process specimens of various temperatures. For example, some specimens must be frozen at temperatures of –80°C or even stored in liquid nitrogen. Other specimens may need to be placed in a heated water bath. Care must be taken to use appropriate equipment, such as thermal gloves and hot mitts, when handling heated or cooled specimens (see Figure 2-9).

Safety awareness is also important when using the vacuum systems that are found in most hospitals. These systems are used to transport pneumatic tubes to and from the laboratory. The suction in these systems is strong and can cause injury if used inappropriately. Caution must be used when opening these tubes, as the specimen container may have broken on its way to the lab, creating a biohazard (see Figure 2-10). The use of the pneumatic tube system must be validated for every analyte intended to be tested on specimens transported to the laboratory

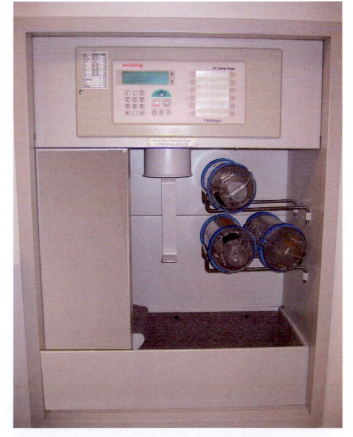

Figure 2-10 Vacuum system pneumatic tube station.

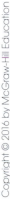

by this method. The facility's S.O.P. should contain the types of specimens approved for pneumatic tube transport, along with how they are to be wrapped or cushioned in the transport tubes.

Ergonomics is the practice of adapting a job task or equipment so that you can perform the task safely and productively. In phlebotomy, this includes sitting rather than standing and bending to perform a blood collection, lowering a bedrail to provide full access to the patient's arm (remember to replace the bedrail to its original position when you are finished), and placing equipment close to the procedure area to avoid reaching. Most healthcare employees use the computer to record and/or process patient information. Adjusting the height of the chair, the angle of the computer screen, and the position of your wrist when using a mouse will help you avoid the long-term physical effects of computer use.

Ergonomic principles should also be used when lifting objects. Bend your knees and use your leg muscles when lifting awkward or heavy objects to help prevent back strain. If you are in doubt about whether an object is too heavy to lift by yourself, ask a coworker to help you.

Allergen Exposure

Allergen exposure to products used in the healthcare setting is not uncommon. For example, healthcare providers may come into contact with latex routinely. Natural rubber latex (NRL) may be found in equipment used in phlebotomy, such as gloves, tourniquets, bandages, and tape. Healthcare employees and patients who are allergic to latex may experience symptoms ranging from itchy, red, watery eyes to chest tightness, shortness of breath, and shock. Latex can also cause bumps, sores, or red, raised areas on the part of the skin exposed to latex. Powdered gloves are especially dangerous because, when the gloves are removed, the powder disperses into the air. Powdered latex gloves should *never* be used for phlebotomy. Instead, use only powder-free, non-latex gloves.

Because latex can be found in several types of items, latex allergies are not to be taken lightly. Severe allergic reactions and even deaths have resulted from latex allergies. If you suspect that you are allergic to latex, you may consider undergoing specialized immunologic evaluations, such as skin tests and blood testing. However, the simplest way to avoid an allergic reaction is to avoid latex entirely. Most facilities now provide non-latex equipment and supplies routinely.

In rare cases, patients and healthcare employees may develop allergies to non-latex gloves and to the alcohol used in alcohol prep pads. Being aware of any possible allergy is essential for preventing allergic reactions.

Electrical Hazards

Electrical hazards include any contact with electrical equipment or the failure of equipment that creates a dangerous condition, which can result in electric shock, burn, electrocution, or even an explosion. These events are caused when electrical potentials move across a person. Ways to minimize electrical hazards include the following:

- Use fuses, circuit breakers, and ground fault interrupters properly to prevent circuit overload.
- Use three-pronged, grounded plugs to avoid short-circuits between incoming electricity, lab instruments, and the person(s) touching the instruments.
- Avoid touching electrical equipment that is wet from spilled liquids.
- Do not touch equipment with wet hands.
- If equipment is damaged, malfunctions, smells unusual, or makes a loud noise, turn it off.
- Do not stretch electrical cords.

- Do not use extension cords.
- Do not use equipment with damaged electrical cords until they are repaired.
- Turn off electrical equipment during a power failure to avoid a surge when power is restored.

In the event that you encounter a victim of electrical shock, always disconnect the power before attempting to rescue the victim.

Fire and Explosive Hazards

Fire and explosive hazards include situations in which a likelihood of fire or explosions exists. Fire hazards also include blocked fire escapes that prevent evacuation if a fire occurs. Fires and explosions can occur due to overloaded electrical circuits, the misuse of chemicals, a lack of training, or carelessness. Your participation in fire training and fire drills helps speed up the escape process in the event of a real fire. As the phlebotomist, you may be the first one to notice a fire as you enter a patient's room.

All healthcare employees should be trained in proper rescue procedures and the use of fire extinguishers. If a fire does occur, perform the four basic steps in fire emergency response, which is abbreviated "RACE" (Rescue, Alarm, Contain, and Extinguish). The RACE procedure includes:

R: Rescue those who need immediate help.

A: Activate the fire alarm or phone in the alarm.

C: Contain the fire as much as possible.

E: Extinguish, if possible.

These steps should be shared among several responders to speed the process. Everyone should be evacuated from the area of the fire quickly. Becoming familiar with the types of fire extinguishers available will help you select the correct one for each and every situation. See Table 2-4.

The most probable fire that healthcare workers may encounter is the trashcan fire. After performing the first three steps in the RACE response sequence, you may be able to attempt extinguishing the fire. Using the acronym PASS will help you remember the correct sequence in using a fire extinguisher. (1) Pull out the pin. (2) Aim (at the base of the fire, not at the flames). (3) Squeeze the trigger. (4) Sweep the base of the fire (see Figure 2-11).

Chemical Hazards

Chemical hazards include harmful or potentially harmful chemicals used by healthcare employees. Chemicals such as strong acids and bases can burn unprotected skin or cause serious damage if splashed in the eyes. For example, in some

TABLE 2-4 Classes of Fires and Extinguishers to Use

Class	Type of Fire	Type of Extinguisher
A	Ordinary combustibles such as cloth, paper, or wood; in a healthcare setting, this might be a trashcan fire.	Pressurized water, dry chemical
B	Flammable liquids such as oils, alcohol, and grease; in the medical laboratory, many liquid chemicals are flammable.	Dry chemical, carbon dioxide
C	Electrical equipment and its wiring, such as appliances and electronic devices; many electronic devices and instruments are used in healthcare settings and in the laboratory.	Dry chemical, carbon dioxide, halon
D	Combustible metals, which are not usually found in the healthcare setting.	Sand or special extinguishing agent

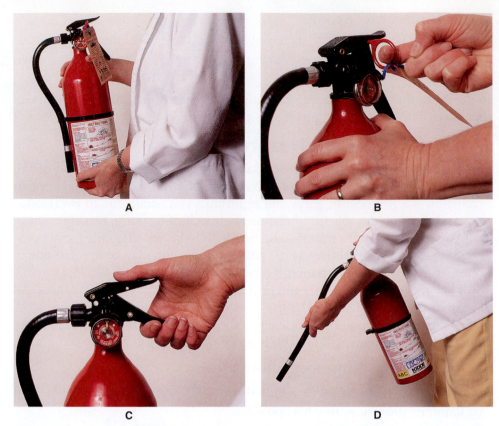

Figure 2-11 Extinguish fires by sweeping the base of the fire.

healthcare settings, phlebotomists may need to add preservatives to 24-hour urine collection containers used for collecting these specimens. As these preservatives contain potentially harmful chemicals, handling chemicals properly is of the utmost importance. Guidelines for handling chemicals include the following:

- Use glassware appropriate for the task.
- Use PPE and engineering controls and never pipet by mouth. PPE for handling chemicals include a lab coat, gloves, and a face shield or goggles.
  - When diluting an acid, add the acid to water. Never add water to an acid. Adding water to an acid can generate a great amount of heat and may cause a burn.
  - Observe state and federal regulations when storing or disposing of chemicals. Some chemicals need to be stored in a flameproof metal cabinet (see Figure 2-12).
  - Compressed gas cylinders must be chained to the wall or to a handcart during transport. Dropping a gas cylinder may prove fatal, as it can have explosive pressure and become a destructive projectile.

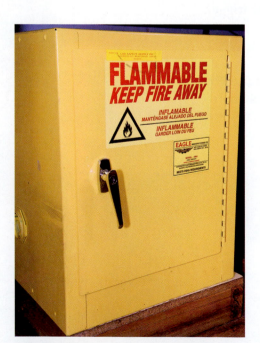

Figure 2-12 Chemical safety cabinet.

Regulations require that chemicals be labeled with the contents of the container, the date of purchase or preparation, and the initials of the preparer. In addition, OSHA recommends that all containers with hazardous chemicals be marked with a hazard symbol that contains their level of risk.

Recently, OSHA modified its Hazard Communication Standard (HCS) to include the **Globally Harmonized System (GHS).** The GHS is an internationally agreed-upon system for communicating chemical hazards in order to improve safety and health in the workplace. The GHS provides detailed criteria for determining a chemical's hazardous effects, standardized labeling criteria, and

a harmonized format for safety data sheets. Hazard classifications are definitions of hazards that are grouped under health hazards and physical hazards. Under the current Hazard Communication Standard (HCS), the label must include the identity of the chemical and the appropriate hazard warnings by displaying a harmonized signal word, a pictogram, and a hazard statement. A **pictogram** is a symbol (including border and background color) that is intended to convey specific information about the hazards of a chemical. The GHS has nine pictograms. See Figure 2-13 for these pictograms. A **signal word**

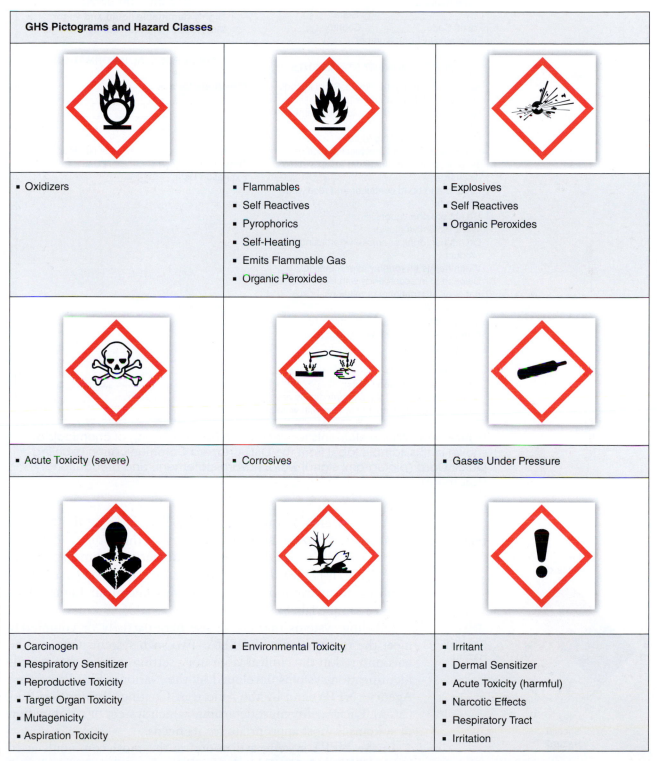

GHS Pictograms and Hazard Classes

■ Oxidizers	■ Flammables ■ Self Reactives ■ Pyrophorics ■ Self-Heating ■ Emits Flammable Gas ■ Organic Peroxides	■ Explosives ■ Self Reactives ■ Organic Peroxides
■ Acute Toxicity (severe)	■ Corrosives	■ Gases Under Pressure
■ Carcinogen ■ Respiratory Sensitizer ■ Reproductive Toxicity ■ Target Organ Toxicity ■ Mutagenicity ■ Aspiration Toxicity	■ Environmental Toxicity	■ Irritant ■ Dermal Sensitizer ■ Acute Toxicity (harmful) ■ Narcotic Effects ■ Respiratory Tract ■ Irritation

Figure 2-13 Pictograms included in the Global Harmonization System for chemical hazard communication (as found on the OSHA website).

SAMPLE LABEL

PRODUCT IDENTIFIER

CODE _____

Product Name _____

SUPPLIER IDENTIFICATION

Company Name_____

Street Address _____
City _____ State _____
Postal Code _____ Country _____
Emergency Phone Number _____

PRECAUTIONARY STATEMENTS

Keep container tightly closed. Store in cool, well ventilated place that is locked.
Keep away from heat/sparks/open flame. No smoking.
Only use non-sparking tools.
Use explosion-proof electrical equipment.
Take precautionary measure against static discharge.
Ground and bond container and receiving equipment.
Do not breathe vapors.
Wear Protective gloves.
Do not eat, drink or smoke when using this product.
Wash hands thoroughly after handling.
Dispose of in accordance with local, regional, national, international regulations as specified.

In Case of Fire: use dry chemical (BC) or Carbon dioxide (CO2) fire extinguisher to extinguish.

First Aid
If exposed call Poison Center.
If on skin (on hair): Take off immediately any contaminated clothing. Rinse skin with water.

HAZARD PICTOGRAMS

SIGNAL WORD

Danger

HAZARD STATEMENT

Highly flammable liquid and vapor.
May cause liver and kidney damage.

SUPPLEMENTAL INFORMATION

Directions for use
_____
_____
_____

Fill weight: _____ Lot Number _____
Gross weight: _____ Fill Date: _____
Expiration Date: _____

Figure 2-14 All the elements required by OSHA for labeling of chemicals are shown in this sample label from the OSHA Hazard Communication Labeling Quick Card (pictogram, signal word, hazard statement, and precautionary statement).

(either "danger" or "warning") is used on the label to indicate the hazard's relative level of severity. A **hazard statement** describes the nature and degree of the chemical's hazard(s). A **precautionary statement,** on the other hand, lists measures to minimize or prevent adverse effects resulting from exposure to a hazardous chemical. Figure 2-14 shows a sample label.

Labeling systems that are in use may partially or completely meet the requirements of OSHA. Two such systems that may be encountered in the clinical laboratory setting include the hazards identification systems developed by the National Fire Protection Agency (NFPA) and by the American Coatings Association, Inc. (ACA). Each facility must determine which system or combination of systems is most appropriate for its needs.

In the NFPA system, a diamond is the most commonly used symbol (Figure 2-15). Table 2-5 outlines the meaning of each part of the NFPA diamond. The NFPA diamond is designed for use

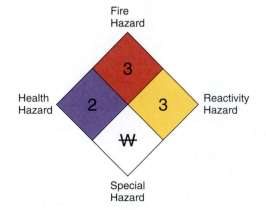

Figure 2-15 NFPA diamond hazard symbol.

TABLE 2-5 National Fire Protection Agency Chemical Hazard Code

Color	Location	Meaning
RED	Upper quadrant	Indicates a chemical's degree of flammability hazard.
		Numbers represent relative flash point in degrees Fahrenheit.
		0—will not burn
		1—not exceeding 200°F
		2—above 100°F
		3—below 100°F
		4—below 73°F
BLUE	Left middle quadrant	Indicates the level of hazard the chemical poses to health.
		0—no health concerns
		1—slightly hazardous
		2—hazardous
		3—extreme danger
		4—deadly
YELLOW	Right middle quadrant	Indicates the chemical's reactivity or stability at certain temperatures
		0—stable
		1—unstable if heated
		2—violent chemical change
		3—shock and heat
		4—may detonate
WHITE	Lower quadrant	Indicates the existence of additional hazards.
		Abbreviations are used to indicate
		ACID—acid
		ALK—alkali
		COR—corrosive
		OXY—oxidizer
		P—polymerization
		W—reacts with water
		Radiation symbol indicates radiation hazard.

in emergency situations where quick access to information about the effects of short or acute exposure is needed.

To meet the requirements of the OSHA Hazard Communication Standard, the ACA developed a Hazardous Materials Identification System (HMIS) that is being adopted by some healthcare facilities. The HMIS uses a color bar (Figure 2-16) that is similar to the NFPA diamond. However, the purpose of the HMIS color bar is not for emergencies; rather it conveys information about broader health warnings. Table 2-6 outlines the meaning of each color bar of the HMIS. Hazards are rated from 0 (minimum) to 4 (severe) and recommended PPEs are shown using pictograms (Figure 2-17).

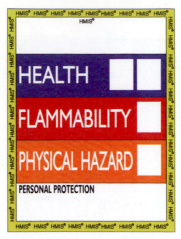

Figure 2-16 The HMIS label uses similar colors as the NFPA diamond. The white bar is different in meaning in that it conveys the type of protective equipment to be used. In addition, newer labels have replaced yellow with orange. The HMIS® trademark and related content are used under license of the American Coatings Association.

TABLE 2-6 HMIS Color Bar Meanings

Color	Location	Meaning
BLUE	Top bar	Indicates the level of hazard the chemical poses to health.
RED	Second bar	Indicates a chemical's degree of flammability hazard.
YELLOW or ORANGE	Third bar	Indicates the chemical's level of physical hazard.
WHITE	Bottom bar	Indicates the types of personal protection needed.

If a chemical contacts the skin or eyes, the best first aid is immediate flushing with large amounts of water. Emergency showers and eyewashes are located throughout the medical laboratory (Figure 2-18). Be sure you know their locations and how to use them. Contaminated clothing should be removed as soon as possible. Chemical spill kits (Figure 2-19) are available to neutralize chemicals spilled on laboratory surfaces and to help minimize exposure.

OSHA mandates that healthcare facilities develop and implement plans to protect healthcare workers from exposure to various hazards. These plans include a **chemical hygiene plan,** a biohazard exposure control plan, and a plan for handling **hazardous materials (HAZMATS).** State "right to know documents" and OSHA document 29 CFR 1910 set standards for chemical hazard communication (HAZCOM) to educate employees about their work environment and to keep them informed of potential hazards.

OSHA requires employers to provide **safety data sheets (SDS),** formerly called material safety data sheets (MSDS), for every chemical purchased by or

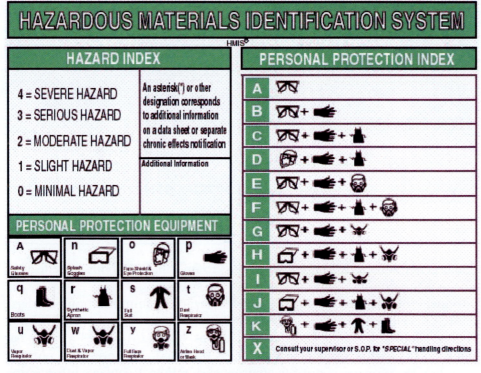

Figure 2-17 The HMIS uses a 0 to 4 rating scale for the hazard index and a variety of pictograms to indicate the recommended PPEs to use when handling the chemical. The HMIS® trademark and related content are used under license of the American Coatings Association.

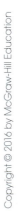

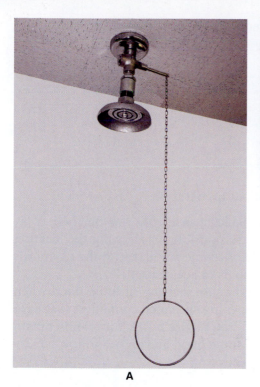

A

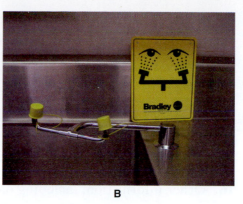

B

Figure 2-18 (A) Emergency shower. (B) Emergency eyewash.

kept in a facility (see Figure 2-20). These data sheets, developed by the chemical suppliers, provide important information about proper handling and storage of the chemicals, specific hazards associated with them, first-aid measures, and personal protection required as well as other relevant information. As outlined by the GHS, safety data sheets must include the following information:

1. Identification
2. Hazard(s) identification
3. Composition/information on ingredients
4. First-aid measures
5. Firefighting measures
6. Accidental release measures
7. Handling and storage

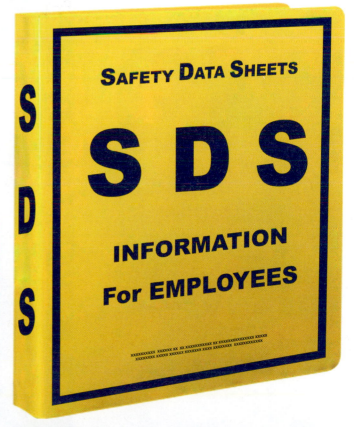

Figure 2-20 Safety data sheets may be stored in a clearly marked binder and placed where easy to find.

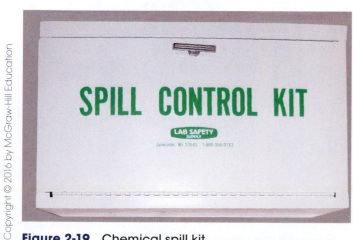

Figure 2-19 Chemical spill kit.

8. Exposure controls/personal protection
9. Physical and chemical properties
10. Stability and reactivity
11. Toxicological information
12. Ecological information
13. Disposal considerations
14. Transport information
15. Regulatory information
16. Other information, including date of preparation or last revision

Employers should ensure SDS are available in print copy or on their company's employee website. Employees are responsible for knowing the location of the SDS for the chemicals they handle. Become familiar with the chemicals you use and know what to do in case of spills or accidents.

Laboratory and other healthcare workers use a chemical fume hood when handling hazardous chemicals or when opening specimen containers that have hazardous preservatives, such as formalin (see Figure 2-21). You should obtain proper training on the use of a chemical fume hood and always follow facility procedures for handling hazardous materials.

Radioactive Hazards

A **radioactive hazard** exists where ionizing radiation is present. Radiation is energy traveling through space. Ionizing radiation can destabilize molecules within cells and lead to tissue damage. Sources of radiation can be found in

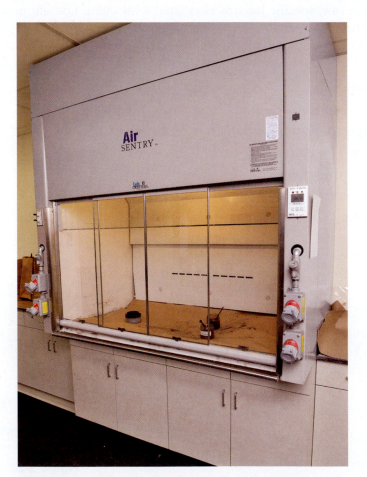

Figure 2-21 Chemical fume hood.

several areas of healthcare settings. The radiation symbol is used as a visual warning of this hazard.

Radiation is used for diagnostic imaging and radiation therapy. However, the medical laboratory may also have sources of radiation because some laboratory tests use radioactive compounds. Laboratory personnel who work with radioactive materials are required to wear a film badge or use a dosimeter to monitor their exposure to radiation. As a phlebotomist, you will need to be aware of those areas where radiation is used and limit the time you stay in those areas. In addition to limiting your exposure time, keeping a safe distance and using appropriate radiation shielding will help minimize your exposure to radiation. Follow the policies and procedures established at your facility.

Reporting Hazards

Most facilities have an office of Risk Management, Safety and Security, or another office to which hazards concerns should be reported. When an incident does occur, an incident report is filed. Employees of healthcare facilities follow a specific process when filing an incident report for any event involving a patient's or their own safety. Phlebotomists should become familiar with the process for addressing safety concerns and occurrences of incidents at their facilities, including reporting hazards and incidents and completing or assisting in the completion of incident reports when appropriate.

Emergency Preparedness

Providing safety for patients, personnel, and visitors is mandatory and becomes critical during emergencies and extreme conditions. These include situations such as a weather disaster, bioterrorist attack, mass casualties, or severe emergencies caused by chemicals, radiation, or fire. Healthcare professionals should maintain a state of professional readiness. Additional training at your place of employment about how to handle each type of emergency may be required, including cardiopulmonary resuscitation (CPR) and first aid. In all cases, during an emergency you should remember to stay calm and think through each situation in order to respond appropriately and create the best outcome.

In order to respond and react appropriately to emergencies, you should be aware of certain signs, symbols, and labels that are found in healthcare facilities. See Table 2-7. Additionally, the hospital association in each state has developed a standard set of color and word codes to represent various types of emergencies. Currently, a nationwide standard for these codes does not exist. Table 2-8 displays the emergency codes used by one hospital. The codes used by other facilities may be different. Therefore, healthcare professionals must be aware of the emergency codes used at their facility.

Evacuation and Shelter-in-Place Plans

Every healthcare facility should have evacuation and shelter-in-place plans in the event of an emergency. For evacuation, maps of the facility with escape routes clearly marked should be posted at visible locations for your reference. "Shelter-in-place" refers to an interior room or rooms within your medical facility with few or no windows that could be used as a refuge. Employees are trained in evacuation and shelter-in-place procedures and periodic practice drills should be performed. Evacuation and shelter-in-place protocols differ and you should be aware of the proper alert to implement the correct procedure.

TABLE 2-7 Signs, Symbols, and Labels

SIGN, SYMBOL, OR LABEL	TITLE	MEANING
CAUTION BIOHAZARD / SHARPS DISPOSAL ONLY	Biohazard	Indicates the actual or potential presence of a biohazard including equipment, containers, rooms, and materials that present a risk or potential risk. The biohazard symbol is black. The background is typically fluorescent orange, orange-red, or other contrasting color.
IN CASE OF FIRE DO NOT USE ELEVATORS USE EXIT STAIRWAYS	Fire Safety	A fire extinguisher sign is placed at the location of the extinguisher. An exit sign like this one indicates the appropriate method of exit in case of a fire. Elevators and escalators are not typically in use during an emergency.
FIRST AID / A E D	First Aid and Automated External Defibrillator (AED)	The sign would indicate a first-aid kit and an automated external defibrillator is available for use. These are placed at the location of the equipment.
NOTICE STOP WASH YOUR HANDS	Wash Your Hands	Hands should be washed frequently. This is a reminder. Usually placed in locations where contamination to hands can occur and available handwashing equipment is nearby.
(Handicap symbol)	Handicap	This symbol indicates the route a handicapped person should take. Consider this for patients who are unable to walk or need to avoid steps for any reason.
EMERGENCY EYE WASH STATION	General Safety Signs	Provide notices of general practice and rules relating to health, first aid, medical equipment, sanitation, housekeeping, and suggestions relative to general safety measures. For example, an eye wash station is used when chemicals, blood, or other foreign items get in the eye.
(Radiation symbol)	Radiation Hazard	Indicates radiation in use that is damaging to cells. Limit exposure or wear protective gear. If working in these areas, wear a film badge or dosimeter to measure amount of exposure.

TABLE 2-8 Emergency Code Colors and Definitions

Codes	Emergency Code Definitions
FIRE	RED—Procedures staff should follow to protect patients, staff, visitors, themselves, and property from a confirmed or suspected fire.
MEDICAL EMERGENCY	BLUE—Facilitate the arrival of equipment and specialized personnel to the location of an adult medical emergency. Provide life support and emergency care.
INFANT/CHILD ABDUCTION	PINK—Activate response to protect infants and children from removal by unauthorized persons, and identify the physical descriptions and actions of someone attempting to kidnap an infant from the medical facility.
COMBATIVE ASSAULT PERSON	GRAY—Activate facility and staff response when staff members are confronted by an abusive/assaultive person.
BOMB THREAT	GREEN—Activate response to a bomb threat or the discovery of a suspicious package.
PERSON WITH WEAPONS OR HOSTAGE	SILVER—Activate facility and staff response to event in which staff members are confronted by persons brandishing a weapon or who have taken hostages in the medical facility.
HAZARDOUS MATERIAL SPILL	YELLOW—Identify unsafe exposure conditions, safely evacuate an area, and protect others from exposure due to a hazardous materials spill release. Perform procedures to be taken in response to a minor or major spill.
INTERNAL DISASTER	TRIAGE INTERNAL—Activate response to incidents that require or may require significant support from several departments in order to continue patient care.
EXTERNAL DISASTER	TRIAGE EXTERNAL—Activate response to external emergencies that require or may require significant support from several departments in order to continue patient care.
POWER BLACK OUT	CODE EDISON—Activate response to a rolling power failure.

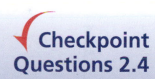

Checkpoint Questions 2.4

1. List at least four types of physical hazards and provide an example of each within a healthcare facility.
2. What is the difference between a chemical spill kit and a biohazard cleanup kit?

Chapter Summary

Learning Outcome	Key Concepts/Examples	Related NAACLS Competency
2.1 Identify the elements in the chain of infection and the ways in which disease can be transmitted. Pages 27–29.	The chain of infection consists of the infectious agent, reservoir, portal of exit, mode of transmission, portal of entry, and susceptible host. Infection can occur if any of these links become compromised. Modes of transmission include contact, droplet, airborne, vehicle-borne, and vector-borne transmission.	2.2
2.2 Demonstrate knowledge of infection control practices and guidelines related to phlebotomy. Pages 29–36.	Infection control practices include using appropriate hand hygiene, following respiratory hygiene and cough etiquette, wearing personal protective equipment (PPE), following Standard Precautions, and following appropriate Isolation Precautions when indicated.	2.00, 2.1, 2.2, 2.3, 2.4
2.3 Implement safety practices to reduce the risk of infection from medical biohazards in compliance with state and federal standards and regulations. Pages 36–38.	Safety practices include compliance with the Bloodborne Pathogens Standard, the Needlestick Safety and Prevention Act, and all other state and federal guidelines for preventing bloodborne and other diseases.	2.1, 2.2, 2.3
2.4 Apply techniques to ensure the physical safety of healthcare workers and patients. Pages 38–51.	Physical hazards found in healthcare settings include exposure to allergy-causing equipment and supplies, including those containing latex; electrical and fire hazards; and exposure to hazardous chemicals and radiation. Many hazards can be avoided by taking commonsense precautions.	2.1, 2.3, 2.4

Chapter Review

A: Labeling

Label the NFPA diamond by indicating each quadrant's color and hazard identification.

1. [LO 2.4] _____

2. [LO 2.4] _____

3. [LO 2.4] _____

4. [LO 2.4] _____

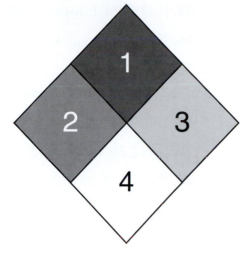

B: Matching

Match the bacteria to the drug-resistant variations that cause illnesses that are difficult to treat using traditional antibiotics.

____**5.** [LO 2.1] *Clostridium difficile*   **a.** MRSA

____**6.** [LO 2.1] Enterococci   **b.** VRE

____**7.** [LO 2.1] *Acinetobacter baumannii*   **c.** C-diff

____**8.** [LO 2.1] *Staphylococcus aureus*   **d.** MDRAB

Match the government agency with its function.

____**9.** [LO 2.2] requires the use of PPE to minimize exposure to bloodborne pathogens   **a.** NIOSH

___**10.** [LO 2.3] publishes recommendations for working with hazardous drugs   **b.** NFPA

___**11.** [LO 2.4] developed a system for chemical hazard identification   **c.** CDC

___**12.** [LO 2.2] developed standards for preventing healthcare-associated infections   **d.** OSHA

C: Fill in the Blank

Complete each statement.

13. [LO 2.2] One of the most critical steps in preventing HAIs is correct

_____.

14. [LO 2.2] When entering a room that has airborne precautions, you should wear a(n)

_____.

D: Sequencing

Indicate the correct order for donning the following PPE.

_____ 15. [LO 2.2] Gloves

_____ 16. [LO 2.2] Goggles

_____ 17. [LO 2.2] Gown

Indicate the correct order for removing the following PPE.

_____ 18. [LO 2.2] Gloves

_____ 19. [LO 2.2] Goggles

_____ 20. [LO 2.2] Gown

What is the correct sequence of action when a fire is encountered?

_____ 21. [LO 2.4] Activate the fire alarm or phone in the alarm.

_____ 22. [LO 2.4] Contain the fire as much as possible.

_____ 23. [LO 2.4] Extinguish the fire if possible.

_____ 24. [LO 2.4] Rescue those who need immediate help.

What is the correct sequence for using a fire extinguisher?

_____ 25. [LO 2.4] Aim the nozzle.

_____ 26. [LO 2.4] Squeeze the trigger.

_____ 27. [LO 2.4] Pull out the pin.

_____ 28. [LO 2.4] Sweep the base of the fire.

E: Case Studies/Critical Thinking

29. [LO 2.1] A patient in an isolation room asks the phlebotomist to take a magazine the patient has just finished reading and return it to the visitor's lounge, where the patient's friend originally found it. How should the phlebotomist handle this request?

30. [LO 2.4] You are opening a tube of blood for testing at a physician office laboratory (POL). The specimen splashes in your face.

   a. What is the health risk of biohazard exposure?

   b. What are the proper steps for handling this incident?

   c. What should have been done to prevent this incident from happening?

31. [LO 2.4] A new electronic instrument is purchased for a POL. It has a 3-foot cord on it. The place that would currently accommodate the instrument is 5 feet away from the nearest electrical outlet. What guidelines should be considered when installing this instrument?

32. [LO 2.4] As a phlebotomist was preparing a 24-hour urine collection container, the preservative splashed into his face.

   a. What is the health risk of hazardous chemical exposure?

   b. What are the proper steps for handling this incident?

   c. What should have been done to prevent this incident from happening?

33. [LO 2.4] A person who is processing specimens first cleans her hands with an alcohol-based sanitizer, then immediately presses the centrifuge's "on" button. She feels a mild shock as the centrifuge turns on.

    a. Why did this electrical hazard event occur?

    b. What should have been done to prevent this incident from happening?

F: Exam Prep

Choose the best answer for each question.

34. [LO 2.1] A phlebotomist enters a room to draw blood on a patient undergoing care for an infected wound. The site of the wound and its bandages are considered which link in the chain of infection?

    a. Infectious agent

    b. Mode of transmission

    c. Portal of exit

    d. Susceptible host

35. [LO 2.1] A fomite is a(n)

    a. alcohol-based foam hand sanitizer.

    b. contaminated object.

    c. sterile container.

    d. type of pathogenic bacterium.

36. [LO 2.1] Which of the following is an example of a healthcare-associated infection (HAI)?

    a. A patient enters the emergency department with suspected food poisoning after eating at a local restaurant.

    b. A patient admitted for a bleeding problem is found to have acute leukemia 2 days after admission.

    c. A phlebotomist develops high blood pressure after having been working at a hospital for three months.

    d. A phlebotomist who has a staph infection does a point-of-care blood draw from a hospital patient, who later develops a staph infection.

37. [LO 2.2] A patient in which type of isolation is the LEAST likely to transmit disease to the phlebotomist?

    a. Airborne

    b. Contact

    c. Droplet

    d. Protective

38. [LO 2.1] For which of the following diseases or conditions might a hospital routinely test patients being admitted to the hospital?

    a. Cancer

    b. MRSA

    c. Ulcer

    d. Arthritis

39. [LO 2.2] A common allergen found in blood collection equipment is

    a. latex.

    b. nitrile.

    c. vitrine.

    d. vinyl.

40. [LO 2.4] Which of the following is a document that summarizes a chemical's characteristics as well as its handling and storage guidelines?

    a. HAZMAT

    b. HEPA

    c. NFPA

    d. SDS

41. [LO 2.2] Double-bagging is

    a. using a bag inside a bag to transport specimens.

    b. placing normal waste into two separate bags.

    c. placing biohazardous material into a bag and then that bag into another bag.

    d. wearing two pairs of gloves while working with biohazardous materials.

42. [LO 2.2] Personal protective equipment includes all of the following EXCEPT

    a. eyewash.

    b. face shields.

    c. gloves.

    d. gown.

43. [LO 2.3] Needlesticks can be prevented by
    a. recapping needles.
    b. cutting needles with a needle cutter.
    c. using a one-handed technique to engage the engineering control.
    d. bending needles before placing them into a sharps container.

44. [LO 2.2] A patient enters an outpatient laboratory for testing. The phlebotomist notices that, after applying alcohol to the patient's skin prior to the blood collection procedure, the skin turned red. What question should the phlebotomist ask the patient?
    a. "Are you allergic to any medications?"
    b. "Do you have any allergies to alcohol or antiseptics?"
    c. "Are you feeling all right?"
    d. No questions are needed. Developing a red color is normal when alcohol touches the skin.

45. [LO 2.4] Physical hazards include all of these EXCEPT
    a. blood and body fluids.
    b. electrical equipment.
    c. latex gloves.
    d. radiation.

46. [LO 2.4] Which of the following is an example of a biohazard?
    a. Touching electrical equipment with wet hands
    b. The potential for a fire to start
    c. Splashing blood when a cap is removed
    d. Spilling a chemical on a countertop

47. [LO 2.4] When is it acceptable to wear dangling jewelry in the healthcare setting?
    a. When long necklaces are tucked underneath clothing
    b. When a surgical cap covers dangling earrings
    c. When a task does not involve hazardous chemicals
    d. Never

48. [LO 2.4] An electronic instrument has a three-pronged cord that is too short to reach the outlet. There is an extension cord in the closet that will only work with a two-pronged plug. What is the safest way to connect power to this instrument?
    a. Cut off the third prong of the instrument plug.
    b. Move the instrument closer to the outlet.
    c. Find a three-pronged extension cord.
    d. Have an electrician change the instrument's plug to two-pronged.

49. [LO 2.4] A physician office laboratory wants to ensure that they are disposing of medical waste properly. Which agency should they consult for medical-waste-handling guidelines?
    a. DHHS
    b. DOT
    c. EPA
    d. OSHA

50. [LO 2.4] What precautions should you take when adding a chemical to a container for at-home specimen collection?
    a. Label the container with the contents, the date, and your initials.
    b. Dilute strong acids by adding them first, then water.
    c. Wear PPE only if the chemical is considered a biohazard.
    d. Laboratory personnel are not responsible for preparing these containers.

51. [LO 2.4] A medical laboratory assistant (MLA) is asked to help unpack a shipment of chemicals for the laboratory. The MLA should first
    a. don all personal protective equipment.
    b. check the NFPA label to see if there is a fire hazard.
    c. read the SDS for storage requirements.
    d. place all the chemicals in the chemical storage cabinet.

52. [LO 2.4] When you are handling a chemical, you notice the NFPA label. What does this label indicate?
    a. Slight health risk
    b. High fire risk
    c. High reactivity risk
    d. Not to be mixed with water

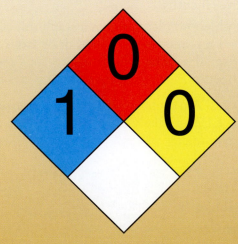

53. [LO 2.1] A woman who has a cold wipes her hands on a dinner napkin and leaves the napkin on the table when she leaves the restaurant. The server who clears the table touches the napkin and later develops a cold. What type of transmission has occurred?

a. Airborne transmission

b. Vector-borne transmission

c. Vehicle-borne transmission

d. Droplet transmission

References

American Coatings Association. (2014) www.paint.org/images/HMIS_PPElist.jpg

Davis, D. (2009). *Laboratory safety: A self-assessment workbook.* Chicago, IL. American Society for Clinical Pathology.

Dudeck, Margaret A., & The Association for Professionals in Infection Control and Epidemiology, Inc. (2009). *National Healthcare Safety Network (NHSN) report: Data summary for 2010, device-associated module.* Retrieved June 13, 2013, from www.cdc.gov/nhsn/PDFs/dataStat/NHSNReport_DataSummaryfor2010.pdf

Loo, V.G., Poirier, L., Miller, M.A., Oughton, M., et al. (2005). A predominantly clonal multi-institutional outbreak of *Clostridium difficile*-associated diarrhea with high morbidity and mortality. *New England Journal of Medicine, 353*(23), 2442–2449. Retrieved February 26, 2011.

Mirza, A., & Steele, R. (2011). Hospital-acquired infections. *Medscape: Drugs, Diseases, and Procedures.* Retrieved July 26, 2011, from http://emedicine.medscape.com/article/967022-overview

Moore, N., & Flaws, M. (2011). Antimicrobial resistance mechanisms in *Pseudomonas aeruginosa. Clinical Laboratory Science, 1,* 47–51.

National Accrediting Agency for Clinical Laboratory Sciences. (2012). *NAACLS entry-level phlebotomist competencies.* Rosemont, IL. NAACLS. Retrieved May 18, 2014, from www.naacls.org/docs/Guide_Approval-section1b-Phleb.pdf

National Fire Protection Agency. (2011). *NFPA 70E: Standard for electrical safety in the workplace.* Retrieved February 26, 2011, from www.nfpa.org.

Occupational Safety & Health Administration. (n.d.). *Safety and health topics: Radiation.* Retrieved February 26, 2011, from www.osha.gov/SLTC/radiation/index.html

Occupational Safety & Health Administration. (n.d.). *The globally harmonized system for hazard communication.* Retrieved February 13, 2014, from www.osha.gov/dsg/hazcom/global.html

Siegel, J. D., Rhinehart, E., Jackson, M., Chiarello, L., & Healthcare Infection Control Practices Advisory Committee. (2007). *Guideline for isolation precautions: Preventing transmission of infectious agents in healthcare settings.* Centers for Disease Control and Prevention. Retrieved June 19, 2013, from www.cdc.gov/hicpac/pdf/isolation/isolation2007.pdf

COMPETENCY CHECKLIST: HAND WASHING

Procedure Steps	Practice			Performed		Master
	1	2	3	Yes	No	
1. Uses paper towel to turn on the water supply.						
2. Discards the paper towel.						
3. Adjusts the water temperature.						
4. Dispenses an appropriate amount of soap into the hand.						
5. Creates a sufficient amount of lather.						
6. Sufficiently removes gross contamination from all skin surfaces.						
7. Rinses off the soap.						
8. Appropriately positions the hands while rinsing them.						
9. Dispenses soap into the palm of the hand.						
10. Cleanses the nail beds of each finger.						
11. Cleanses underneath the nails in an appropriate fashion.						
12. Rinses off the soap.						
13. Appropriately positions the hands while rinsing.						
14. Dries the hands, using paper towels.						
15. Uses paper towel to turn off the water supply.						

COMMENTS: _____
_____
_____
_____

SIGNED

EVALUATOR: _____

STUDENT: _____

NAME: _____ DATE: _____

COMPETENCY CHECKLIST: GOWNING, GLOVING, AND MASKING

Procedure Steps	Practice			Performed		
	1	2	3	Yes	No	Master
Donning PPE						
1. Removes the lab coat.						
2. Washes hands before putting on the protective clothing.						
3. Dons the gown, tying the ties at the neck and waist.						
4. Dons a mask.						
5. Positions the mask with the appropriate side facing out.						
6. Securely fastens the wire at the top of the mask around the nose.						
7. Securely ties the ties high on the head.						
8. Dons gloves.						
9. Positions the gloves with the cuff pulled over the sleeve of the gown.						
Removing PPE						
10. Removes the gloves.						
11. Removes the gloves inside out without contaminating the hands.						
12. Deposits the gloves in the appropriate receptacle.						
13. Removes goggles or face shield.						
14. Only touches the handles or head band when removing the mask.						
15. Deposits the goggles in the appropriate receptacle.						
16. Unties the gown at the waist if ties at the back of the gown.						
17. Unties the gown at the neck.						
18. Removes the gown inside out.						
19. Does not touch the front of the gown with either the hands or the uniform during removal.						
20. Removes the mask by only touching the ties.						
21. Discards the mask.						
22. Properly washes the hands.						

COMMENTS: _____
_____
_____
_____

SIGNED

EVALUATOR: _____

STUDENT: _____

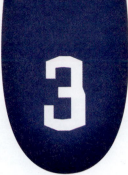

3 Introduction to Medical and Anatomical Terminology

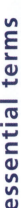

essential terms

abdominopelvic
anatomical position
anatomy
anterior
atoms
brachium
caudal plane
cells
combining vowel
coronal
cranial
deep
deoxyribonucleic acid (DNA)
diaphragm
distal
dorsal
femoral
frontal plane
inferior
lateral
medial

midsagittal plane
molecules
organelles
organism
organs
physiology
posterior
prefix
prone
proximal
ribonucleic acid (RNA)
sagittal plane
suffix
superficial
superior
supine
thoracic
tissues
transverse plane
ventral
word root

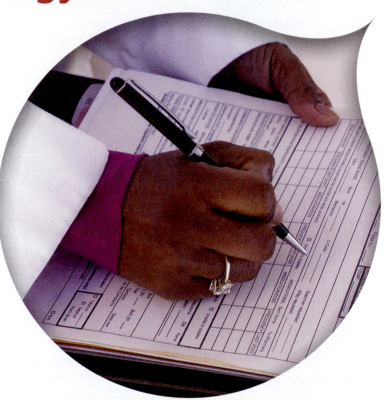

Learning Outcomes

3.1 Recognize commonly used medical terminology.

3.2 Define common medical abbreviations.

3.3 Explain body position, direction, and parts using medical terms.

Related NAACLS Competencies

1.00 Demonstrate knowledge of the healthcare delivery system and medical terminology.

1.7 Use common medical terminology.

3.00 Demonstrate basic understanding of the anatomy and physiology of body systems and anatomic terminology in order to relate major areas of the clinical laboratory to general pathologic conditions associated with the body systems.

Introduction

This chapter is intended to present the basics of how medical words are formed. Emphasis is given to anatomic and medical terminology as well as to abbreviations that phlebotomists are likely to encounter in the health-care setting.

3.1 Medical Language

Medical terminology can often look like a foreign language because its complex-looking terms, rarely used in most of our everyday dialogues, are formed from Greek and Latin words. However, healthcare professionals use this terminology daily when communicating with colleagues. Medical terminology allows healthcare professionals to identify diseases and affected areas of the body much more precisely than if they used our everyday language. To learn medical terminology, you will need to understand the basic word parts and how to build and decode terms in order to "read" them.

Let's start with the root of a word. All medical terms have a **word root** that contains their base meaning. Many terms also have a **suffix** at the end that alters the meaning of the word root. See Table 3-1 for some examples. Since the meanings of the word parts stay consistent, it is easier to learn new terms containing already known word parts—for example:

- *Appendectomy*—the word root *append* refers to "appendix" and the suffix *-ectomy* means "surgical removal." So *appendectomy* means "removal of the appendix."

- *Hysterectomy*—the word root *hystero* means "uterus." Given that *-ectomy* means "surgical removal," *hysterectomy* means "surgical removal of the uterus."

Some terms also contain a **prefix,** which comes at the term's beginning and, like a suffix, alters its meaning. In defining terms, the general rule is to

TABLE 3-1 Medical Terminology Word Parts

Word Part	Description	Term Using Word Part	Term Meaning
Word root	Base meaning of the term	Colostomy	*Colo* = colon; *-stomy* = to cut (or create) a new opening *Colostomy* = to cut a new opening for the colon
Suffix	Ending of term; alters meaning of the word root	Hematology	*Hemat* = blood; *-ology* = study of *Hematology* = study of the blood
Prefix	Beginning of the term; alters the meaning of the word root	Tachycardia	*Tachy-* = rapid; *cardi* = heart; *-ia* = condition of *Tachycardia* = condition of rapid heart (beat)
Combining vowel	Placed between word root and suffix to ease pronunciation	Cardiologist	*Cardi* = heart; *o* = combining vowel to ease pronunciation; *-logist* = specialist in knowledge of *Cardiologist* = specialist in the knowledge of the heart

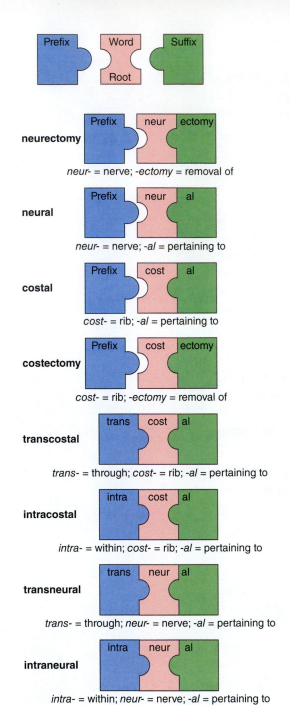

neurectomy

neur- = nerve; *-ectomy* = removal of

neural

neur- = nerve; *-al* = pertaining to

costal

cost- = rib; *-al* = pertaining to

costectomy

cost- = rib; *-ectomy* = removal of

transcostal

trans- = through; *cost-* = rib; *-al* = pertaining to

intracostal

intra- = within; *cost-* = rib; *-al* = pertaining to

transneural

trans- = through; *neur-* = nerve; *-al* = pertaining to

intraneural

intra- = within; *neur-* = nerve; *-al* = pertaining to

Figure 3-1 Word parts are put together like puzzle pieces to create medical terms.

start with the suffix, then add the prefix (if present) and finally the word root(s). The terms *premenstrual* and *postmenstrual* are broken down as follows:

- The suffix *-al* means "pertaining to."
- The prefix *pre-* means "before."
- The prefix *post-* means "after."

The word root *menstru* refers to "menstrual period"; therefore *premenstrual* means "pertaining to before the menstrual period" and *postmenstrual* is "pertaining to after the menstrual period."

For terms whose suffix begins with a consonant, a **combining vowel** (often *o*) is used between the word root and the suffix to ease pronunciation—for example,

- *Gastroparesis*—The word root *gastr* ("stomach") is joined to the suffix *-paresis* ("paralysis"). Here, the letter *o* is inserted between the two to make pronunciation easier. Unlike prefixes and suffixes, combining vowels do not change the term's meaning.

Medical terms are built just like a puzzle, using the prefix, the word root, and the suffix. Don't forget the combining vowel when needed.

Figure 3-1 shows the building of some common medical terms.

Phlebotomy Terminology

Once you understand how medical terms are built from word parts, you will begin to develop your own medical terminology vocabulary. As a phlebotomist, you must recognize and use medical terms every day. Many of these important terms are identified as essential terms at the beginning of each chapter and then bolded throughout the text. The *Medical Terms* appendix contains a list of the prefixes, suffixes, and word roots most commonly used in the language of medicine. In addition, Table 3-2 provides a list of some common prefixes, word roots, suffixes, and terms used in phlebotomy.

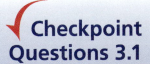

Checkpoint Questions 3.1

1. When determining the meaning of an unknown medical term, in what order would you generally decipher the meaning of the word root, combining vowel, prefix, and suffix?
2. What is the purpose of a combining vowel?
3. Referring to the appendix *Medical Terms*, build a word that means low blood sugar level.
4. What does the word *cyanosis* mean?

TABLE 3-2 Phlebotomy Terminology Common Examples

Prefix	Definition	Example
a-	Without	Asepsis—*without* sepsis (an infectious disease)
ante-	Before	Antecubital—*before* or in front of the elbow
anti-	Against	Anticoagulant—substance that works *against* coagulation (clotting)
bio-	Life	Biology—the study of *life*
cyan-	Blue	Cyanosis—a condition of blueness of the skin
dia-	Through	Dialysis—cleansing the blood by passing it *through* a special machine
endo-	Internal, within	Endothelial cells—cells that line the lumen (*inside* surface) of the blood vessels
epi-	On, above	Epidermis—the outer layer of skin, which is *on* or *above* the dermis
erythro-	Red	Erythrocyte—*red* blood cell
hyper-	Increased	Hypertension—*increased* blood pressure
hypo-	Below	Hypodermic—an area *below* the skin
inter-	Between	Intercellular—located *between* cells
leuk-	White	Leukemia—increased *white* blood cells in the blood
micro-	Small	Microscope—instruments used to view *small* objects
mono-	One, single	Monocyte—a white blood cell with a *single* characteristic nucleus
per-	Through	Percutaneous—*through* the skin
peri-	Around	Pericardium—membrane *around* the heart
poly-	Many	Polymorphonuclear—white blood cell that appears to have *many* nuclei
post-	After	Postprandial—*after* a meal
pre-	Before	Prenatal—*before* delivery of an infant
sub-	Below, under	Subcutaneous—*under* the skin
tachy-	Rapid	Tachycardia—*rapid* heart beat

Word Root	Definition	Example
arterio	Artery	Arterial—pertaining to an *artery*
bili	Bile	Bilirubin—substance formed during breakdown of hemoglobin
cardi	Heart	Pericardial—pertaining to around the *heart*
cephal	Head	Cephalic vein—the vein that runs along the lateral side of the arm to the head
cyt	Cell	Cytology—study of *cells*
derm	Skin	Dermis—inner layer of skin
estr	Female	Estrogen—*female* hormone
gastr	Stomach	Gastritis—inflammation of the *stomach*
hem	Blood	Hemolysis—the breakdown of red *blood* cells
hemat	Blood	Hematoma—an accumulation of *blood* beneath the skin
gluc	Sugar, glucose	Glucose—the *sugar* in a patient's blood
glyc	Sugar, glucose	Glycemia—increased amount of *glucose* in the blood
hepat	Liver	Hepatitis—inflammation of the *liver*
lip	Fat	Lipemic—appears to have an increased amount of *fat*
onc	Tumor	Oncogenic—producing a *tumor*

(continued)

TABLE 3-2 Phlebotomy Terminology Common Examples *(Continued)*

path	Disease	Pathogen—produces *disease*
ped	Child	Pediatric—referring to *children*
phleb	Vein	Phlebitis—inflammation of a *vein*
scler	Hard	Sclerosis—a state of *hardness*
thromb	Clot	Thrombocyte—a cell involved in *clotting*
ven	Vein	Venipuncture—puncture of a *vein*
Suffix	**Definition**	**Example**
-algia	Pain	Neuralgia—nerve *pain*
-ase	Enzyme	Lipase—an *enzyme* that breaks down lipids (fats)
-cyte	Cell	Leukocyte—white blood *cell*
-emia	Blood	Hypoglycemia—low *blood* sugar
-ist	One who specializes in	Phlebotomist—*one who specializes in* phlebotomy
-itis	Inflammation of	Arteritis—*inflammation of* an artery
-logist	Specialist	Microbiologist—*specialist* who studies microorganisms
-logy	Study of	Etiology—*study of* the cause of a disease
-lysis	Breakdown, destruction	Glycolysis—*breakdown* of glucose
-osis	Condition of	Ecchymosis—*condition of* skin discoloration
-ous	Having	Infectious—*having* infection
-pathy	Disease	Myopathy—*disease* of the muscles
-stasis	Stoppage	Hemostasis –*stoppage* of blood or bleeding
-tomy	Cutting into	Phlebotomy—*cutting into* a vein
-ule	Small	Venule—a *small* vein

3.2 Medical Abbreviations

In healthcare, medical abbreviations and symbols—sometimes derived from Greek or Latin terms—help shorten the information that needs to be recorded. As a phlebotomist, you should be able to recognize common abbreviations and symbols related to specimens and to the laboratory tests that you perform. These are used in

- Medical records
- Prescriptions
- Medical orders
- Bills for medical procedures

You may have seen a sign in a patient's hospital room that said "NPO," which stands for "nil per os," or "nothing by mouth." Some abbreviations consist of the letters of the words they represent. This type of abbreviation is called an *acronym*. For example, "ABG" is the acronym for "arterial blood gases." With most medical abbreviations related to the body systems, a good rule to follow is "When in doubt, spell it out." Some abbreviations, symbols, and acronyms are prone to misinterpretation and have resulted in a significant number of errors. For this reason, The Joint Commission (TJC) and the Institute for Safe Medication

Practice (ISMP)—two healthcare organizations whose mission includes the promotion of patient safety—have identified abbreviations that should not be used. An example of an error-prone abbreviation is U (for unit). When handwritten, U can be mistaken for a zero. Another example is the abbreviation "q1d," which means "everyday," versus "q.i.d.," which means "four times a day." These and other abbreviation mistakes have unfavorable effects on patient care. To help prevent mistakes, healthcare facilities have approved abbreviation lists that do not include those identified by TJC and ISMP. All employees must follow these rules to ensure consistency. For a complete list of error-prone abbreviations, visit the ISMP online at www.ismp.org. In addition, the appendix *Medical Abbreviations* contains a list of common abbreviations and symbols used in medical practice.

Laboratory tests also regularly use abbreviations in orders and in reports. Table 3-3 shows some examples of laboratory test abbreviations. The appendix

TABLE 3-3 Examples of Laboratory Test Abbreviations*

CBC	Complete blood count test includes • RBC (red blood cell count) • HCT (hematocrit) • Hgb (hemoglobin) • WBC (white blood cell count) • MCV (mean corpuscular volume) • MCH (mean corpuscular hemoglobin) • MCHC (mean corpuscular hemoglobin concentration) • Plat (platelet count)
BMP	Basic metabolic panel blood test includes • Glu (glucose or sugar) • Na (sodium) • K (potassium) • Ca (calcium) • Cl (chloride) • CO_2 (carbon dioxide) • HCO_3 (bicarbonate) • BUN (blood urea nitrogen) • Creat (creatinine)
CK	• Creatine kinase *(Part of blood enzyme test. Tested with troponin to check for muscle breakdown.)*
Lipid panel	Blood lipids (fats) test includes • Chol (total cholesterol) • LDL (low-density lipoprotein or "bad" cholesterol) • HDL (high-density lipoprotein or "good" cholesterol) • Trig (triglycerides)
UA	Urinalysis test of the urine includes • pH (measure of acidity or basicity) • Sp Gr (specific gravity or density) • Prot (protein) • Glu (glucose or sugar) • Ket (ketones) • Nit (nitrite) • Leuk (leukocytes or white blood cells)

*See the appendix *Laboratory Tests*, for additional information and examples.

Laboratory Tests contains a detailed list of laboratory tests, their abbreviations, specimen requirements, and the laboratory section responsible for performing each test.

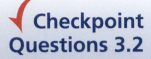

Checkpoint Questions 3.2

1. If you receive an order to draw blood for testing Na, Ca, K, and Cl, what tests will be performed on the blood?
2. A patient has come in to have her blood drawn for a fasting glucose test, but the patient drank a soft drink before coming to the laboratory. How can the word "glucose" be abbreviated in the notes to the lab staff concerning this?
3. A job advertisement states that a "PRN" phlebotomist position is available. What does this mean?

3.3 Anatomical Terminology

Anatomy is the scientific study of body *structure*. Anatomically, you would describe the heart as a hollow, cone-shaped organ that is an average of 14 centimeters long and 9 centimeters wide. Understanding anatomy also allows you to comprehend the normal position of body structures. For example, as a phlebotomist, you will need to know the normal position of the veins and arteries. The term **physiology** refers to the study of the *function* of the body's organs. For example, the function of blood vessels is to transport blood throughout the body. Anatomy and physiology are commonly studied together because they are always related. This knowledge will help you understand the procedures you will perform as a phlebotomist.

Organization of the Body

The human body is complex in its structure and function. It is organized from the chemical level (the simplest level) all the way up to the organ system level. Figure 3-2 illustrations the organization of the human body from the simplest to the most complex level.

At the chemical level, the body is comprised of billions of atoms and molecules that make up chemicals such as acids, proteins, and sugars. **Atoms** are the simplest units of all matter. Matter is anything that takes up space and has weight—any solid, liquid, or gas. The four most common atoms in the human body are carbon, hydrogen, oxygen, and nitrogen. **Molecules** are units of matter formed from at least two atoms. Proteins and carbohydrates are examples of molecules that consist of hundreds of atoms. Molecules join together to form **organelles,** which are essentially cell parts. Organelles, such as nuclei, lysosomes, and mitochondria, combine to build various types of cells, including

- Leukocytes (white blood cells)
- Erythrocytes (red blood cells)
- Neurons (nerve cells)
- Adipocytes (fat cells)

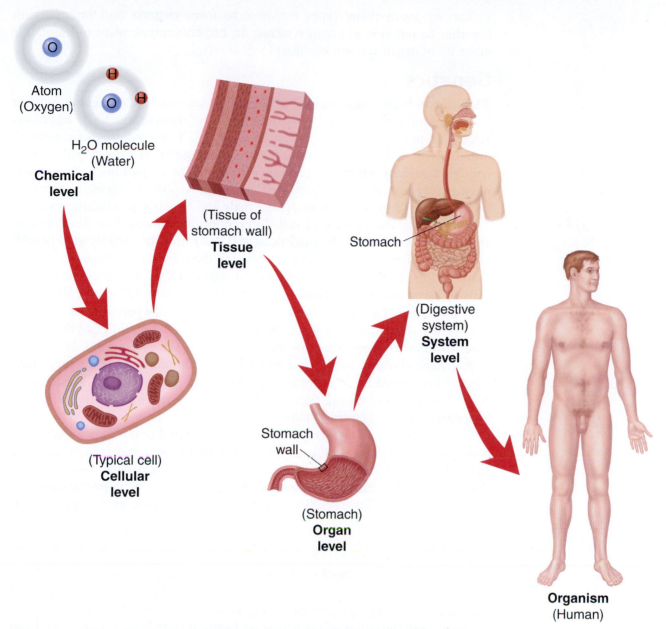

Atom
(Oxygen)

H_2O molecule
(Water)
**Chemical
level**

(Typical cell)
**Cellular
level**

(Tissue of
stomach wall)
**Tissue
level**

Stomach
wall

(Stomach)
**Organ
level**

Stomach

(Digestive
system)
**System
level**

Organism
(Human)

Figure 3-2 The human body is organized into levels, beginning with the chemical level and progressing through the cellular, tissue, organ, organ system, and organism (whole body) levels.

Cells are considered to be the smallest living units in the body. When the same types of cells organize together, they form **tissues.** The four major types of body tissue are epithelial, connective, nervous, and muscle, and their functions are as follows:

- Epithelial tissue provides a covering for organs, such as the skin and the linings of the body's various passages, like inside the mouth.

- Connective tissue, found in bone and blood, supports other tissues and binds them together.

- Nervous tissue is made up of nerve cells; it carries "messages" to and from various parts of the body.

- Muscle tissue includes striated (voluntary) muscles that move the skeleton and smooth (involuntary) muscles that perform tasks automatically, such as the stomach muscle, which helps digest food.

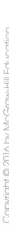

Two or more tissue types combine to form **organs** and organs work together to function as organ systems. An **organism** (any plant or animal) is made up of organ systems essential to its survival.

Genetics

The human body is an organism. The organ systems of the human body, or body systems, carry out vital body functions. For example, the heart and blood vessels unite to form the cardiovascular system. The cardiovascular system's organs circulate blood throughout the body to ensure that all body cells receive enough nutrients. There are 12 body systems in the human body: the integumentary, skeletal, muscular, lymphatic, immune, respiratory, digestive, nervous, endocrine, cardiovascular, urinary, and male and female reproductive systems.

Controlling the process of cell differentiation, growth, and development are molecules of **deoxyribonucleic acid (DNA)** and **ribonucleic acid (RNA).** DNA holds the genetic code that contains all the information needed for these body processes. RNA assists cells in translating DNA messages, prompting cells to carry out specific tasks. Genes are sequences of DNA and RNA that code for a type of protein or for an RNA chain that has a particular function in the body. Laboratory testing for these genes or their function can determine paternity as well as genetic disorders.

A genetic disorder is a disease caused by an altered form of a gene. Many cancers are caused by an alteration in a gene or a group of genes in a person's cells. These alterations can occur randomly or as a result of an environmental exposure, such as cigarette smoke.

Certain genetic disorders are inherited. A mutated (altered) gene is passed down through a family and each generation of children may inherit the gene that causes the disease. One such genetic disorder is hemophilia. Other genetic disorders develop due to problems with the number of gene packages, called chromosomes. In Down syndrome, for example, there is an extra copy of chromosome 21.

Anatomical Terms

Anatomical terms are used to describe the locations of body parts and body regions. To use these terms correctly, assume that the body is in the **anatomical position**—standing upright and facing forward. The arms are at the sides of the body, and the palms of the hands are facing forward (see Figure 3-3). Even if patients are lying down, for consistency and correct communication when using anatomical terms, always refer to patients as if they were in the anatomical position. A patient lying on his back is in **supine** position, but not in anatomical position if his hands are not facing upward. A patient lying face down is in **prone** position.

Directional Anatomical Terms

The directional anatomical terms are **cranial, caudal, ventral, dorsal, medial, lateral, proximal, distal, superficial,** and **deep.** They are used to identify the position of body structures compared to other body structures. You would say that the eyes are medial to (in the middle of) the ears but lateral to (at the side of) the nose. The skin is superficial and the heart is deep. See Table 3-4 and Figure 3-4 for an explanation and illustration of these important directional terms.

Anatomical Terms Used to Describe Body Sections

Sometimes, in order to study internal body parts, it helps to imagine the body as being divided into sections. Medical professionals often use terms such as

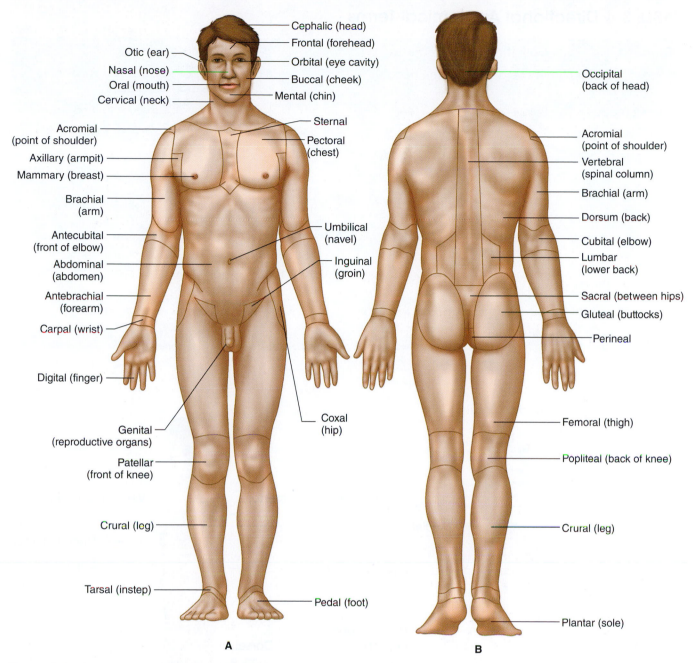

Figure 3-3 Numerous anatomical terms are used to describe regions of the body: (A) anterior view anatomical position and (B) posterior view anatomical position.

sagittal, *transverse*, and *frontal* (*coronal*) to describe how the body is divided into sections. The following list outlines these terms, and Figure 3-5 illustrates the relevant planes:

- A **sagittal plane** divides the body into left and right portions.
- A **midsagittal plane** runs lengthwise down the midline of the body and divides it into equal left and right halves.
- A **transverse plane** divides the body into **superior** (upper) and **inferior** (lower) portions.
- A **frontal**, or **coronal**, **plane** divides the body into **anterior** (frontal) and **posterior** (rear) portions.

TABLE 3-4 Directional Anatomical Terms

Term	Definition	Example
Superior (cranial)	Above or close to the head	The thoracic cavity is superior to the abdominal cavity.
Inferior (caudal)	Below or closer to the feet	The neck is inferior to the head.
Anterior (ventral)	Toward the front of the body	The nose is anterior to the ears.
Posterior (dorsal)	Toward the back of the body	The brain is posterior to the eyes.
Medial	Close to the midline of the body	The nose is medial to the ears.
Lateral	Farther away from (or to the side of) the midline of the body	The ears are lateral to the nose.
Proximal	Close to a point of attachment or to the trunk of the body	The knee is proximal to the toes.
Distal	Farther away from a point of attachment or from the trunk of the body	The fingers are distal to the elbow.
Superficial	Close to the surface of the body	Skin is superficial to muscles.
Deep	More internal	Bones are deep to skin.

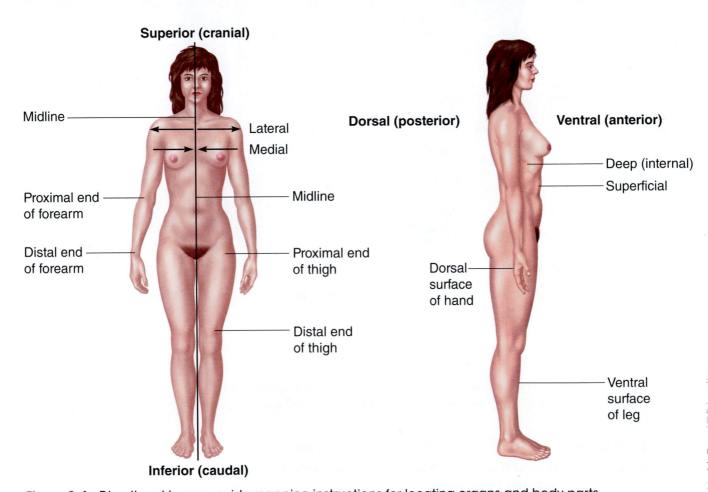

Figure 3-4 Directional terms provide mapping instructions for locating organs and body parts.

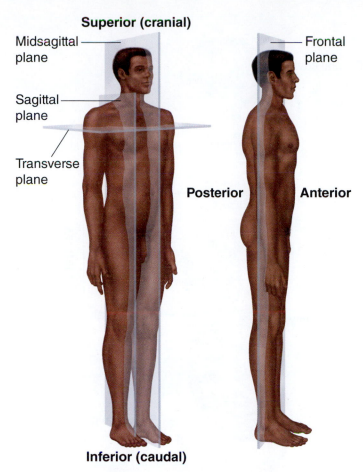

Superior (cranial)

Midsagittal plane

Sagittal plane

Transverse plane

Frontal plane

Posterior   Anterior

Inferior (caudal)

Figure 3-5 Spatial terms are based on imaginary planes dividing the body.

Anatomical Terms Used to Describe Body Parts

Many other anatomical terms are used to describe different regions or parts of the body. For example, the term **brachium** refers to the arm and the term **femoral** refers to the thigh. Figure 3-3 illustrates many of the common anatomical terms used to describe body parts.

Body Cavities and Abdominal Regions

The largest body cavities are the dorsal cavity and the ventral cavity. The dorsal cavity is divided into the cranial cavity and the spinal cavity. The cranial cavity houses the brain and the spinal cavity contains the spinal cord. The ventral cavity is divided into the **thoracic** cavity and the **abdominopelvic** cavity. The muscle called the **diaphragm** separates the thoracic and abdominopelvic cavities. The lungs, heart, esophagus, and trachea are contained in the thoracic cavity. The abdominopelvic cavity is divided into a superior abdominal cavity and an inferior pelvic cavity. The stomach, small and large intestines, gallbladder, liver, spleen, kidneys, and pancreas are all located in the abdominal cavity. The bladder and internal reproductive organs are located in the pelvic cavity. Figure 3-6 depicts these cavities. The abdominal area can be further divided into nine regions or four quadrants, which are illustrated in Figure 3-7.

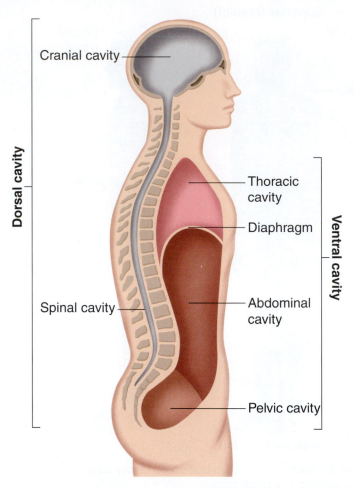

Figure 3-6 The two main body cavities are the dorsal and ventral cavities.

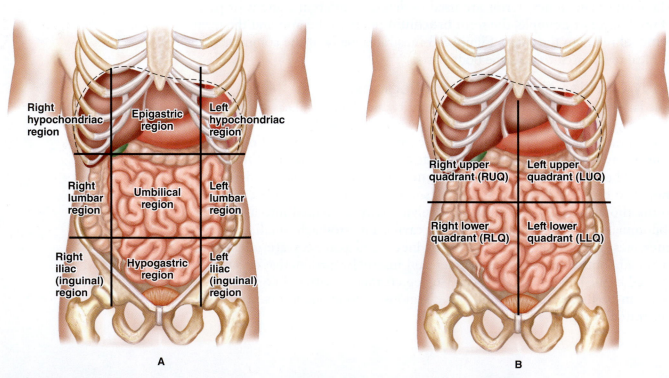

A

B

Figure 3-7 The abdominal area is divided into (A) nine regions or (B) four quadrants.

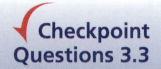

1. Describe the anatomical position.
2. Which organs are located in the abdominal cavity?
3. How do the terms "deep" and "superficial" relate to phlebotomy?

Checkpoint Questions 3.3

Chapter Summary

Learning Outcome	Key Concepts/Examples	Related NAACLS Competency
3.1 Recognize commonly used medical terminology. Pages 61–64.	Medical terminology comes from Greek and Latin words. Medical terms consist of a word root, a prefix and/or suffix, and sometimes a combining vowel. Building and decoding word parts will help you recognize and understand medical terminology.	1.00, 1.7
3.2 Define common medical abbreviations. Pages 64–66.	Abbreviations and symbols help shorten and simplify the information communicated in medical settings. Certain medical abbreviations are prone to errors and should not be used. Check the meaning of abbreviations carefully in practice. Some medical abbreviations are derived from Latin or Greek terms.	1.7
3.3 Explain body position, direction, and parts using medical terms. Pages 66–73.	Specific anatomical medical terms are used to identify body parts, planes, and positions. Knowing these terms will help the phlebotomist perform his or her job more efficiently.	1.00, 3.00

Chapter Review

A: Labeling

Label each body plane in the following figure.

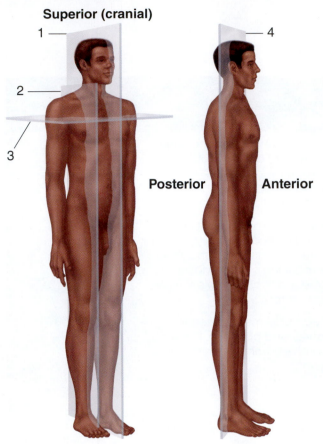

1. [LO 3.3] _____

2. [LO 3.3] _____

3. [LO 3.3] _____

4. [LO 3.3] _____

B: Matching

Match the following terms with their correct description or definition. Refer to the appendix *Medical Terms* as needed.

_____**5.** [LO 3.1] adipo-

_____**6.** [LO 3.1] aero-

_____**7.** [LO 3.1] ambi-

_____**8.** [LO 3.1] bracheo-

_____**9.** [LO 3.1] circum-

_____**10.** [LO 3.1] cryo-

_____**11.** [LO 3.1] -ectomy

_____**12.** [LO 3.1] encephalo-

_____**13.** [LO 3.1] hypo-

_____**14.** [LO 3.1] -itis

_____**15.** [LO 3.1] laparo-

_____**16.** [LO 3.1] -lysis

_____**17.** [LO 3.1] oculo-

_____**18.** [LO 3.1] ortho-

_____**19.** [LO 3.1] -pathy

_____**20.** [LO 3.1] -plasia

_____**21.** [LO 3.1] -sepsis

_____**22.** [LO 3.1] stomato-

_____**23.** [LO 3.1] thoraco-

_____**24.** [LO 3.1] trans-

_____**25.** [LO 3.1] vaso-

a. abdomen
b. across
c. arm
d. around
e. both
f. brain
g. chest
h. cold
i. cutting out
j. disease
k. disintegration
l. eye
m. fat
n. formation
o. infection
p. inflammation of
q. mouth
r. straight
s. under
t. vessel
u. with oxygen

C: Fill in the Blanks

Write in the word(s) to complete the statement or answer the question.

26. [LO 3.1] Medical terminology is formed from _____ and _____ words.

27. [LO 3.1] The main part of a medical word is called the _____.

28. [LO 3.3] A molecule that contains genetic code is a(n) _____.

29. [LO 3.3] The smallest living unit is the _____.

30. [LO 3.3] Body _____ hold vital organs, such as the brain, lungs, and kidneys.

D: Sequencing

Place the level of structures that comprise the human body in order from simplest to most complex.

31. [LO 3.3] _____ cells

32. [LO 3.3] _____ chemicals

33. [LO 3.3] _____ organelles

34. [LO 3.3] _____ organism

35. [LO 3.3] _____ organs

36. [LO 3.3] _____ tissues

E: Case Studies/Critical Thinking

37. [LO 3.2] An order for medication was written "q.o.d.," but the person reading the order thought the order said "q.i.d." What are the implications of this misinterpretation? How could this mistake have been avoided?

38. [LO 3.3] Just before you enter a patient's room to collect a specimen, the nurse asks you to make sure that when you leave the patient she is not supine. What does this mean?

39. [LO 3.2] When performing a venipuncture on a patient who has an intravenous (IV) line in his arm, you must always locate a site distal to the IV site. What does this mean?

F: Exam Prep

Choose the best answer for each question.

40. [LO 3.1] Which of the following is a prefix?

   a. Aero   **b.** Itis

   c. Osis   **d.** Tomy

41. [LO 3.1] Which of the following is a suffix?

   a. Anti   **b.** Dys

   c. Hypo   **d.** Pathy

42. [LO 3.1] This is used in the center of medical words to ease in their pronunciation.

   a. Combining vowel   **b.** Prefix

   c. Suffix   **d.** Word root

43. [LO 3.1] The study of body structures and their functions is

   a. anatomy and pathology.

   b. physiology and anatomy.

   c. pathology and physiology.

   d. anatomy and physiology.

44. [LO 3.3] You have been told to attempt your first blood draw in the most distal portion of the arm. Where would you look for a vein?

   a. Elbow   **b.** Forearm

   c. Wrist   **d.** Hand

45. [LO 3.3] Tissues are formed from

   a. similar cells.   **b.** organs.

   c. organelles.   **d.** molecules.

46. [LO 3.3] Which of the following is NOT one of the four major types of body tissue?

   a. Connective   **b.** Nervous

   c. Muscular   **d.** Vascular

47. [LO 3.3] Which set of words contains opposites?

   a. Cranial and caudal

   b. Dorsal and back

   c. Lateral and outside

   d. Proximal and close

48. [LO 3.3] Which plane divides the body into upper and lower sections?

   a. Frontal   **b.** Midsagittal

   c. Sagittal   **d.** Transverse

49. [LO 3.3] The frontal plane divides the body

   a. from top to bottom.

   b. from side to side.

   c. from front to back.

   d. down the middle.

50. [LO 3.3] Which of the following cavities is included in the dorsal cavity?

    a. Abdominal   b. Pelvic

    c. Spinal   d. Thoracic

51. [LO 3.3] If a body structure is found in front of another body structure, it is said to be _____ to that structure.

    a. anterior   b. inferior

    c. posterior   d. superior

52. [LO 3.3] When asked to draw blood from a vein inferior to the bend at the elbow, you would draw blood from a site _____ the bend at the elbow.

    a. above   b. below

    c. behind   d. next to

53. [LO 3.1] The term *brachium* refers to the

    a. arm.   b. ear.

    c. foot.   d. leg.

54. [LO 3.3] The diaphragm is a muscle that separates which two body cavities?

    a. Cranial and spinal

    b. Dorsal and pelvic

    c. Dorsal and ventral

    d. Thoracic and abdominopelvic

55. [LO 3.3] The heart is found in the

    a. abdominal cavity.   b. dorsal cavity.

    c. pelvic cavity.   d. thoracic cavity.

56. [LO 3.3] Organs that are found in the thoracic cavity include the

    a. stomach.   b. esophagus.

    c. kidneys.   d. liver.

57. [LO 3.2] Which laboratory test is part of a CBC?

    a. Na   b. LDL

    c. pH   d. WBC

58. [LO 3.2] Which laboratory test is part of a lipid panel?

    a. HDL   b. CBC

    c. MCHC   d. K

59. [LO 3.3] Organs that are found in the abdominal cavity include all of the following EXCEPT the

    a. spleen.   b. lungs.

    c. kidneys.   d. intestines.

connect

Enhance your learning by completing these exercises and more at connect.mheducation.com.

References

Booth, K. A. (2013). *Healthcare science technology* New York: McGraw-Hill.

Booth, K. A., Whicker, L. G., & Wyman, T. D. (2014). *Medical assisting: Administrative and clinical procedures with anatomy and physiology* (5th ed.). New York: McGraw-Hill.

National Accrediting Agency for Clinical Laboratory Sciences. (2013). *NAACLS entry-level phlebotomist competencies.* Retrieved June 27, 2013, from www.naacls.org/docs/Guide_Approval-section1b-Phleb.pdf

Sheir, D. (2011). *Hole's essentials of human anatomy & physiology* (11th ed.). New York: McGraw-Hill.

Thierer, N. (2010). *Medical terminology: Language for healthcare* (3rd ed.). New York: McGraw-Hill.

4

Body Systems and Related Laboratory Tests

essential terms

autoimmune disease
cardiovascular system
digestive system
endocrine system
external respiration
female reproductive
  system
immune system
integumentary system
internal respiration

ligaments
lymphatic system
male reproductive
  system
muscular system
nervous system
respiratory system
skeletal system
tendons
urinary system

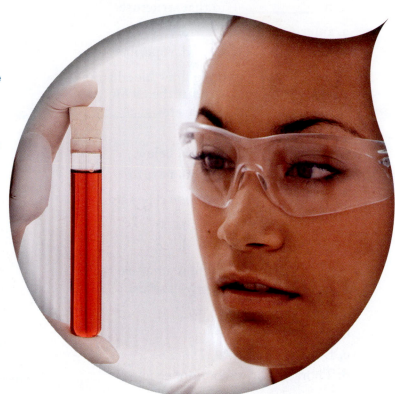

Learning Outcomes

4.1 Describe the functions of the integumentary system, common diseases and disorders that affect this system, and related laboratory tests.

4.2 Describe the functions of the skeletal system, common diseases and disorders that affect this system, and related laboratory tests.

4.3 Describe the functions of the muscular system, common diseases and disorders that affect this system, and related laboratory tests.

4.4 Describe the functions of the lymphatic and immune systems, common diseases and disorders that affect these systems, and related laboratory tests.

4.5 Describe the functions of the respiratory system, common diseases and disorders that affect this system, and related laboratory tests.

4.6 Describe the functions of the digestive system, common diseases and disorders that affect this system, and related laboratory tests.

4.7 Describe the functions of the nervous system, common diseases and disorders that affect this system, and related laboratory tests.

4.8 Describe the functions of the endocrine system, common diseases and disorders that affect this system, and related laboratory tests.

4.9 Describe the functions of the cardiovascular system, common diseases and disorders that affect this system, and related laboratory tests.

4.10 Describe the functions of the urinary system, common diseases and disorders that affect this system, and related laboratory tests.

4.11 Describe the functions of the female and male reproductive systems, common diseases and disorders that affect these systems, and related laboratory tests.

Related NAACLS Competencies

1.00 Demonstrate knowledge of the healthcare delivery system and medical terminology.

1.6 Describe how laboratory testing is used to assess body functions and disease.

3.00 Demonstrate basic understanding of the anatomy and physiology of body systems and anatomical terminology in order to relate major areas of the clinical laboratory to general pathologic conditions associated with the body systems.

3.1 Describe the basic functions of each main body system, and demonstrate basic knowledge of the circulatory, urinary, and other body systems necessary to perform assigned specimen collection tasks.

Introduction

Body systems are the organ systems formed when organs join together to carry out vital body functions. For example, the heart and blood vessels unite to form the cardiovascular system. The cardiovascular system's organs circulate blood throughout the body to ensure that all body cells receive enough nutrients. There are 12 body systems: the integumentary, skeletal, muscular, lymphatic, immune, respiratory, digestive, nervous, endocrine, cardiovascular, urinary, and male and female reproductive systems.

The diseases and disorders that affect the human body can be classified according to the body system or systems they affect. For example, a bladder infection can be classified as a disease of the urinary system. Physicians diagnose diseases and disorders by examining the patient's physical symptoms and by ordering laboratory and other diagnostic tests. Therefore, one method of classifying laboratory tests is to organize them according to body system. This chapter contains a brief review of each body system, followed by common diseases and disorders that affect that system and the laboratory tests used to diagnose or monitor them.

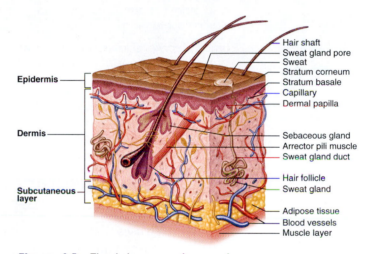

Figure 4-1 The integumentary system.

4.1 Integumentary System

The **integumentary system** is unique in that it encloses and protects all of the other body systems. It consists of the skin (*derm/o, dermat/o, cutane/o*), hair (*trich/o*), nails (*onych/o, ungu/o*), and sweat glands. The integumentary system provides protection, regulates temperature, and prevents water loss. When sunlight hits the skin, it converts the substance 7-dehydrocholesterol to vitamin D. The skin, which is the largest organ of the body, also helps in sensory perception. Sensory perception is the interpretation or awareness of sensory stimulation. Touch is one of your senses. In the skin, there are nerve endings that create your sense of touch. See Figure 4-1.

TABLE 4-1 Tests for Common Integumentary Diseases and Disorders

Tests	Description of Test	Related Diseases and Disorders
Blood Tests		
Antibody titers	Measures level of antibodies to specific antigens. Commonly used to determine whether a patient has (or has had in the past) certain diseases.	Rubella, rubeola, chickenpox, shingles, mononucleosis, viral hepatitis, systemic lupus erythematosus (SLE); also used to check for immune deficiencies and autoimmune disease
Immunoglobulin levels	Measures immunoglobulin levels; high level of immunoglobulin A (IgA) or E (IgE) indicates an allergic response	Seasonal allergies, immunodeficiencies
Other Tests to Assess the Integumentary System		
Wet prep	Microscopic evaluation of skin or nail scraping	Fungal infections of the skin or nails
Culture of scraping	Skin scraping is grown on a culture medium and examined under a microscope to diagnose infections caused by *Staphylococcus aureus* and other bacterial, fungal, and parasitic infections	*Staphylococcus* ("staph") infection Athlete's foot Ringworm Fingernail or toenail infection
Skin biopsy	Small piece of skin tissue is removed and examined under a microscope	Skin cancer
Urine melanin	Urine is tested for level of melanin, a skin pigment that may be found in urine if melanoma is present	Skin cancer (melanoma)

Integumentary System Disorders and Associated Lab Tests

Viruses that affect the skin, such as rubella, rubeola, and herpes zoster, which causes chickenpox and shingles, are common integumentary system disorders. Some allergies also cause skin disorders, such as rashes. Fungal infections are a common problem for toenails, fingernails, and skin. One of the more serious integumentary system disorders is skin cancer. The three major types of skin cancer are squamous cell carcinoma, basal cell carcinoma, and melanoma. Of the three, melanoma is the most serious. Table 4-1 lists common laboratory tests used to diagnose these and other disorders of the integumentary system.

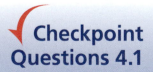

Checkpoint Questions 4.1

1. List at least four functions of the integumentary system.
2. What is the purpose of antibody titers?

4.2 Skeletal System

The **skeletal system** consists of bones (*oste/o*), associated cartilages (*chondr/o*), ligaments, and joints (*arthr/o, articul/o*). The skeletal system provides the body with protection and support. The ribs protect the heart and lungs. The bones support the soft tissues of the body and provide a place for muscles to attach. They produce blood cells and store minerals and fat. The bones can also store excess calcium (*calc/i*). See Figure 4-2 for the common bones of the skeletal system.

Skeletal System Disorders and Associated Lab Tests

Diseases and disorders that affect the skeletal system include osteoporosis, osteoarthritis and rheumatoid arthritis, gout, osteosarcoma (bone cancer), and various disorders related to nutritional deficiencies or poor posture. Many of these disorders are diagnosed based on symptoms and diagnostic images, such as x-rays, but the phlebotomist may be asked to draw blood for several different diagnostic tests, as described in Table 4-2.

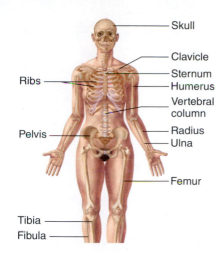

Figure 4-2 The skeletal system.

TABLE 4-2 Tests for Common Skeletal System Diseases and Disorders

Tests	Description of Test	Related Diseases and Disorders
Blood Tests		
Alkaline phosphatase (ALP)	Screens for abnormal bone growth	Bone tumors, Paget's disease (abnormal bone enlargement and deformation)
Calcium (Ca)	Screens for abnormal blood calcium levels	Rickets (children) or osteomalacia (adults); these diseases involve softening of the bones and serum calcium levels tend to be decreased
Uric acid	Measures the level of uric acid in the blood to determine whether the body is breaking it down properly	Gout (a type of arthritis in which the body does not break down uric acid adequately)
Vitamin D	Screens for adequate Vitamin D to help maintain bone calcium	Rickets or osteomalacia
Erythrocyte sedimentation rate (ESR)	Measures the rate at which erythrocytes settle at the bottom of a calibrated tube; elevated levels indicate the presence of inflammation	Some types of arthritis, including rheumatoid arthritis
Rheumatoid factor (RF)	Tests for the autoantibody that is present in rheumatoid arthritis	Present in rheumatoid arthritis but not juvenile-type rheumatoid arthritis
Other Tests to Assess the Skeletal System		
Synovial fluid analysis	Battery of tests that includes visual analysis; microscopic analysis; measurement of glucose proteins, LDH, and uric acid; and bacterial culture	Gout, other types of arthritis, joint infections
Bone marrow biopsy	A needle biopsy to remove bone marrow for diagnostic tests	Multiple myeloma (cancer that starts in bone marrow)

1. Which blood tests might be ordered if a healthcare provider suspects that a child has rickets?
2. Which tests might be ordered if a patient is suspected of having rheumatoid arthritis?

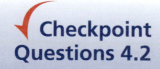

Checkpoint Questions 4.2

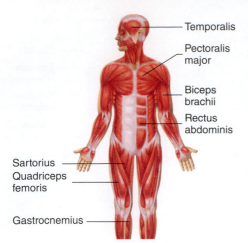

Temporalis
Pectoralis major
Biceps brachii
Rectus abdominis
Sartorius
Quadriceps femoris
Gastrocnemius

Figure 4-3 The muscular system.

4.3 Muscular System

The **muscular system** produces body movements, such as the abduction, adduction, extension, and flexion of the bones in the skeletal system. Muscle tissue (*my/o, muscul/o*) contracts, or shortens, to move parts of the skeleton, vessels, and internal organs (*viscer/o*). Muscles also produce body heat. Some muscles stay partially contracted to help maintain posture. For example, the muscles in the back tighten to keep the spine straight. Muscles receive direction from the nervous system to contract or relax.

The muscular system consists of the muscles and connective tissue, including tendons and ligaments. **Tendons** attach muscles to bones and **ligaments** attach bones to other bones. Figure 4-3 shows some of the major muscles in the muscular system.

Muscular System Disorders and Associated Lab Tests

Muscles are subject to strains and sprains, including some that involve serious muscle damage. Tendonitis is a painful inflammation of a tendon, usually due to either a sports injury or repetitive activities such as using a computer. Other common disorders include torticollis ("wry neck"), fibromyalgia, myasthenia gravis, and muscular dystrophy. Laboratory tests used to assess the muscular system are described in Table 4-3.

TABLE 4-3 Tests for Common Muscular System Diseases and Disorders

Tests	Description of Test	Related Diseases and Disorders
Blood Tests		
Autoimmune antibodies	Screens for abnormal antibody levels that may indicate various autoimmune diseases	Myasthenia gravis, polymyalgia rheumatica
Creatine kinase (CK)	Measures the level of the enzyme creatine kinase in the blood; CK-MM is specific to skeletal muscle damage, while CK-MB will also be affected by skeletal muscle disorders	General muscle damage, muscular dystrophy, skeletal muscle disease, muscle damage due to myocardial infarction (heart attack)
Lactate/lactic acid	Monitors production of lactic acid during muscle activity or due to certain medications	Heart failure
Lactate dehydrogenase (LH/LDH)	Measures the level of the protein LDH in the blood; often performed when tissue damage is suspected	Muscle injury, muscular dystrophy, blood flow deficiency (ischemia)
Myoglobin	Measures the level of the protein myoglobin in the blood; myoglobin is released into the bloodstream when muscle tissue is damaged	Skeletal muscle inflammation or trauma, myocardial infarction, muscular dystrophy, rhabdomyolysis (breakdown of muscle fibers)
Other Tests to Assess the Muscular System		
Urine myoglobin	Measures myoglobin presence in urine; myoglobin enters the urine when kidneys filter it out of the blood	Skeletal muscle inflammation or trauma, myocardial infarction, muscular dystrophy, rhabdomyolysis (breakdown of muscle fibers)
Muscle biopsy	Removal of a small piece of tissue through a biopsy needle for examination	Trichinosis, toxoplasmosis, or other muscle infections; muscular dystrophy; muscle atrophy or necrosis (tissue death); polymyositis

1. Name two autoimmune diseases that affect the muscular system and the blood test that may be ordered to diagnose them.
2. Which tests might be ordered to help determine the extent of a given muscle injury?

Body Mechanics

Safety & Infection Control

Body mechanics can be defined as the positions and movements used to maintain proper posture and to avoid muscle and bone injuries. Preventing strains helps you avoid injury to the body, especially the back. As a phlebotomist, you will often need to lift, move, and carry objects. On occasion, you may need to lift, transfer, or position patients.

As a phlebotomist, you should use good body mechanics. Consider the following techniques:

- Maintain good posture: keep your back straight and your feet about shoulder-width apart.
- Avoid reaching: move close to the patient or the object you will be lifting.
- Avoid twisting while lifting: Face the patient or object directly.
- Lift correctly: use the strong muscles of your legs by bending your hips and knees. Avoid using the muscles of your back to lift.
- Carry carefully: avoid lifting heavy objects or patients. Ask for assistance. Carry objects close to your body.

4.4 Lymphatic and Immune Systems

The **immune system** (*immun/o*) is responsible for protecting the body against bacteria, viruses, fungi, toxins, parasites, and cancer. It provides protection by circulating white blood cells (*cyt/o*) and antibodies throughout the body. Antibodies are formed by the white blood cells when a foreign substance invades the body. Once produced, the antibodies remain in the body, so if the same foreign substance invades the body a second time, the antibodies are already there to do their job. Therefore, if someone gets sick with a disease such as chickenpox, that person typically does not get sick from it again.

The immune system works with the organs of the **lymphatic system** (*lymph/o*) to clear the body of disease-causing agents. It removes foreign substances from the blood and lymph the way a filter removes solids from a liquid. The lymphatic system helps maintain tissue fluid balance and absorbs fats from the digestive tract; it returns excess fluid and proteins from the tissues to the bloodstream. The lymphatic vessels (*angi/o, vas/o, vascul/o*), lymph nodes, glands (*aden/o*), tonsils, thymus, and spleen make up this system. The organs of the lymphatic and immune systems are shown in Figure 4-4.

Lymphatic and Immune Disorders and Associated Lab Tests

The purpose of the lymphatic and immune systems is to help fight disease, but these systems can be the focus of diseases and disorders, just like all the other body systems. Mononucleosis, chronic fatigue

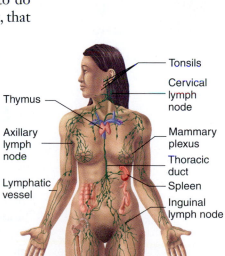

Figure 4-4 Organs of the lymphatic and immune systems.

TABLE 4-4 Tests for Common Lymphatic and Immune System Diseases and Disorders

Tests	Description of Test	Related Diseases and Disorders
Blood Tests		
Antinuclear antibody panel (ANA)	Measures levels of the antibodies produced by the immune system that attack body tissues	Rheumatoid arthritis, systemic lupus erythematosus, scleroderma, thyroid disease
Complete blood count (CBC)	Count of red and white blood cells and platelets, amount of hemoglobin in the blood, and hematocrit (the fraction of blood composed of red blood cells); often performed with a differential (CBC/diff) to count the various types of white blood cells	Allergies, infections, anemia
Monospot	Checks for two antibodies that appear in the blood when a person has mononucleosis	Mononucleosis
Other Tests to Assess the Lymphatic and Immune Systems		
Biopsy of lymph node or other lymphatic tissues	Removal of a small piece of lymph tissue through a biopsy needle for examination	Cancer, sarcoidosis, tuberculosis
Lymphatic fluid culture	Lymphatic fluid is placed in a culture medium to encourage growth of microorganisms; cultured microorganisms are examined under a microscope	Various bacterial infections

syndrome, HIV/AIDS, and lymphedema (blockage of the lymphatic vessels) are examples of disorders associated with these systems. Allergies are the result of an immune response to dust, smoke, pollen, or hundreds of other stimulants.

In some cases, the immune system makes a mistake and attacks the body itself. This is known as an **autoimmune disease**. Rheumatoid arthritis, ulcerative colitis, and myasthenia gravis are examples of autoimmune diseases. Common laboratory tests related to the lymphatic and immune systems are described in Table 4-4.

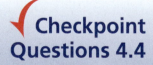

Checkpoint Questions 4.4

1. Briefly describe how the lymphatic and immune systems work together to protect the body from harmful microorganisms.
2. Name four diseases that can be diagnosed using an antinuclear antibody panel (ANA).

4.5 Respiratory System

The **respiratory** (*pneum/o, pneumon/o, pneumat/o*) **system** provides oxygen (*ox/o, oxia*) to body cells and removes carbon dioxide (*capnia*). Respiration, or breathing (*pnea, spir/o*), is the process of taking in oxygen and giving off carbon dioxide. Oxygen enters the lungs and is transferred to hemoglobin on the red blood cells. The red blood cells transport the oxygen to the tissues of the body. The blood also picks up waste gases, including carbon dioxide, in the tissues and carries them to the lungs. The gases leave the blood cells and are removed from the body when the person exhales. **Internal respiration** is the gas exchange between the blood and body cells. **External respiration** is the exchange of air between the lungs (*pulm/o, pulmon/o*) and the outside environment.

The respiratory system includes the lungs and the airways (trachea, bronchi, and bronchioles) as well as the nasal and oral cavities. The lungs are surrounded by a cavity enclosed in a membrane. This cavity normally contains a small amount of fluid, called pleural fluid. These structures are shown in Figure 4-5.

Respiratory System Disorders and Associated Lab Tests

Many diseases and disorders can impact the respiratory system. They include mild problems such as upper respiratory infections, laryngitis, bronchitis, and sinusitis as well as more serious diseases. Influenza, asthma, pneumonia, tuberculosis, chronic obstructive pulmonary disease (COPD, which includes chronic bronchitis and emphysema), Legionnaire's disease, cystic fibrosis, and lung cancer are examples of serious respiratory disorders. Atelectasis, or collapsed lung, generally occurs as a result of trauma but can be the result of COPD or other medical problems.

Diagnostic tests of the respiratory system are generally related to the presence of various gases in the blood, most notably oxygen and carbon dioxide, or the identification of disease-causing microorganisms. Table 4-5 describes laboratory tests related to the respiratory system.

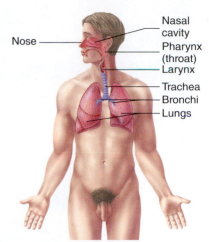

Figure 4-5 The respiratory system.

TABLE 4-5 Tests for Common Respiratory Diseases and Disorders

Tests	Description of Test	Related Diseases and Disorders
Blood Tests		
Arterial blood gases (ABG)	Measures levels of oxygen, carbon dioxide, and bicarbonate as well as the pH (acidity or alkalinity) in arterial blood	Acidosis, alkalosis, emphysema
Electrolytes (Na, K, Cl, CO_2)	Measures blood levels of sodium, potassium, chloride, and carbon dioxide (in the form of bicarbonate (CHO_3-)), and sometimes calcium, magnesium, and phosphorus as well	Electrolyte imbalances; Cushing syndrome; COPD; acute disorders such as ketoacidosis, methanol poisoning, or aspirin overdose
Complete blood count (CBC)	Count of red and white blood cells and platelets, amount of hemoglobin in the blood, and hematocrit (the fraction of blood composed of red blood cells)	Various infections (elevated WBC count may indicate that the body is fighting an infection)
DNA study	Analyzes DNA sample to look for genetic sequences that suggest specific diseases	Cystic fibrosis
Other Tests to Assess the Respiratory System		
Bronchial washing	The patient's respiratory tract is flushed with a saline solution, which is then analyzed and examined under a microscope for the presence of foreign particles	Asbestosis and other environment-related respiratory disorders; lung cancer
Sputum culture	Secretions from the lungs and bronchi are placed on culture medium; any microbial growth is examined microscopically; often includes sensitivity testing (culture and sensitivity or C&S) to determine effectiveness of various antibiotics	Bronchitis, lung abscess, pneumonia, tuberculosis
Throat culture	Material swabbed from the back of the patient's throat is placed on a culture medium; any microbial growth is examined microscopically; often includes sensitivity testing	Various bacterial infections
Pleural fluid analysis	Analysis of fluid that has collected in the pleural cavity	Lung cancer, infection

Checkpoint Questions 4.5

1. What is the difference between internal respiration and external respiration?
2. Which four electrolyte levels are most commonly tested to detect an electrolyte imbalance that could indicate a respiratory disease?

4.6 Digestive System

The **digestive system** is responsible for the intake and digestion of food, the absorption of nutrients, and the removal of solid waste. The organs of the digestive system can be divided into two categories: organs of the alimentary canal and accessory organs. The alimentary canal is the long tube that transports what we eat. The organs of the alimentary canal extend from the mouth (*or/o*) to the anus (*an/o*). They are the mouth, pharynx (*pharyn/o*), esophagus, stomach, small intestine, large intestine, rectum, and anus. The accessory organs are the teeth, tongue, salivary glands, liver, gallbladder, and pancreas.

Digestion is the chemical and mechanical breakdown of foods into forms that your body can absorb (nutrients). Chemical digestion starts when the enzyme amylase, secreted in the mouth, begins breaking down food. The tongue (*gloss/o*) and teeth (*odent/o*, *dent*) assist in the mechanical breakdown of food. Pepsin/pepsinogen in the stomach also provide chemical breakdown. Nutrients are passed to various body cells and waste products are removed through the rectum. Nutrients and waste are both products of digestion. The organs of the digestive system are shown in Figure 4-6.

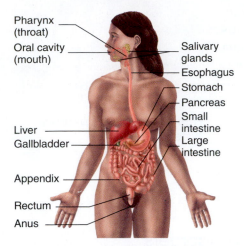

Figure 4-6 The digestive system.

Labels: Pharynx (throat), Oral cavity (mouth), Salivary glands, Esophagus, Stomach, Pancreas, Small intestine, Liver, Gallbladder, Large intestine, Appendix, Rectum, Anus

Digestive System Disorders and Associated Lab Tests

Many digestive system disorders are specific to individual organs. For example, Type 1 diabetes mellitus is a disorder in which the pancreas does not produce enough insulin. Ulcers generally occur in the stomach (*gastr/o*) or intestines. Hepatitis is an inflammation of the liver. Other disorders involve more than one organ or even the digestive system in general. For example, gastroesophageal reflux disease (GERD) affects both the stomach and the esophagus. Because all of the organs of the digestive system work together in the digestive process, laboratory tests are frequently needed to isolate the cause of symptoms related to this system. Table 4-6 describes some of these tests.

TABLE 4-6 Tests for Common Digestive Diseases and Disorders

Tests	Description of Test	Related Diseases and Disorders
Blood Tests		
Nutritional analysis	Measures the blood levels of various vitamins	Malnutrition, nutritional imbalance or deficiency
Carotene	Determines the level of carotene in the blood	Vitamin A deficiency
Carcinoembryonic antigen (CEA)	Detects CEA in the blood; CEA is an antigen that is found in the blood when certain types of cancers are present	Intestinal, pancreatic, thyroid, lung, and breast cancer, as well as cancers of the reproductive and urinary tracts

TABLE 4-6 Tests for Common Digestive Diseases and Disorders (Continued)

Tests	Description of Test	Related Diseases and Disorders
Glucose	Measures the amount of glucose (sugar) in the blood	Type 2 diabetes, overactive or underactive thyroid gland, pancreatic cancer, pancreatitis
Glucose tolerance test (GTT)	Measures the amount of glucose (sugar) in the blood over a specific length of time	Type 2 diabetes, gestational diabetes, Cushing syndrome
Ceruloplasmin	Measures the level of ceruloplasmin (a copper-containing protein) in the blood	Chronic liver disease, Wilson's copper storage disease, infections, lymphoma, rheumatoid arthritis
Hepatic function panel (liver function tests)	Tests included may vary in different laboratories, but in general, this panel measures the blood level of chemicals such as albumin, LDH, bilirubin, alanine aminotransferase (ALT), aspartate aminotransferase (AST), gamma-glutamyl transferase (GGT), alkaline phosphatase (ALP), total protein; these tests may also be ordered individually	Hepatitis, cirrhosis, other chronic liver diseases
Amylase	Measures the amount of the enzyme amylase in the blood	Pancreatic disorders
Lipase	Measures the amount of the enzyme lipase in the blood	Pancreatic disorders
Ammonia (NH_3)	Measures ammonia buildup in the blood	Hepatic encephalopathy
Other Tests to Assess the Digestive System		
Fecal fat	Measures amount of fat in the feces to determine how well fat is being absorbed by the body	Pancreatitis, gallstones, Crohn's disease, pancreatic cancer, celiac disease
Fecal occult blood	Determines whether red blood cells are present in the feces	Colon cancer, other gastrointestinal cancers, esophagitis, gastritis, hemorrhoids, inflammatory bowel disease
Fecal white blood cells	Checks for white blood cells in the feces to help determine the cause of inflammatory diarrhea	Ulcerative colitis, salmonellosis, shigellosis
Stool for ova and parasites (O&P)	Stool specimen is examined microscopically to determine whether certain parasites or their ova (eggs) are present	Amebiasis, giardiasis, and other parasitic infections
Stool culture	Stool sample is placed on culture medium; any microbial growth is examined microscopically	Bacterial gastroenteritis, infections caused by *E. coli, C. difficile*, and other bacteria
Urine chemistries	Measures levels of glucose, ketones, protein, and other chemicals in the urine	Gastrointestinal infections, Type 1 diabetes, anorexia, malnutrition, hyperthyroidism
Biopsies of various gastrointestinal organs	Removal of a small piece of tissue through a biopsy needle for examination	Cancers associated with the individual organs
Gastric fluid analysis	Determines the pH and content of residual gastric fluid in the stomach	Gastric ulcer, gastric cancer, tuberculosis, pernicious anemia
Peritoneal fluid analysis	Examines fluid taken from the abdominal cavity (peritoneal space) for presence of albumin, protein, and red and white blood cells	Peritonitis, cirrhosis of the liver, lymphoma, other gastrointestinal cancers

1. Name the organs of the digestive system and the accessory organs.
2. What tests are generally included in a hepatic function panel?

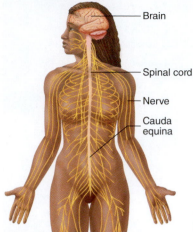

Brain

Spinal cord

Nerve

Cauda equina

Figure 4-7 The nervous system.

4.7 Nervous System

The **nervous system** is responsible for conscious actions, such as voluntary muscle movements, and unconscious actions, such as breathing. The two major divisions are the central nervous system (CNS) and the peripheral nervous system (PNS). The CNS consists of the brain (*encephal/o*) and the spinal cord (*myel/o*), whereas the cranial (*crani/o*) nerves (*neur/o*) and the spinal nerves make up the PNS. The nervous system functions by transmitting electrical impulses. Neurons, or nerve cells, make up the conducting tissue of the nervous system. The tissue that supports and protects the nervous tissue is the neuroglia, which forms a web around nervous tissue. The nervous system includes the brain, spinal cord, and peripheral nerves. See Figure 4-7.

Nervous System Disorders and Associated Lab Tests

Diseases and disorders of the nervous system range from headaches to complex conditions such as epilepsy and amyotrophic lateral sclerosis (ALS, Lou Gehrig's disease). Some, such as cerebrovascular accident (CVA, stroke), Alzheimer's disease, and meningitis, are associated specifically with the brain. Other disorders, including multiple sclerosis, sciatica, and Guillain-Barré syndrome, are linked with the nerve cells. Table 4-7 describes laboratory tests used to diagnose or monitor diseases and disorders of the nervous system.

TABLE 4-7 Tests for Common Nervous System Diseases and Disorders

Tests	Description of Test	Related Diseases and Disorders
Blood Tests		
Acetylcholine receptor antibody	Determines presence or absence of acetylcholine receptor antibody	Myasthenia gravis
Drug levels	Measures the blood levels of various therapeutic drugs to monitor patient response and to help determine therapeutic levels	Epilepsy, other brain disorders
Creatine kinase brain/smooth muscle isoenzyme (CK-BB)	Measures the level of creatine kinase BB isoenzyme in the blood	Cerebrovascular accident (CVA, stroke), lung cancer
Other Tests to Assess the Nervous System		
Cerebrospinal fluid (CSF) analysis	Measures levels of proteins, glucose, antibodies, and other components in CSF (components tested vary)	Meningitis, encephalitis, cancer, Reye syndrome
CSF culture	CSF is placed on culture medium; any microbial growth is examined microscopically; often includes sensitivity (C&S)	Aseptic meningitis, tuberculosis, cryptococcosis, fungal infections
CSF immunoglobulin levels	Measures immunoglobulin G (IgG) level in the CSF	Acute bacterial meningitis

1. Name two diseases or disorders associated specifically with the brain and two that are associated with the nerve cells.
2. Which isoenzyme of creatine kinase may be ordered if a patient shows signs and symptoms of stroke?

4.8 Endocrine System

The **endocrine system** (*endo*, "within," and *crine*, "to secrete") includes the organs of the body that secrete hormones directly into body fluids, including the blood. Hormones help regulate the chemical reactions within cells. The endocrine system influences body tissue by secreting hormones that react with specific receptors located within the various tissues. The receptors are stimulated or inhibited by the hormone, and the tissue reacts accordingly. For example, the hormone insulin is secreted by the pancreas to cause a decrease in blood glucose level. The hormone oxytocin is secreted by the pituitary gland when a woman is breast-feeding, causing milk production.

Essentially, the endocrine system controls the functions of organs and tissues at the cellular level. Unlike the nervous system, which controls the body immediately through nerves, the endocrine system controls the body over time using hormones.

The endocrine system is made up of a number of glands, which secrete many hormones. See Figure 4-8 for the glands in the endocrine system. Table 4-8 describes the hormones secreted by these glands.

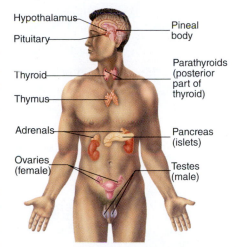

Figure 4-8 The endocrine system.

TABLE 4-8 Endocrine Glands: Their Hormones and Actions

Gland	Hormone	Action Produced
Hypothalamus (produces)	Antidiuretic hormone (ADH)	Stored and released by posterior pituitary; stimulates kidneys to retain water
	Oxytocin (OT)	Stored and released by posterior pituitary; stimulates uterine contraction for labor and delivery
Anterior pituitary	Growth hormone (GH)	Promotes growth and tissue maintenance
	Melanocyte-stimulating hormone (MSH)	Stimulates pigment regulation in epidermis
	Adrenocorticotropic hormone (ACTH)	Stimulates adrenal cortex to produce its hormones
	Thyroid-stimulating hormone (TSH)	Stimulates the thyroid to produce its hormones
	Follicle-stimulating hormone (FSH)	(F) Stimulates ovaries to produce ova and estrogen
		(M) Stimulates testes to produce sperm and testosterone
	Luteinizing hormone (LH)	(F) Stimulates ovaries for ovulation and estrogen production
		(M) Stimulates testes to produce testosterone
	Prolactin (PRL)	(F) Stimulates breasts to produce milk
		(M) Works with and complements LH

(continued)

TABLE 4-8 Endocrine Glands: Their Hormones and Actions *(Continued)*

Gland	Hormone	Action Produced
Posterior pituitary (releases)	Antidiuretic hormone (ADH)	Stimulates kidneys to retain water
	Oxytocin (OT)	Stimulates uterine contraction for labor and delivery
Pineal body	Melatonin	Regulates biological clock; links to onset of puberty
Thyroid	Triiodothyronine (T3) and thyroxine (T4)	Protein synthesis and increased energy production for all cells
	Calcitonin	Increases bone calcium and decreases blood calcium
Parathyroid	Parathyroid hormone (PTH)	Agonist to calcitonin; decreases bone calcium/increases blood calcium
Thymus	Thymosin and thymopoietin	Both hormones stimulate the production of T-lymphocytes
Adrenal cortex	Aldosterone	Stimulates body to retain sodium and water
	Cortisol	Decreases protein synthesis; decreases inflammation
Adrenal medulla	Epinephrine and norepinephrine	Prepares body for stress; increases heart rate, respiration, and blood pressure
Pancreas (islets of Langerhans)	Alpha cells: glucagon	Increases blood sugar; decreases protein synthesis
	Beta cells: insulin	Decreases blood sugar; increases protein synthesis
Gonads: ovaries (female)	Estrogen and progesterone	Secondary sex characteristics; female reproductive hormone
Gonads: testes (male)	Testosterone	Secondary sex characteristics; male reproductive hormone

Endocrine System Disorders and Associated Lab Tests

Most endocrine disorders are caused by glands either over-secreting or under-secreting their hormones. Probably the most common and best-known endocrine disorder is diabetes mellitus. In Type 1 diabetes, the pancreas does not produce insulin. In Type 2 diabetes, either the body does not produce enough insulin or the body cells do not use it efficiently. A third type of diabetes—gestational diabetes—occurs only during pregnancy.

Other endocrine disorders include over- or under-secretion of growth hormone, resulting in giantism or dwarfism, and over- or under-secretion of ACTH, resulting in Addison's disease and Cushing's syndrome, respectively. Table 4-9 lists commonly ordered laboratory tests for the endocrine system.

TABLE 4-9 Tests for Common Endocrine System Diseases and Disorders

Tests	Description of Test	Related Diseases and Disorders
Blood Tests		
A1c (glycated hemoglobin)	Determines the patient's average blood glucose level over the past 2 to 3 months	Types 1 and 2 diabetes mellitus, prediabetes
Adrenocorticotropic hormone (ACTH)	Measures the level of the ACTH hormone in the blood	Addison's disease, Cushing's syndrome, tumor of the adrenal gland, hypopituitarism

Tests	Description of Test	Related Diseases and Disorders
Antidiuretic hormone (ADH)	Measures the blood level of ADH, which is produced by the hypothalamus in the brain	Diabetes insipidus, primary polydipsia, brain tumor, brain infection, certain types of lung cancer, stroke
Aldosterone (Ald)	Measures the level of aldosterone in the blood	Addison's disease, congenital adrenal hyperplasia
Cortisol	Measures the level of the steroid hormone cortisol in the blood	Addison's disease, Cushing's syndrome, tumor of the adrenal gland, hypopituitarism, acute adrenal crisis
Fasting blood glucose (also called fasting blood sugar or FBS)	Measures the level of glucose in the blood after the patient has fasted for at least 8 hours	Prediabetes, Type 2 diabetes, overactive or underactive thyroid gland, pancreatic cancer, pancreatitis
Follicle-stimulating hormone (FSH)	Measures the level of FSH in the blood	Female: menopause, polycystic ovary syndrome, ovarian cysts, infertility, anorexia, Turner syndrome Male: Klinefelter syndrome, infertility
Luteinizing hormone (LH)	Measures the level of LH in the blood	Female: menopause, polycystic ovary syndrome, ovarian cysts, Turner syndrome Male: anorchia, hypogonadism, Klinefelter syndrome
Glucagon	Measures the level of the hormone glucagon in the blood	Diabetes, Cushing's syndrome, cirrhosis of the liver, hypoglycemia, pancreatitis
Glucose tolerance test (GTT)	Determines how well the body breaks down glucose over a 2- to 3-hour period	Prediabetes, Type 2 diabetes, gestational diabetes
Growth hormone (GH)	Measures the level of GH in the blood	Acromegaly, giantlism, dwarfism, pituitary tumor
Insulin	Measures the level of insulin in the blood	Diabetes
Renin	Measures the level of renin in the blood	Hypertension (high blood pressure), kidney disorders
Thyroid function panel	Measures the level of T3, T4, and TSH; often includes a thyroid scan with a radioactive iodine tracer as well	Thyroid cancer, goiter, overactive or underactive thyroid gland, Graves' disease, hypopituitarism, thyroid nodule
Other Tests to Assess the Endocrine System		
Urine ketones	Measures the level of ketones in the urine	Type 2 diabetes
Tissue biopsy of individual glands	Removal of a small piece of tissue through a biopsy needle for examination	Cancer of the various glands

1. What is the major function of the endocrine system?
2. Name four blood tests that might be ordered to diagnose or monitor diabetes mellitus.

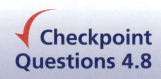

✓ **Checkpoint Questions 4.8**

4.9 Cardiovascular System

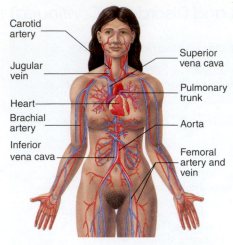

Carotid artery
Jugular vein
Heart
Brachial artery
Inferior vena cava
Superior vena cava
Pulmonary trunk
Aorta
Femoral artery and vein

Figure 4-9 The circulatory system.

The **cardiovascular system**, sometimes called the *circulatory system*, is responsible for sending blood to the lungs to pick up oxygen and to the digestive system to collect nutrients and then for delivering the oxygen and nutrients throughout the body. It also gathers waste products throughout the body and delivers them to the organ systems that remove them from the body. For example, urea is a waste product that forms when the body breaks down proteins. The blood collects urea throughout the body and circulates it through the kidneys, where it is separated from the blood and eliminated from the body in urine.

The cardiovascular system consists of the heart (*cardi/o*) and the blood vessels. Blood (*hem/o, hemat/o*) travels through the vessels (*angi/o, vas/o, vascul/o*) to take oxygen (*ox/o, oxia*) and food to all the cells. Figure 4-9 shows the major vessels of the cardiovascular system. The full chapter on the system includes more detail on the cardiovascular system and how it works.

Cardiovascular System Disorders and Associated Lab Tests

Diseases and disorders of the cardiovascular system include those related to the heart as well as those related to the vascular system, or blood vessels. Laboratory tests are commonly performed to assess three major aspects of cardiovascular health:

- Heart and circulation
- Blood vessels and hemostasis (control of blood flow in blood vessels)
- Red blood cells (RBC)
  - Concentration as determined by the red blood cell count and hematocrit, which is the portion or percent of RBCs in whole blood
  - Size as reported by the mean corpuscular volume (MCV)
  - Hemoglobin, the oxygen-carrying protein found in RBCs, which is measured directly and its value used to calculate the mean corpuscular hemoglobin (MCH), the amount of hemoglobin in an average RBC, and the mean corpuscular hemoglobin concentration (MCHC), which reflects how "full" the RBC is of hemoglobin
  - RBC distribution width (RDW), a measure of the difference in size from the patient's smallest RBC to the patient's largest RBC
  - RBC morphology, the blood smear observation of RBC size and shape variation
  - White blood cells (WBC)
  - Concentration as determined by the WBC count
  - Distribution of types as determined by a differential count, which reflects the number and percent of the different types of white blood cells (explained further in the chapter on the cardiovascular system)
  - Platelets
  - Concentration as determined by the platelet count
  - Platelet morphology, the blood smear observation of platelet size variation

Table 4-10 describes tests that are commonly performed to diagnose or monitor diseases and disorders of the cardiovascular system.

TABLE 4-10 Tests for Cardiovascular Diseases and Disorders

Tests	Description of Test	Related Diseases and Disorders
Tests Related to the Heart and Circulation		
B-type natriuretic peptide (BNP)	Determines the blood level of B-type natriuretic peptide	Heart failure
Creatine kinase (CK)	Measures the level of CK-MB (the creatine kinase isoenzyme found mostly in the heart); CK-MM is also affected during myocardial infarction	Myocardial infarction, heart trauma, myocarditis
Lipid profile	Measures levels of total cholesterol, including its components of • low-density lipoprotein (LDL) • high-density lipoprotein (HDL) • very low-density lipoprotein (VLDL) Triglycerides are also part of the lipid profile.	Heart disease, cerebrovascular accident (stroke), and conditions related to blocked arteries
Troponin I/ Troponin T	Measures the amount of troponin in the blood, which elevates when the heart muscle is damaged.	Myocardial infarction
Tests Related to the Blood Vessels and Hemostasis		
Electrolytes (Na, K, Cl, CO_2)	Measures blood levels of sodium, potassium, chloride, and carbon dioxide (in the form of bicarbonate), and sometimes calcium, magnesium, and phosphorus as well	Congestive heart failure; monitoring of diuretic medications
Bleeding time	Measures the time it takes small blood vessels in the skin to stop bleeding (this test is no longer recommended)	Thrombocytopenia, platelet aggregation defects, Von Willebrand disease
Clotting factor assays	Determines the levels of specific clotting proteins; performed when PT or APTT test results are abnormal	Hemophilia, Von Willebrand disease
Clotting inhibitor and antibody studies	Detects and measures inhibitors to various coagulation (clotting) factors in the blood	Congenital factor deficiencies, cancer, immunologic disorders
Platelet count	Determines the number of platelets in the blood to diagnose or monitor disease	Disseminated intravascular coagulation, hemolytic anemia, leukemia, polycythemia vera, thrombocythemia
Platelet function studies	Assess various functions of the platelets	Coronary artery disease, unstable angina, myocardial infarction
Prothrombin time (PT)	Measures the time it takes blood plasma to clot	Clotting factor deficiencies, vitamin K deficiency, disseminated intravascular coagulation
D-dimer and other fibrin degradation products (FDP/FSP)	Measures the blood levels of the byproducts generated when the body breaks down blood clots	Deep vein thrombosis, pulmonary embolism
Tests Related to the Blood Cells		
ABO, Rh factor	Determines the presence of specific antigens on red blood cells	Blood typing

(continued)

TABLE 4-10 Tests for Cardiovascular Diseases and Disorders *(Continued)*

Tests	Description of Test	Related Diseases and Disorders
Tests Related to the Blood Cells		
Complete blood count (CBC)	Measures the following components of the blood: • White blood cells (WBC) • Red blood cells (RBC) • Hemoglobin (Hgb) • Hematocrit (Hct) • Mean corpuscular volume (MCV) • Mean corpuscular hemoglobin (MCH) • Mean corpuscular hemoglobin concentration (MCHC) • Red cell distribution width (RDW) • Platelet count (Plat)	Blood clotting problems, anemia, systemic lupus erythematosus, leukemia and other blood cancers
Differential	Determines the percentage of individual types of white blood cells—neutrophils, lymphocytes, monocytes, eosinophils, and basophils—as well as hematopoietic cells such as nucleated RBCs and early stages of WBCs	Myelocytic leukemia, aplastic anemia, septicemia
Erythrocyte sedimentation rate (ESR)	Measures the rate at which red blood cells fall to the bottom of a specially calibrated tube; an increase of plasma proteins during times of inflammation and other disorders causes RBCs to fall more quickly	Anemia, lymphoma, multiple myeloma, autoimmune disorders, infections, inflammation, arthritis
Iron studies (Fe and TIBC)	Series of tests to measure the level of iron in the serum, the blood's total iron-binding capacity, unsaturated iron-binding capacity, and the amount of iron stored in the body	Iron deficiency, iron-deficient anemia
Malaria test	Microscopic examination of the blood to detect malaria parasites; in some cases, the individual species of parasite is determined	Malaria
Reticulocyte count (Retic)	Measures the percentage of immature red blood cells (reticulocytes) in the blood	Bone marrow failure, erythroblastosis fetalis, hemolytic anemia, aplastic anemia, pernicious anemia, vitamin B_{12} deficiency
Other Tests to Assess the Cardiovascular System		
Blood culture	Determines whether bacteria or other microorganisms are present in the blood	Septicemia
Bone marrow analysis	Ordered when blood counts are abnormal	Anemia, leukopenia, leukocytosis, polycythemia, thrombocytopenia, cancer of the blood or bone marrow, hemochromatosis
Pericardial fluid analysis	Evaluates pericardial fluid (the fluid in the pericardium that lubricates the movement of the heart) to determine the cause of increased fluid levels	Congestive heart failure, lymphoma, mesothelioma, metastatic cancer, pericarditis

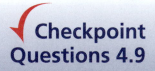

Checkpoint Questions 4.9

1. What three aspects of cardiovascular health do laboratory tests generally measure?

2. Which blood tests are included in a lipid profile?

4.10 Urinary System

The kidneys (*nephr/o, ren/o*), ureters (*ureter/o*), bladder (*cyst/o, vesic/o*), and urethra (*urethr/o*) make up the **urinary system**. The urinary (*ur/o, uria*) system is responsible for

- removing metabolic waste from the blood
- maintaining proper balance of water (*hydro*), salts, and acids in the body fluids
- removing excess fluids from the body

The kidneys are the functional units of the urinary system. They filter and remove metabolic waste products from the blood. The kidneys combine these metabolic wastes with water and ions to form urine (*urin/o*). The urine is transported through the ureters to the bladder, where it is stored until it is excreted. The bladder empties into the urethra, which transports the urine outside the body. Figure 4-10 shows the major organs of the urinary system.

The kidneys also secrete the hormone erythropoietin, which stimulates the bone marrow to produce red blood cells, and the hormone renin, which helps regulate blood pressure. The functions of the kidneys are important in maintaining a balanced, stable state in the body's internal environment, a state called *homeostasis*.

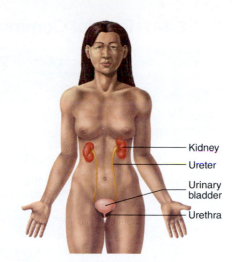

Figure 4-10 The urinary system.

Urinary System Disorders and Associated Lab Tests

Most of the metabolic processes that take place in the body result in waste products. Because the purpose of the urinary system is to remove wastes from the body, diseases and disorders associated with the urinary system may result in an increase in waste products in the blood. Examples of urinary system disorders include acute or chronic renal (kidney) failure, polycystic kidney disease, kidney stones, glomerulonephritis, pyelonephritis, and cystitis (bladder infection). Laboratory tests that are commonly ordered to diagnose or monitor diseases and disorders of the urinary system are listed in Table 4-11.

TABLE 4-11 Tests for Common Urinary System Diseases and Disorders

Tests	Description of Test	Related Diseases and Disorders
Blood Tests		
Albumin	Measures the level of albumin in blood serum	Chronic renal failure, glomerulonephritis
Blood urea nitrogen (BUN)	Measures the level of urea nitrogen in the blood; urea nitrogen is formed when proteins break down	Glomerulonephritis, acute tubular necrosis, pyelonephritis, kidney failure, urinary tract obstruction, acute nephritic syndrome, medullary cystic kidney disease
Creatinine	Measures the level of creatinine in the blood; creatinine is formed when creatine in the muscles breaks down	Acute tubular necrosis, glomerulonephritis, urinary tract obstruction, diabetic nephropathy, hemolytic-uremic syndrome

(continued)

Tests	Description of Test	Related Diseases and Disorders
Blood Tests		
Glomerular filtration rate	Provides an estimate of how much blood passes through the glomeruli in the kidneys per minute; glomeruli are the structures in the kidneys that filter waste products from the blood	Chronic renal failure, acute renal failure
Serum osmolality	Measures the amounts of chemicals in blood serum to determine water balance in the body	Uremia
Other Tests to Assess the Urinary System		
Urinalysis	Examination of physical and chemical properties of urine, including microscopic examination	Acute nephritic syndrome, acute tubular necrosis, atheroembolic renal disease, bladder stones, chronic glomerulonephritis, chronic renal failure, cystinuria, enuresis, acute pyelonephritis, urethritis
Creatinine clearance	Compares the level of creatinine in the blood and urine; requires both a blood sample and a urine sample	Acute tubular necrosis, bladder obstruction, end-stage renal failure, glomerulonephritis, renal ischemia
Urine culture	Urine is placed in a culture medium; any microbial growth is examined microscopically; often includes sensitivity (C&S)	Urinary tract infections

---

✓ **Checkpoint Questions 4.10**

1. Name the three main functions of the urinary system.
2. What tests might be ordered if a physician suspects that a patient has glomerulonephritis?

4.11 Female and Male Reproductive Systems

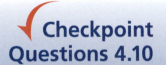

The **female reproductive system** consists of the ovaries, vagina, uterus, mammary glands, and associated structures. This system produces oocytes, which develop into female sex cells called *ova* (eggs; singular: *ovum*), and is the site of fertilization and fetal development. It produces milk for the newborn and hormones that influence sexual function and behaviors. If an ovum is fertilized by a male sex cell (sperm), the female system nurtures the fertilized ovum until birth. Figure 4-11 shows the organs of the female reproductive system.

In the male, several organs are parts of both the reproductive and the urinary systems. The organs in the **male reproductive system** include the testes, accessory structures, ducts, and penis. The male reproductive system produces and transports sperm. It also generates hormones that influence sexual functions and behaviors. Figure 4-12 shows the organs of the male reproductive system.

Mammary gland (in breast)
Uterine tube
Ovary
Uterus
Vagina

Figure 4-11 The female reproductive system.

Reproductive System Disorders and Associated Lab Tests

Disorders of the reproductive systems include infertility, sexually transmitted infections (STIs), and infections as well as cancers of the various reproductive organs. Some diseases, such as epididymitis, prostate cancer, and ovarian cancer, are gender-specific. Others, including most STIs, can occur in both males and females. STIs include chlamydia, gonorrhea, syphilis, herpes simplex, HIV/AIDS, trichomoniasis, and condyloma acuminatum (genital warts). Table 4-12 lists laboratory tests that are commonly ordered to diagnose diseases and disorders of the reproductive systems.

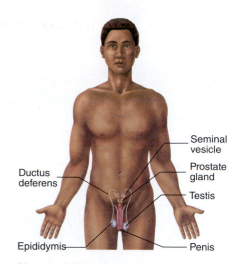

Figure 4-12 The male reproductive system.

TABLE 4-12 Tests for Common Reproductive System Diseases and Disorders

Tests	Description of Test	Related Diseases and Disorders
Blood Tests		
Estradiol	Measures the amount of estradiol (a form of estrogen) in the blood	Abnormal sexual development, ovarian cancer, menstrual abnormalities, Turner syndrome
Follicle-stimulating hormone (FSH)	Measures the level of FSH in the blood	Abnormal sexual development, menopause, polycystic ovary syndrome, ovarian cysts, infertility
Human chorionic gonadotropin (hCG)	Qualitative test determines whether the hormone is present; quantitative test measures the level of hCG in the blood	Normal pregnancy, miscarriage, ectopic pregnancy, ovarian cancer, hydatidiform mole of the uterus, uterine cancer, testicular cancer
Luteinizing hormone (LH)	Measures the level of LH in the blood	Males: anorchia, hypogonadism, Klinefelter syndrome
		Females: menopause, polycystic ovary disease, Turner syndrome
Progesterone	Measures the level of progesterone in the blood	Pregnancy, ovarian cancer, amenorrhea, ectopic pregnancy, adrenal cancer
Prolactin	Measures the level of prolactin in the blood	Galactorrhea, headaches, infertility, erectile dysfunction
Prostate-specific antigen (PSA)	Measures the level of PSA in the blood	Prostate cancer
Rapid plasma reagin (RPR) and VDRL tests	Determine whether antibodies are present to *Treponema pallidum*, the organism that causes syphilis	Syphilis
Testosterone	Measures the level of testosterone in the blood	Cancer of the testes or ovaries
Other Tests to Assess the Reproductive Systems		
Microbiology cultures	Performed on semen and other secretions to isolate and identify infection-causing bacteria	Cystitis, epididymitis, other reproductive system infections
PAP smear	Cells scraped from the opening of the cervix are examined microscopically	Cervical cancer

(continued)

TABLE 4-12 Tests for Common Reproductive System Diseases and Disorders *(Continued)*

Tests	Description of Test	Related Diseases and Disorders
Other Tests to Assess the Reproductive Systems		
Semen analysis	Measures the amount and quality of semen and sperm	Infertility, Klinefelter syndrome
Tissue biopsy	Removal of a small piece of tissue through a biopsy needle for examination	Cancer of various reproductive organs
Tumor markers	Determines whether substances called tumor markers are present in blood or body fluids that indicate a specific type of tumor	Cancer of various reproductive organs

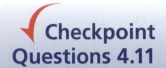 **Checkpoint Questions 4.11**

1. List the organs of the male and female reproductive systems.
2. Which laboratory tests might be ordered if a female shows signs of abnormal sexual development?

Chapter Summary

Learning Outcome	Summary	Related NAACLS Competency
4.1 Describe the functions of the integumentary system, common diseases and disorders that affect this system, and related laboratory tests. Pages 79–80.	The integumentary system consists of the skin, hair, and nails. Common disorders include viruses that affect the skin, allergies, and cancer. Commonly ordered laboratory tests are listed in Table 4-1.	1.00, 1.6, 3.00, 3.1
4.2 Describe the functions of the skeletal system, common diseases and disorders that affect this system, and related laboratory tests. Pages 80–81.	The skeletal system consists of bones, associated cartilages, ligaments, and joints. Common disorders include osteoporosis, osteoarthritis and rheumatoid arthritis, gout, osteosarcoma, and nutritional deficiencies. Commonly ordered laboratory tests are listed in Table 4-2.	1.6, 3.00, 3.1
4.3 Describe the functions of the muscular system, common diseases and disorders that affect this system, and related laboratory tests. Pages 82–83.	The muscular system consists of the muscles and connective tissue, including tendons and ligaments. Common disorders include strains and sprains, tendonitis, torticollis, fibromyalgia, myasthenia gravis, and muscular dystrophy. Commonly ordered laboratory tests are listed in Table 4-3.	1.6, 3.00, 3.1
4.4 Describe the functions of the lymphatic and immune systems, common diseases and disorders that affect these systems, and related laboratory tests. Pages 83–84.	The organs of the lymphatic and immune systems include the thymus, lymph nodes, lymphatic vessels, glands, tonsils, and spleen. The immune system protects the body against harmful microorganisms by producing antibodies against specific antigens. The lymphatic system removes foreign substances from the blood and lymph. Mononucleosis, HIV/AIDS, and lymphedema are examples of diseases that affect these systems. Commonly ordered laboratory tests are listed in Table 4-4.	1.6, 3.00, 3.1

Learning Outcome	Summary	Related NAACLS Competency
4.5 Describe the functions of the respiratory system, common diseases and disorders that affect this system, and related laboratory tests. Pages 84–86.	The respiratory system includes the lungs, trachea, bronchi, bronchioles, and nasal and oral cavities. Common disorders include upper respiratory infections, bronchitis, pneumonia, lung cancer, and chronic obstructive pulmonary disease (COPD). Commonly ordered laboratory tests are listed in Table 4-5.	1.6, 3.00, 3.1
4.6 Describe the functions of the digestive system, common diseases and disorders that affect this system, and related laboratory tests. Pages 86–88.	The digestive system organs are the mouth, pharynx, esophagus, stomach, small intestine, large intestine, rectum, and anus; the accessory organs are the teeth, tongue, salivary glands, liver, gallbladder, and pancreas. Common disorders include diabetes mellitus, ulcers, gastroesophageal reflux disease (GERD), and hepatitis. Commonly ordered laboratory tests are listed in Table 4-6.	1.6, 3.00, 3.1
4.7 Describe the functions of the nervous system, common diseases and disorders that affect this system, and related laboratory tests. Pages 88–89.	The central nervous system consists of the brain and the spinal cord; the peripheral nervous system consists of the cranial nerves and spinal nerves. Disorders of the nervous system include cerebrovascular accident (CVA, stroke), Alzheimer's disease, and sciatica. Commonly ordered laboratory tests are listed in Table 4-7.	1.6, 3.00, 3.1
4.8 Describe the functions of the endocrine system, common diseases and disorders that affect this system, and related laboratory tests. Pages 89–91.	The endocrine glands include the hypothalamus, pituitary, pineal body, thyroid, parathyroid, thymus, adrenal cortex, adrenal medulla, pancreas, ovaries, and testes. Most disorders of the endocrine system are caused by glands either over-secreting or under-secreting their hormones. Commonly ordered laboratory tests are listed in Table 4-9.	1.6, 3.00, 3.1
4.9 Describe the functions of the cardiovascular system, common diseases and disorders that affect this system, and related laboratory tests. Pages 92–94.	The cardiovascular system consists of the heart and the blood vessels. Common diseases and disorders include heart failure, myocardial infarction (heart attack), and coronary artery disease. Commonly ordered laboratory tests are listed in Table 4-10.	1.6, 3.00, 3.1
4.10 Describe the functions of the urinary system, common diseases and disorders that affect this system, and related laboratory tests. Pages 95–96.	The urinary system includes the kidneys, bladder, ureters, and urethra. Common diseases and disorders include renal failure, glomerulonephritis, urinary tract infections, kidney stones, and cystitis. Commonly ordered laboratory tests are listed in Table 4-11.	1.6, 3.00, 3.1
4.11 Describe the functions of the female and male reproductive systems, common diseases and disorders that affect these systems, and related laboratory tests. Pages 96–98.	The female reproductive system consists of the ovaries, vagina, uterus, mammary glands, and associated structures. The male reproductive system consists of the testes, accessory structures, ducts, and penis. Common diseases and disorders include infertility, sexually transmitted infections (STIs), and cancer of the various organs. Commonly ordered laboratory tests are listed in Table 4-12.	1.6, 3.00, 3.1

Chapter Review

A: Labeling

Label the parts of the respiratory and cardiovascular systems in the following images.

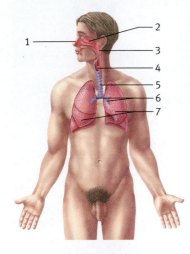

1. [LO 4.5] _____

2. [LO 4.5] _____

3. [LO 4.5] _____

4. [LO 4.5] _____

5. [LO 4.5] _____

6. [LO 4.5] _____

7. [LO 4.5] _____

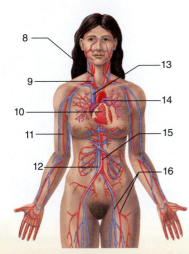

8. [LO 4.9] _____

9. [LO 4.9] _____

10. [LO 4.9] _____

11. [LO 4.9] _____

12. [LO 4.9] _____

13. [LO 4.9] _____

14. [LO 4.9] _____

15. [LO 4.9] _____

16. [LO 4.9] _____

B: Matching

Match the following organs with their corresponding body system.

___**17.** [LO 4.8] adrenals

___**18.** [LO 4.3] biceps

___**19.** [LO 4.10] bladder

___**20.** [LO 4.7] brain

___**21.** [LO 4.11] epididymis

___**22.** [LO 4.2] femur

___**23.** [LO 4.1] hair

___**24.** [LO 4.9] heart

___**25.** [LO 4.5] larynx

___**26.** [LO 4.6] liver

___**27.** [LO 4.11] penis

___**28.** [LO 4.5] pharynx

___**29.** [LO 4.3] quadriceps

___**30.** [LO 4.6] salivary glands

___**31.** [LO 4.2] skull

___**32.** [LO 4.7] spinal cord

___**33.** [LO 4.4] spleen

___**34.** [LO 4.4] tonsils

___**35.** [LO 4.10] ureter

___**36.** [LO 4.11] uterus

___**37.** [LO 4.11] vagina

a. cardiovascular

b. digestive

c. endocrine

d. integumentary

e. lymphatic

f. muscular

g. nervous

h. reproductive

i. respiratory

j. skeletal

k. urinary

C: Fill in the Blank

Write in the word(s) to complete each statement.

38. [LO 4.5] The organ in which gas exchange takes place is the _____.

39. [LO 4.10] Liquid wastes are stored in and eliminated by the _____.

40. [LO 4.1] The largest organ in the body is the _____.

41. [LO 4.11] Reproductive organs specific to the female include the _____.

42. [LO 4.11] Reproductive organs specific to the male include the _____.

D: Sequencing

In what sequence does food pass through the digestive system? Put the following organs in chronological order from numbers 1 through 7.

_____43. [LO 4.6] anus

_____44. [LO 4.6] esophagus

_____45. [LO 4.6] large intestine

_____46. [LO 4.6] oral cavity

_____47. [LO 4.6] rectum

_____48. [LO 4.6] small intestine

_____49. [LO 4.6] stomach

E: Case Studies/Critical Thinking

50. [LO 4.7] A patient cannot feel any pain when you draw her blood. She explains that she does not feel light sensations or pressure when touched on her arms or legs. A disorder in which body system(s) may be causing this issue?

51. [LO 4.3] An elderly patient, living a sedentary lifestyle (lack of activity), is feeling very cold and does not produce much of his own body heat. Explain which body system may be contributing to this and why.

52. [LO 4.1,4.3, 4.7, 4.9] Which body systems does a phlebotomist use when drawing blood? Explain the reasons for each system in your answer.

53. [LO 4.1, 4.7, 4.9] When drawing blood on a patient, with which of the patient's body systems does the equipment come in contact?

F: Exam Prep

Choose the best answer for each question.

54. [LO 4.6] Which of the following blood tests aids in the evaluation of the digestive system?

   a. Albumin
   b. Creatinine
   c. Hemoglobin
   d. Uric acid

55. [LO 4.10] The renal tubules are part of which body system?

   a. Cardiovascular
   b. Digestive
   c. Respiratory
   d. Urinary

56. [LO 4.5] One of the blood tests used primarily to evaluate the respiratory system is abbreviated

   a. ABG.
   b. BNP.
   c. CBC.
   d. EPO.

57. [LO 4.2] Cartilage and ligaments are part of which body system?

   a. Cardiovascular
   b. Muscular
   c. Respiratory
   d. Skeletal

58. [LO 4.3] Connective tissue and tendons are part of which body system?

 a. Cardiovascular

 b. Muscular

 c. Respiratory

 d. Skeletal

59. [LO 4.5] *Oxia*, *capnia*, *pnea*, and *spiro* are word parts that refer to which body system?

 a. Cardiovascular

 b. Endocrine

 c. Respiratory

 d. Urinary

60. [LO 4.6] The liver and gallbladder are part of which body system?

 a. Digestive

 b. Endocrine

 c. Respiratory

 d. Urinary

61. [LO 4.6] A panel of tests used to assess liver function may include all of these EXCEPT

 a. ammonia.

 b. bilirubin.

 c. creatine kinase.

 d. lactate dehydrogenase.

62. [LO 4.8] Laboratory tests used to assess the endocrine system include all of these EXCEPT

 a. aldosterone.

 b. B-type natriuretic peptide.

 c. cortisol.

 d. erythropoietin.

63. [LO 4.7] Word parts that refer to the nervous system include all of these EXCEPT

 a. *cranio*.

 b. *encephalo*.

 c. *myo*.

 d. *neuro*.

64. [LO 4.1] Regulation of body heat occurs in the

 a. cardiovascular system.

 b. digestive system.

 c. integumentary system.

 d. muscular system.

65. [LO 4.2] You receive an order to draw blood on a patient for alkaline phosphatase, calcium, phosphorus, and vitamin D. The physician is most likely concerned about the patient's

 a. cardiovascular system.

 b. digestive system.

 c. muscular system.

 d. skeletal system.

66. [LO 4.5] The trachea and bronchi are part of the

 a. cardiovascular system.

 b. lymphatic system.

 c. respiratory system.

 d. skeletal system.

67. [LO 4.5] A sputum culture will detect infections in the

 a. digestive system.

 b. endocrine system.

 c. lymphatic system.

 d. respiratory system.

68. [LO 4.9] The body system responsible for carrying oxygen, nutrients, and waste products is the

 a. cardiovascular system.

 b. digestive system.

 c. respiratory system.

 d. urinary system.

69. [LO 4.8] Other body systems are influenced by chemicals and hormones produced in the organs of the

 a. cardiovascular system.

 b. endocrine system.

 c. lymphatic system.

 d. respiratory system.

70. [LO 4.7] Providing communication via a series of electrical impulses is the main function of the

 a. digestive system.

 b. integumentary system.

 c. muscular system.

 d. nervous system.

71. [LO 4.10] Maintaining a balance of water, salts, and acids is the function of the

    a. digestive system.

    b. integumentary system.

    c. respiratory system.

    d. urinary system.

72. [LO 4.1] Dermatitis and athlete's foot are disorders of the

    a. digestive system.

    b. integumentary system.

    c. reproductive system.

    d. skeletal system.

73. [LO 4.10] If the function of the urinary system is in question, the tests that would be most helpful include all of these EXCEPT

    a. BUN.

    b. creatinine.

    c. glucose.

    d. osmolality.

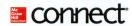

Enhance your learning by completing these exercises and more at connect.mheducation.com.

References

Booth, K.A. (2013). *Healthcare science technology.* New York: McGraw-Hill.

Booth, KA., Whicker, L.G., & Wyman, T.D. (2014). *Medical assisting: Administrative and clinical procedures with anatomy and physiology* (5th ed.). New York: McGraw-Hill.

National Accrediting Agency for Clinical Laboratory Sciences. (2013). *NAACLS entry-level phlebotomist competencies.* Retrieved June 27, 2013, from www.naacls.org/docs/Guide_Approval-section1b-Phleb.pdf

Sheir, D. (2011). *Hole's essentials of human anatomy & physiology* (11th ed.). New York: McGraw-Hill.

Thierer, N. (2010). *Medical terminology: Language for healthcare* (3rd ed.). New York: McGraw-Hill.

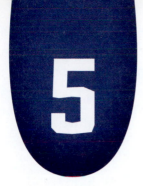

5

The Cardiovascular System

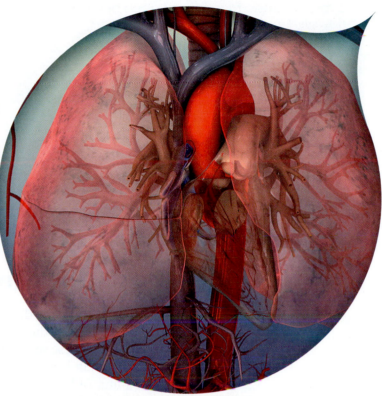

Learning Outcomes

5.1 Describe circulation and the purpose of the vascular system.

5.2 Identify and describe the structures and functions of the different types of blood vessels.

5.3 Locate and name the veins most commonly used for phlebotomy procedures.

5.4 Identify the major components of blood and describe the major functions of each.

5.5 Define hemostasis and describe the basic coagulation process.

5.6 Describe how ABO and Rh blood types are determined.

Introduction

Knowledge of the circulatory system will help phlebotomists understand the effects blood collection procedures can have on results obtained for tests. This chapter takes a deeper look into the circulatory system and its components and functions as well as its impact on blood tests specifically done for the circulatory system.

5.1 The Heart and Circulation

As discussed in Chapter 4, the cardiovascular system is responsible for circulating blood throughout the body. The heart, the blood vessels, and the blood that flows through these structures make up this system.

The average adult has about 8 to 12 pints of blood. A pint is about the same amount as a unit of blood. This is the usual amount of blood given during a blood transfusion. Eight pints equal a gallon. Think of a gallon jug of milk. Your body contains at least this much blood at any given time.

The blood is continually distributed through more than 70,000 miles of tubes (blood vessels), collectively known as the vascular system. If these tubes were lined up end to end, they would reach between New York City and San Francisco over 24 times.

The phlebotomist must have an understanding of the circulation of blood, as well as its composition and functions. In addition to blood's cellular and liquid composition, the phlebotomist must also understand how the closed circuit of blood vessels transports blood. Knowing the location of blood vessels, especially the most commonly used veins, and the composition of blood is essential to performing venipuncture.

Circulation and the Vascular System

The vascular system consists of several tubelike structures called blood vessels. These tubes, which vary in size and structure, are all interconnected, forming a closed circuit. This closed circuit, along with the heart, is responsible for the circulation of blood throughout the body.

The heart is a large muscle that pumps blood through the vascular system. The heart performs as a dual pump system, propelling both oxygenated and deoxygenated blood. A look inside the heart reveals a wall of muscle, called a **septum,** that divides it down the middle into left and right sides. The right side of the heart carries deoxygenated blood. The left side carries oxygenated blood. Another wall separates the rounded top part of the heart from the cone-shaped

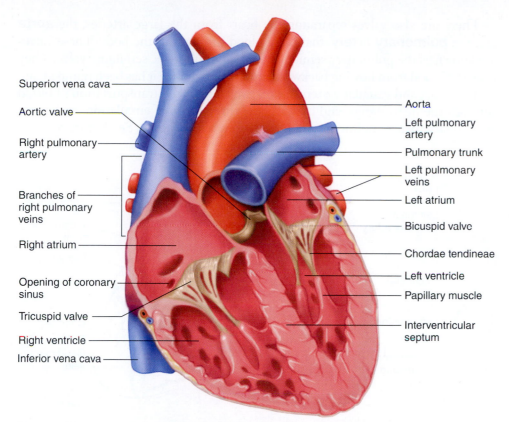

Figure 5-1 The heart is a muscular pump with four chambers; it distributes the blood to the lungs and the body.

bottom part. Thus, there are four chambers (spaces) inside the heart. Each top chamber is called an **atrium** (plural: **atria**). The bottom chambers are called **ventricles.** See Figure 5-1.

The heart consists of three layers. The inside layer is the endocardium. It is lined with endothelial cells similar to the lining of blood vessels. The myocardium is the muscular middle layer. The left ventricle has the thickest myocardium since it is responsible for pumping blood to the rest of the body. The outermost layer is the epicardium. This layer consists of two membranes: the inner, serous visceral membrane attached to the heart and the outer, fibrous parietal membrane. Between these two membranes is the pericardial fluid, which is secreted by the visceral (serous) membrane. The two membranes and the fluid within are known as the pericardial sac. See Figure 5-2.

Blood flows from the atria down into the ventricles because there are openings in the walls that separate the ventricles. These openings are called **valves** because they open in one direction—like trapdoors—to let the blood pass through. Then they close, so that the blood cannot flow backward into the atria. The valve between the right atrium and right ventricle is the tricuspid valve. The valve between the left atrium and left ventricle is the mitral (bicuspid) valve. With this system, blood flows in only one direction inside the heart.

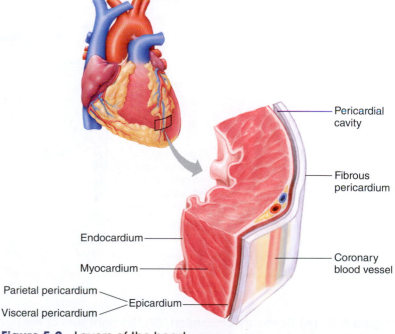

Figure 5-2 Layers of the heart.

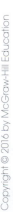

There are also valves separating the heart from the large arteries, the **aorta** and the **pulmonary artery,** that carry blood throughout the body. These valves are known as the pulmonary semilunar valve and the aortic semilunar valve. They keep the blood from flowing backward into the heart once it has been pumped out.

The heart and vascular system are responsible for the transportation of blood through the heart, lungs, and body. These three types of circulation are known as coronary (heart), pulmonary (lungs), and systemic (body). See Figure 5-3.

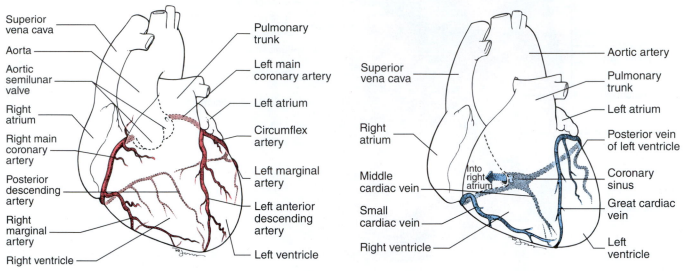

1. Branches of the coronary arteries supply blood to the heart tissue.

2. Branches of the cardiac veins drain blood from the heart tissue.

A

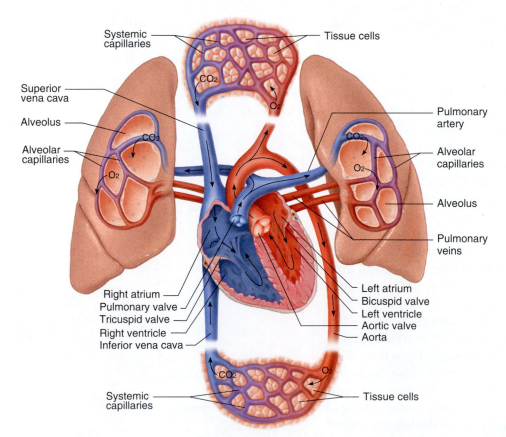

B

Figure 5-3 (A) Coronary circulation. (B) The right side of the heart pumps blood to the lungs (pulmonary circulation). The left side of the heart delivers blood to the body (systemic circulation).

Coronary Circulation

Coronary circulation provides blood supply to the heart. Oxygenated blood travels from the left ventricle, through the aorta, and directly into the coronary arteries. There are two main coronary arteries (left and right). The left main artery has more branches because the left side of the heart is more muscular and requires a larger blood supply. Once the oxygen is distributed to the heart, the blood without oxygen travels through the coronary veins and is collected in the coronary sinus. The coronary sinus is a group of coronary veins joined together. This sinus empties the blood directly into the right atrium.

Pulmonary Circulation

Blood from the body enters the heart through the right atrium. This blood is **deoxygenated** and has a high concentration of carbon dioxide, a waste gas that it picks up from the body's cells. Pulmonary circulation consists of the path the blood takes through the lungs to become **oxygenated.** From the right atrium, the blood travels to the right ventricle and then through the pulmonary arteries to the lungs. In the lungs, it picks up oxygen and releases carbon dioxide, which is then exhaled. This process takes place in the alveoli (air sacs) of the lungs. The oxygenated blood flows through the pulmonary veins to the left atrium of the heart. This oxygenated blood supply is ready to be pumped throughout the body. Figure 5-4 shows the path of the blood in pulmonary circulation.

Systemic Circulation

Systemic circulation is responsible for delivering nutrient-rich, oxygenated blood to all other parts of the body. It starts in the left atrium, with oxygenated blood provided from the lungs. The blood travels through the left ventricle, which pumps it out through the aorta to all of the body tissues. In the digestive tract, it picks up essential nutrients such as carbohydrates, proteins, and vitamins. The blood then distributes these nutrients, along with oxygen, to all of the body's cells. It also picks up waste products, such as urea and carbon dioxide, from the body cells. As the blood passes through the kidneys, urea and other liquid wastes are filtered out to form urine. The deoxygenated blood returns to the right atrium of the heart, where pulmonary circulation begins.

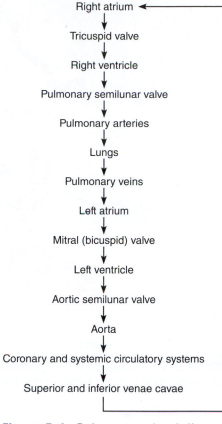

Figure 5-4 Pulmonary circulation blood pathway.

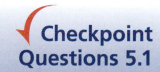

Checkpoint Questions 5.1

1. Briefly describe the purpose of the three types of circulation in the human body.
2. Describe the basic structure of the heart.

5.2 Blood Vessels

The three main types of blood vessels are arteries, veins, and capillaries. **Arteries** are vessels that transport blood away from the heart. All arteries except the pulmonary arteries contain oxygenated blood, and all veins except the pulmonary veins carry deoxygenated blood. The pulmonary arteries transport deoxygenated blood away from the heart to the lungs. The pulmonary veins carry oxygenated blood from the lungs back to the heart. The important fact to remember is that all arteries carry blood away from the heart and all veins transport blood toward the heart.

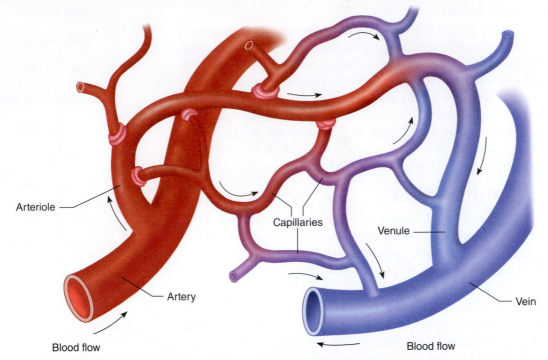

Arteriole

Capillaries

Venule

Artery

Vein

Blood flow

Blood flow

Figure 5-5 Arteries carry oxygen-rich blood through capillaries, where gas exchange occurs. Veins carry deoxygenated blood back to the heart.

The largest artery, the aorta, transports oxygenated blood from the heart. The aorta branches into smaller arteries, which divide further to become even smaller **arterioles,** until they reach the capillaries. The **capillaries** are the smallest of all the blood vessels; they are also the most numerous blood vessels in the human body. Capillaries serve as the connecting points between the arterioles and the **venules** (small veins). They deliver oxygen from the blood to the tissues. Capillaries then join together to form venules, which in turn gather together to form larger **veins.** Finally, the largest veins—the superior and inferior **venae cavae**—return the deoxygenated blood to the right atrium of the heart. This cycle continues over and over again, with blood traveling through each of the body's blood vessels, forming a circular vascular network. See Figure 5-5.

Structure of Blood Vessels

Blood vessels are structured to perform specific functions according to their type. Arteries and veins are composed of the following three layers of tissue (see Figure 5-6):

- **Tunica intima**—the innermost, smooth layer in direct contact with the blood
- **Tunica media**—the middle, thickest layer, capable of contracting and relaxing
- **Tunica adventitia**—the outer covering, which protects and supports the vessel

Capillaries, the smallest blood vessels, have only one layer of tissue. This single-layer vessel is so small that blood cells have to pass through it in single file.

Arteries

Arteries are considered *efferent* vessels because they carry blood away from the heart. Artery walls are elastic, muscular, and much thicker than the walls of veins and capillaries. They must be thicker and stronger to withstand the

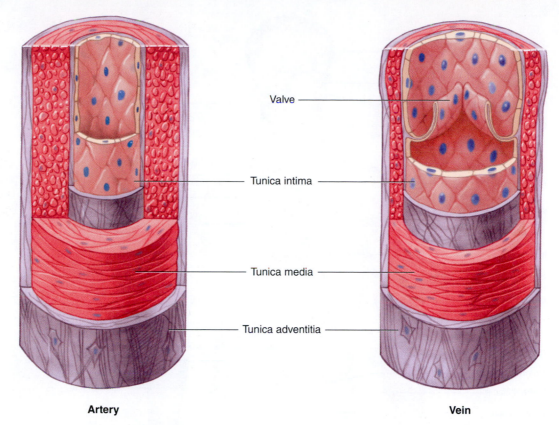

Valve

Tunica intima

Tunica media

Tunica adventitia

Artery   **Vein**

Figure 5-6   Arteries and veins are composed of three layers of tissue.

pressure with which blood is pumped from the heart. Each time the heart "beats," or contracts, it pushes blood through the arteries under high pressure. This results in the pulse that can be felt at specific sites on the body, including the radial pulse at the wrist and the carotid pulse at the neck. Because most arteries carry oxygenated blood, arterial blood is a bright red. Many arteries are paired, meaning that there is a left and a right artery with the same name. See Figure 5-7.

Capillaries

Capillaries are the smallest blood vessels; they provide a link from arterioles to venules. All gas exchange occurs at this level. Capillaries can only be seen through a microscope. Their walls are made up of a single layer of cells to allow for selective permeability, so substances can pass into and out of the blood. Nutrients, molecules, and oxygen pass out of the capillaries and into surrounding cells and tissues.

Waste products, such as carbon dioxide and nitrogenous waste, pass from the body's cells and tissues back into the bloodstream for excretion by means of the respiratory, urinary, integumentary, and digestive systems.

Veins

As veins carry blood toward the heart, they are considered *afferent* vessels. See Figure 5-8. Large veins usually have the same names as the arteries they run beside.

The pressure from the heart is diminished by the time the blood reaches the veins; therefore, the force is not as great as it is in the arteries. Muscle movement helps push blood through the veins. However, veins flow against gravity in many areas of the body. To prevent blood from flowing backward

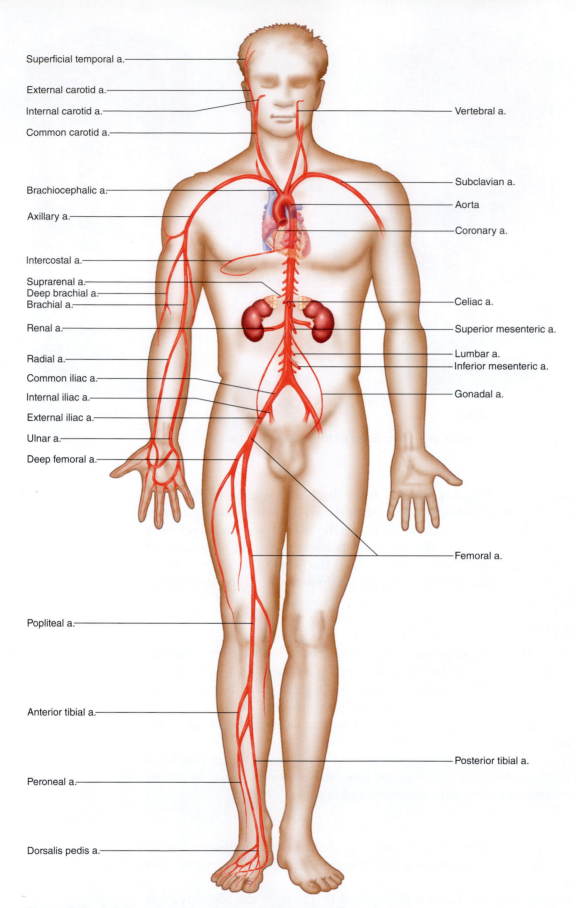

Superficial temporal a.

External carotid a.

Internal carotid a.

Common carotid a.

Vertebral a.

Brachiocephalic a.

Axillary a.

Subclavian a.

Aorta

Coronary a.

Intercostal a.

Suprarenal a.

Deep brachial a.

Brachial a.

Celiac a.

Renal a.

Superior mesenteric a.

Radial a.

Lumbar a.

Inferior mesenteric a.

Common iliac a.

Internal iliac a.

Gonadal a.

External iliac a.

Ulnar a.

Deep femoral a.

Femoral a.

Popliteal a.

Anterior tibial a.

Posterior tibial a.

Peroneal a.

Dorsalis pedis a.

Figure 5-7 Arteries carry blood away from the heart.

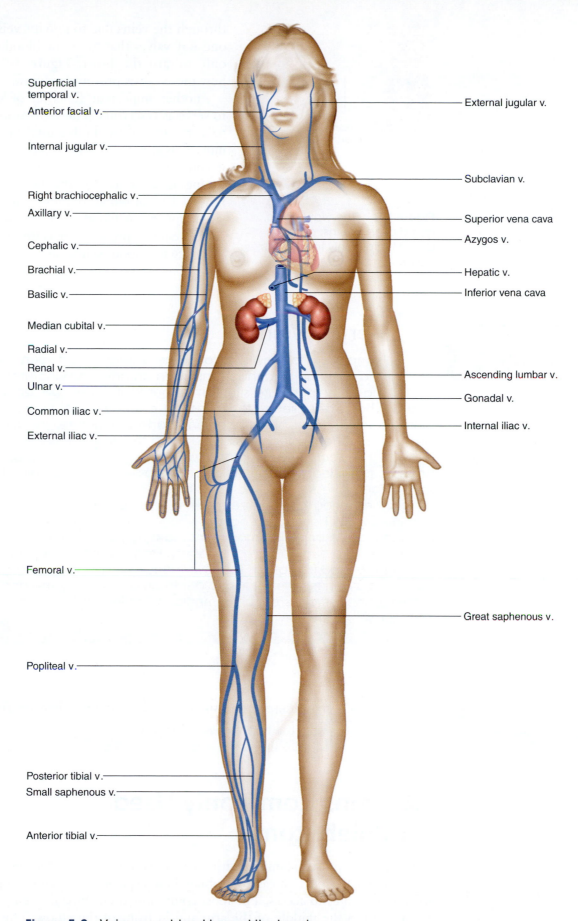

Superficial temporal v.

Anterior facial v.

Internal jugular v.

Right brachiocephalic v.

Axillary v.

Cephalic v.

Brachial v.

Basilic v.

Median cubital v.

Radial v.

Renal v.

Ulnar v.

Common iliac v.

External iliac v.

Femoral v.

Popliteal v.

Posterior tibial v.

Small saphenous v.

Anterior tibial v.

External jugular v.

Subclavian v.

Superior vena cava

Azygos v.

Hepatic v.

Inferior vena cava

Ascending lumbar v.

Gonadal v.

Internal iliac v.

Great saphenous v.

Figure 5-8 Veins carry blood toward the heart.

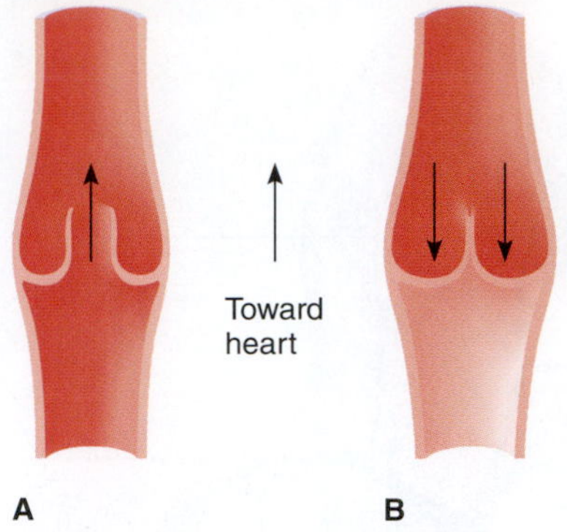

Figure 5-9 One-way valves, found only in veins, permit blood to flow only toward the heart.

Toward heart

A   B

through the veins due to gravity, veins have one-way valves that force the blood to flow only toward the heart. Figure 5-9 shows how these valves prevent backflow.

Another important function of veins is to serve as reservoirs. The veins store about 65% to 70% of the body's total blood volume. This blood is a darker red color because it contains less oxygen. It flows in a slow, oozing manner, unlike the fast, pulsating flow of arterial blood. Because veins store a large amount of blood, have thinner walls, and have lower pressure, they are the vessels of choice for blood collection.

Critical Thinking

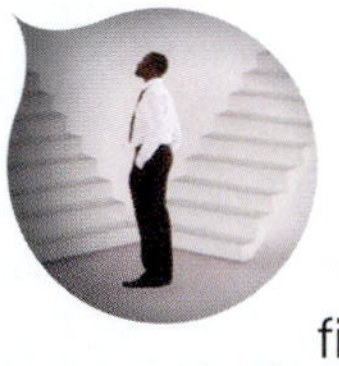

Artery or Vein?

It is important to know how to tell the difference between an artery and a vein and what happens when an artery is punctured. When finding a venipuncture site, remember that a vein will feel bouncy and will have a resiliency to it, and an artery will feel firmer and will pulsate. In the event of an accidental artery puncture, the blood will appear bright red instead of dark red and the flow will usually be more forceful. If this occurs, immediately withdraw the needle and apply firm pressure for at least 5 minutes. Once the bleeding has stopped, apply a taut gauze dressing. Instruct the patient to keep the arm relatively still for a short period to minimize the flow of blood. This will help prevent a **hematoma.** A hematoma occurs when blood collects under the skin, forming a black and blue mass. A hematoma forms as a result of inserting a needle through a vein or an artery. Fragile veins can also be a factor in hematoma formation. To prevent accidental arterial puncture, do not select a vein that lies over or close to an artery. When an accidental arterial puncture does occur, immediately notify a nurse (or supervisor, in the case of outpatient draws).

✓ Checkpoint Questions 5.2

1. Why are veins considered more suitable for phlebotomy than arteries?
2. Name and describe the three types of blood vessels.

5.3 Veins Commonly Used for Phlebotomy

Phlebotomists must be familiar with the veins commonly used for phlebotomy. Such knowledge makes it easier to obtain blood specimens, even from patients with limited sites to access. The most commonly used veins for venipuncture are located in the middle of the arm and in front of the elbow. This area is called the **antecubital fossa** and is the site of the three most preferred veins for venipuncture (see Figure 5-10).

Site Selection

Selecting the perfect vein is not always easy. The patient may have only one arm available for use and the skin on that arm may be sensitive to touch. In the event of dermatitis (inflammation of the skin in which the area is red and may contain skin lesions) or other conditions, and when there are no other sites available, you may use the arm, but do not place the tourniquet directly on the arm. Instead, place the tourniquet over the patient's gown or clothing, or wrap the arm in gauze and then apply the tourniquet. Do not draw blood from an arm that has an intravenous infusion (IV) because the contents of the infusion will alter the blood specimen results. In addition, for patients who have had a mastectomy (breast removal) or stroke, do not draw blood from the arm on the affected side of the body. Signs should be posted in the room that read "NO BLOOD PRESSURES OR VENIPUNCTURES" for the affected arm.

The most commonly used vein for venipuncture is the **median cubital vein,** located in the middle of the forearm. The median cubital vein is the largest and best-anchored, or least-moving, vein in the forearm, making it the favored site for venipuncture.

The next-best site is the **cephalic vein,** which is also well anchored; however, it may be harder to palpate (feel). When the body is in the anatomical position, the cephalic vein lies lateral to the median cubital vein.

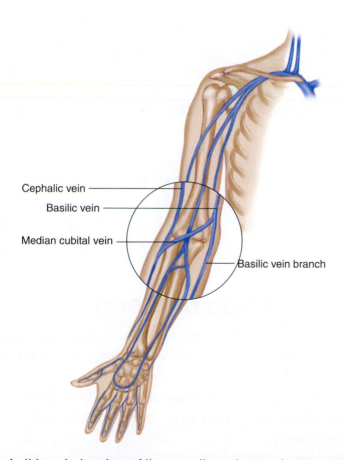

Cephalic vein

Basilic vein

Median cubital vein

Basilic vein branch

Figure 5-10 In this anterior view of the arm, the veins most commonly used for venipuncture are located in the middle of the arm and in front of the elbow.

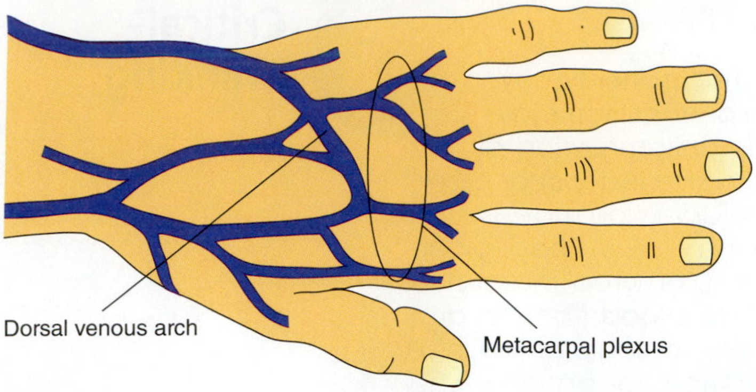

Dorsal venous arch

Metacarpal plexus

Figure 5-11 Veins in the back of the hand are sometimes used for venipuncture when the antecubital veins are not accessible.

The third choice is usually the **basic vein.** This site, though easier to palpate, is not well anchored. It tends to roll when touched, making it more difficult to access. When the body is in the anatomical position, the basilic vein lies medial to the median cubital vein. Additionally, the basilic vein lies close to the median nerve and the brachial artery, which must be avoided during venipuncture procedures because these structures might be accidentally punctured or damaged.

Other sites for venipuncture, such as veins in the back of the hand (dorsal arch), are used when the antecubital veins are not accessible (see Figure 5-11). These hand veins are smaller, less anchored, and sometimes require the use of a smaller-gauge needle, usually a butterfly needle (explained in the chapter *Blood Collection Equipment*). Using hand veins for venipuncture can also be more painful for the patient.

Although physicians sometimes need to obtain blood from blood vessels in the head, legs, or feet, these sites are not acceptable for venipuncture by phlebotomists. More sites for phlebotomy are discussed later in this textbook.

Law & Ethics

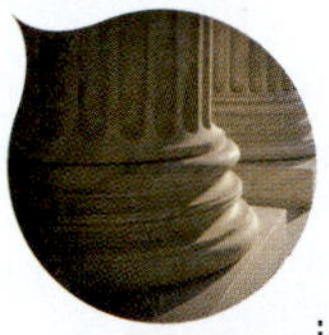

Selecting a Vein

The phlebotomist must use correct technique after properly selecting the vein. Accidental puncture of the median nerve could result in temporary or permanent loss of function in that arm. This would constitute an act of negligence, and there are cases in which patients have been awarded millions of dollars to compensate them for their losses. The best way to prevent injuring this nerve is to avoid "probing around" at the site.

✓ Checkpoint Questions 5.3

1. What are the two most common locations for venipuncture?
2. List the three most commonly used veins in venipuncture in order of preference from most to least preferred, and explain why they are ranked in this order.

5.4 Composition of Blood

Blood is the primary transporting fluid of the body. Its composition is complex and essential to sustaining life. Blood has many important functions and plays a role in numerous body functions:

- Blood transports oxygen and nutrients to the body's cells and tissues.
- It transports hormones to their target area, so that the body can function in its proper capacity.
- It eliminates waste materials from the body's cells.
- It maintains water balance for the body's cells and tissues.

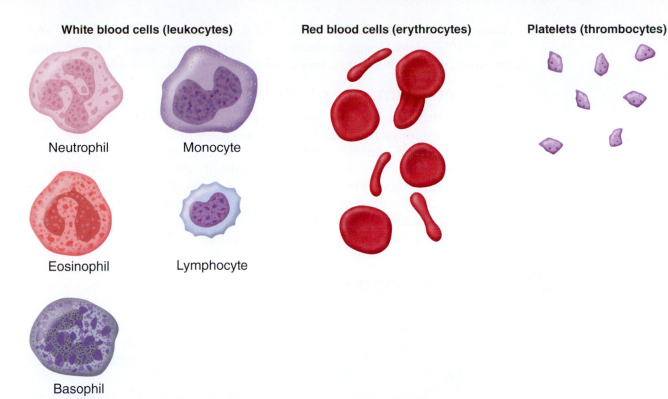

White blood cells (leukocytes)

Neutrophil

Monocyte

Eosinophil

Lymphocyte

Basophil

Red blood cells (erythrocytes)

Platelets (thrombocytes)

Figure 5-12 The formed elements of blood include white blood cells, red blood cells, and platelets.

- It transports antibodies and protective substances throughout the body, so that they can attack pathogens (disease-producing microorganisms).
- It assists with regulating body temperature.
- It helps maintain acid-base balance.

When a tube of anticoagulated blood (blood kept from clotting) stands undisturbed, it will separate into two parts, or components. One part is cellular (formed elements) and the other is liquid (plasma). Formed elements include red blood cells (erythrocytes), white blood cells (leukocytes), and platelets (thrombocytes). See Figure 5-12.

Formed elements make up about 45% of blood's total volume. Almost 99% of the circulating cells are red blood cells. Blood cells originate mostly from inside the bone marrow. See Table 5-1. The liquid component, or plasma, is a straw-colored or pale yellow fluid that is mostly water. Plasma makes up

TABLE 5-1 Cellular Components of Blood

Blood Cells	Normal Quantity*	Description
Erythrocytes (red blood cells)	M. 4.5–6.2 million/mm³ F. 4.2–5.4 million/mm³	Contain hemoglobin; transport oxygen and carbon dioxide
Leukocytes (white blood cells)	5,000–10,000/mm³	Protect against infections
Thrombocytes (platelets)	150,000–450,000/mm³	Aid in blood clotting

*Blood cell ranges vary according to lab reference materials.

about 55% of blood's total volume, and it contains 90% to 92% water and 8% to 10% *solutes* (dissolved chemicals). These solutes consist of electrolytes, enzymes, glucose, hormones, lipids, proteins, and metabolic substances.

Formed Elements of Blood

The cells that make up the formed elements of the blood arise from stem cells (cells from which specific body cells are formed). Two such stem cells are found in separate **hematopoietic** (blood-forming) compartments: **myeloid** (developed from bone marrow) and **lymphoid** (developed from the lymphatic system). Blood cells formed by myeloid stem cells include the red blood cells, platelets, granulocytes, and monocytes. Blood cells formed by lymphoid stem cells include two different types of lymphocytes, B cells and T cells. See Figure 5-13 for the differentiation of blood cells.

Life Span Considerations

Fetal Blood Formation

Blood cells first arise from the yolk sac during the embryonic stages of human development. The liver and spleen form blood cells during the fetal stage and are the primary sites of blood formation until the bones develop and begin to take over the process. At birth, bone marrow is the primary site of blood cell formation.

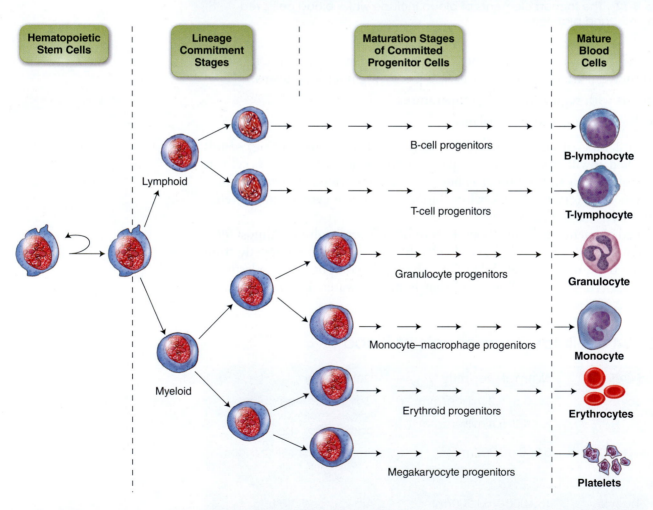

Figure 5-13 Blood cells originate from stem cells. Cells developing in the lymphoid tissues become either B-cell or T-cell lymphocytes. Cells developing in the myeloid tissues (such as bone marrow) become granulocytes, monocytes, erythrocytes (red blood cells), or thrombocytes (platelets).

Erythrocytes (Red Blood Cells)

Erythrocytes (red blood cells, or RBCs) originate in the bone marrow and are the most numerous of all the blood cells. On average, a healthy adult has approximately 4.2 to 6.1 million red blood cells per cubic millimeter (mm^3) of blood. The normal range varies, depending on the gender. RBCs average 7 to 8 micrometers (μm) across their diameter, and their average volume is 90 femtoliters (fL). A femtoliter is 10^{-15} liter. At this size, about 18 million RBCs could sit on the head of a pin. When fully mature, erythrocytes resemble the shape of a doughnut without a hole. This appearance is referred to as **biconcave** because both sides of the red blood cell cave inward at the center (see Figure 5-14). This shape allows flexibility, so that the RBCs can pass through blood vessels of various sizes, down to tiny capillaries, in order to perform their functions.

Erythrocytes are constantly being manufactured by the bone marrow. The average life span of a red blood cell is about 120 days. After that, they begin to lose their biconcave shape and ability to carry oxygen. The liver, spleen, and bone marrow sequester (remove), phagocytize (ingest), and destroy old, worn-out red blood cells. Thousands of red blood cells are formed and destroyed daily.

Red blood cells are responsible for carrying oxygen to every cell in the body and for removing carbon dioxide from the cells. This ability to transport oxygen and carbon dioxide occurs as a result of a very important molecule called **hemoglobin.** Hemoglobin is made up of a protein molecule called *globin* and an iron compound called *heme.* A red blood cell contains several million molecules of hemoglobin.

Pediatric Levels: Red Blood Cells

Life Span Considerations

At birth, infants normally have an increased amount of red blood cells and hemoglobin. Within the first several weeks, however, these levels drop. Red blood cell and hemoglobin levels for children are similar to those for females. However, as children reach adulthood, the values for males and females begin to vary.

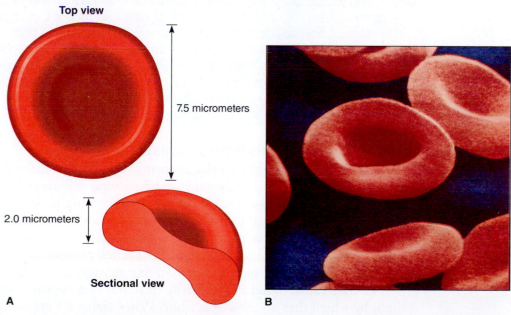

Top view

7.5 micrometers

2.0 micrometers

Sectional view

A

B

Figure 5-14   (A) Red blood cells have a biconcave shape. (B) Scanning electron micrograph of red blood cells.

Excessive blood loss, the destruction of red blood cells, and/or decreased blood cell formation can all affect the supply of hemoglobin. An abnormally low hemoglobin level and/or a decrease in the number of red blood cells is called *anemia*. Symptoms of anemia include weakness, headache, difficulty breathing, and pale skin color. Several conditions can cause a decrease in hemoglobin and/or RBC numbers:

- Sickle cell anemia
- Hemophilia
- Some forms of cancer
- A dietary deficiency of iron, folate, and/or vitamin B_{12}

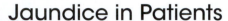

Critical Thinking

Jaundice in Patients

Elevated levels of bilirubin cause the skin and eyes to take on a yellowish color, called jaundice. Because the liver is the organ that processes bilirubin, elevated bilirubin levels can occur as a result of liver problems such as hepatitis, cirrhosis, and obstruction of the ducts in the liver. Blood is drawn on these patients to monitor the bilirubin level. As always, proper technique must be used to ensure accuracy of bilibrubin results.

Bilirubin produced during the breakdown of red blood cells is processed by the liver, deposited in the intestines, and then eliminated. Low levels of bilirubin are normally present in the blood because of the normal cycle of red blood cell production and destruction. However, some forms of anemia cause RBCs to be destroyed prematurely in the bloodstream. This destruction (**hemolysis**) leads to higher levels of bilirubin in the blood and may cause **jaundice** (yellow coloration of the skin and eyes).

Life Span Considerations

Newborn Bilirubin Levels

When the liver breaks down worn-out red blood cells, one of the byproducts is bilirubin. Infants normally are born with an excess of red blood cells and hemoglobin. In some infants, the liver may not be able to keep up with the amount of bilirubin that is being produced by the destruction of RBCs. Excessive amounts of bilirubin may cause damage to organs, such as the brain. Bilirubin is light sensitive, and light can break it down, which is why infants who have elevated bilirubin levels are placed under ultraviolet lamps to help rid their bodies of excess bilirubin. Frequently blood tests are done to monitor the bilirubin level.

Leukocytes (White Blood Cells)
Leukocytes, or white blood cells, are primarily responsible for destroying foreign substances, such as pathogens, and removing cellular debris. Leukocytes are not confined to vascular spaces when performing their duties. They can pass through capillaries' thin walls in a process known as **diapedesis.** Once white blood cells are at the site of foreign invaders, they can surround and destroy these pathogens through a process called **phagocytosis.** In phagocytosis, the leukocytes engulf, or "eat," foreign substances and/or cellular debris.

Leukocytes are round and primarily clear, but they appear white because the light by which they are viewed is white. When stains are applied to leukocytes, they take on various colors based on the cell type. These stains will be explained

Immunocompromised Patients

The phlebotomist may be required to draw blood from patients who are immunocompromised. Immunocompromised patients have a weakened immune system. One such situation is when the patient has an abnormally low neutrophil count and therefore has a low resistance to infections. Even the slightest infection can prove to be life threatening to these patients. In addition to Standard Precautions, immunocompromised patients require extra measures to be taken to prevent the transmission of pathogens. The phlebotomist must perform meticulous hand hygiene and apply sterile personal protective equipment, not only to protect herself but also to protect the patient. Should the phlebotomist have a common cold or other symptoms of illness, she should refrain from entering the patient's room to prevent severe illness and even death in patients with low resistance to infections.

further later in this chapter. The average adult has between 5,000 and 10,000 white blood cells per cubic millimeter (mm^3) of blood, unless an infection or other disorder is present.

During a bacterial infection, the number of white blood cells increases in order to send an army of defender cells to the infection site. Certain diseases, such as leukemia, cause an abnormally elevated number of white blood cells. Other conditions, such as acquired immune deficiency syndrome (AIDS), cause a drastic decrease in the white blood cell count.

There are several ways to classify the many diverse types of white blood cells. One system divides white blood cells into two main categories: *myeloid* cells (**granulocytes, monocytes**) and *lymphoid* cells (**T-cell lymphocytes, B-cell lymphocytes,** and **natural killer (NK) cells,** also known as large granular lymphocytes). Another system categorizes white blood cells into **polymorphonuclear,** cells that have a nucleus that is segmented into two or more lobes, and **mononuclear,** cells that have a single-lobed nucleus. Table 5-2 describes the various types of myeloid and lymphoid white blood cells that are normally seen in the peripheral blood.

A CBC or WBC differential laboratory test is used to determine the percentage of each type of WBC in the blood. If the differential is performed manually, a medical laboratory technician or scientist counts 100 white blood cells on stained slides, keeping track of how many of each type of cell are counted. Automated equipment performs a differential by counting and classifying all of the WBCs in the sample.

The most numerous of all the white blood cells in adults are the **neutrophils,** which average 10 to 16 μm across their diameter and normally have three or four nuclear lobes. The granules in the **cytoplasm** (the area of the cell outside the nucleus) of neutrophils appear tan, pink, or lavender when stained. These granules contain enzymes that are involved in phagocytosis. Neutrophils help defend the body against infections, and their average life span is from 6 hours to a few days. They move quickly to the site of infection and engulf the invader. As the neutrophils kill or neutralize the pathogens, **pus** is formed, which contains neutrophils, pathogens, and parts of the cells at the site of infection or injury.

The second type of granulocytes are the **eosinophils,** which average 10 to 16 μm across their diameter and normally have two nuclear lobes. Eosinophils are present in low numbers compared with neutrophils. Their cytoplasmic granules stain bright red-orange with eosin (an orange-colored dye). The eosinophil's granules contain chemicals that assist in controlling inflammatory reactions to prevent the spread of inflammation. Eosinophils can phagocytize

TABLE 5-2 Types of White Blood Cells

Cell Type	Description	Adult Normal Range % of Total WBC Count	Function
Polymorphonuclear/Granulocytes			
	Neutrophils have distinct nuclei with 3 or 4 lobes. They show neutral staining: tan, lavender, or pink.	60%–70%	Aid in immune system defense; release pyrogens (chemicals produced by leukocytes to cause fever); phagocytize (engulf bacteria); use lysosomal enzymes to destroy bacteria; level increases during infection and inflammation
	Eosinophils have a bilobed nucleus and cytoplasmic granules that stain orange-red.	1%–4%	Assist with inflammatory responses; secrete chemicals that destroy certain parasites; level increases with allergies and parasitic infection
	Basophils have a bilobed nucleus and cytoplasmic granules that stain deep blue.	0%–1%	Assist with inflammatory response by releasing histamine; release heparin (anticoagulant) and produce a vasodilator; count increases with chronic inflammation and during healing from infection
Mononuclear			
	Monocytes have large, kidney-shaped nuclei. They have fine cytoplasmic granules.	2%–6%	Are the largest WBCs; become macrophages; phagocytize dying cells, microorganisms, and foreign substances; levels increase during chronic infections, such as tuberculosis (TB)
	Lymphocytes have round nuclei and a minimum amount of cytoplasm. Lymphocytes may be B cells, T cells, or natural killer (NK) cells.	20%–30%	B-cell lymphocytes assist the immune system by producing antibodies; T-cell lymphocytes assist the immune system through interactions with other leukocytes; NK cells quickly respond to stressed cells; lymphocyte levels increase during viral infections

and destroy parasites, respond to allergic reactions, and help kill tumor cells. Eosinophils live for about 8 to 12 days and increase in number in response to parasitic infections and allergic conditions.

Basophils are the least common granulocytes. Basophils average 10 to 16 μm across their diameter and normally have two nuclear lobes. Basophils contain cytoplasmic granules that stain dark blue or blue-black with basic dyes. Basophils do not phagocytize like eosinophils and neutrophils. Rather, they help to swell a local area in response to an injury or a foreign invader. Basophils release histamine, which is a substance that causes capillary walls to dilate, or expand, allowing blood to enter the infected site. Histamine can accumulate in tissues during an allergic reaction as well. In addition to histamine, basophils also release heparin, which is an **anticoagulant.** Body areas containing large amounts of blood, such as the liver and lungs, have the largest number of basophils. It is believed that the release of heparin in these areas prevents the formation of tiny blood clots.

Monocytes are mononuclear and are the largest of all the circulating white blood cells. They average 12 to 18 μm across their diameter and normally have a round to kidney bean–shaped nucleus. Monocytes' primary function is phagocytosis. They contain fine granules, which play a major role in the destruction of microorganisms. Monocytes are not present in large amounts, but they survive for several months and are effective against chronic infections. They are capable of leaving the bloodstream to move into the tissues, and when they do, they are referred to as *macrophages*. These macrophages are larger cells, and they not only engulf pathogens but they also remove old, worn-out red blood cells when performing their phagocytic actions.

Lymphocytes are also mononuclear but normally do not contain any granules. Lymphocytes average 7 to 15 μm across their diameter and normally have a dense, round nucleus surrounded by very little cytoplasm. Lymphocytes play an important role in the body's immune system. They produce **antibodies** and other substances that help destroy pathogens. The life span of lymphocytes ranges from a few days to several years. Lymphocytes can be divided into three groups: T-cell lymphocytes, B-cell lymphocytes, and NK cells. T cells are formed in the thymus, whereas B cells are formed in the lymphoid compartment of the bone marrow and in the lymph nodes. T-lymphocytes are responsible for directing cell-mediated immune responses (cells helping other cells perform their function). T-lymphocytes can further be subdivided into helper T cells and suppressor T cells. Helper T cells, or CD4 cells, help other cells, such as monocytes, perform their function more efficiently. (T cells are those that are destroyed by the human immunodeficiency virus, or HIV.) Suppressor T cells, or CD8 cells, control or stop another cell's activities. B-cell lymphocytes are responsible for humoral immunity (the production of antibodies). NK cells rapidly respond to stressed or infected cells without the need for antibodies.

Pediatric Levels: White Blood Cells

Life Span Considerations

The distribution of the various white blood cells is different for children than it is for adults. At birth, infants have a very high percentage of neutrophils (up to 80%). Lymphocytes soon dominate the distribution of white blood cells in young children as they begin to encounter the world and all its antigens. Children are constantly being exposed to new things in their environments. The body must be ready to produce antibodies, if needed, with each new molecule that is encountered by the body. Children normally have 40% to 60% lymphocytes and 20% to 30% neutrophils. As they approach adulthood, the white blood cell distribution becomes more like adult levels (see Table 5-2).

B cells help defend the body by transforming into plasma cells, which then synthesize, or combine, and release antibody molecules. The antibodies are made to match the specific antigens that triggered their production. This B-cell response is called the humoral response because immunity is in the humors, or fluids, of the body.

NK cells are lymphocytes that target body cells infected by viruses as well as other types of abnormal cells, including cancer cells. After attaching to a targeted cell, the NK cell breaks through the cell's membrane and injects chemicals that cause the cell to lyse (break up). NK cells are also thought to work with other types of lymphocytes to help control immune responses.

During a suspected infection, it is very helpful for the physician to know the percentages and amounts of each type of white blood cell to assist with diagnosing and treating the patient. For this reason, a CBC with differential is one of the more commonly ordered laboratory tests.

Platelets (Thrombocytes)

Platelets, or **thrombocytes,** are the smallest of all the cellular components, averaging 1 to 4 μm across their diameter. Platelets do not contain a nucleus. Platelets, unlike other blood cells, are not complete cells. Instead, they are fragments of larger cells, megakaryocytes, found in bone marrow. Megakaryocytes are the largest cells in the bone marrow, exhibiting a very large, multiple-lobed nucleus. Each platelet typically remains in circulation for about 9 to 12 days, and the normal adult range is between 150,000 and 450,000 per cubic millimeter (mm^3) of blood.

Platelets play an important role in preventing blood loss because, when an injury occurs, they are the first components to arrive at the site. Platelets stick to the injury site and form a platelet plug, which slows or stops the bleeding. Platelets also secrete a substance called serotonin, which causes the blood vessels to spasm, or narrow, and decreases blood loss until a clot forms. Platelets, along with substances in the liquid composition of blood, are essential for minimizing blood loss due to an injury. Platelets are formed in the bone marrow, and old platelets are trapped and removed by the spleen.

Liquid Component (Plasma)

The liquid portion of whole blood is called **plasma.** Plasma is a pale yellow fluid comprised mostly of water. The ingredients, or constituents, of plasma include the following:

- *Water* is 90% to 92% of plasma. This percentage is monitored by the kidneys and the pituitary gland and affected by the large intestine and the amount of water consumed.

- *Nutrients* are materials passed through the digestive system directly into the bloodstream. These include cholesterols, fatty acids, amino acids, and glucose.

- *Hormones* assist with chemical reactions and allow the body to maintain a constant balance. One example is thymosin, which helps the immune system battle foreign invaders. A more common hormone is insulin, which regulates the amount of sugar in the bloodstream.

- *Electrolytes* include sodium, potassium, calcium, magnesium, and chloride. These are found in food and are used in chemical processes such as the regulation of the body's water.

- *Proteins* such as fibrinogen, globulins, and albumin:
  - **Fibrinogen** is a protein that aids in clotting and is manufactured in the liver.

- *Globulins* are manufactured both in the liver and in the lymphatic system as antibodies, which fight foreign invaders in the body.
- *Albumin* is the most abundant of all plasma proteins. It is a product of the liver and helps pull water into the bloodstream to assist in regulating blood pressure.

- *Waste* is produced as a result of the body's cells undergoing a chemical reaction. Plasma is responsible for carrying waste to the organs that remove or excrete it. Examples of waste products are urea, uric acid, creatinine, and xanthine.
- *Protective substances* include antitoxins, opsonins, agglutinin, and bacteriolysins.

Plasma and serum have a distinct difference. Plasma is the liquid portion of *unclotted* blood, collected in a tube with an anticoagulant, which prevents clotting. The tubes that are most commonly used with an anticoagulant have purple or lavender tops. **Serum** is the liquid portion of *clotted* blood, collected in a tube without an anticoagulant, so that a clot has been allowed to form. A clot forms when fibrinogen converts into fibrin and traps the formed elements of the blood. When the clot forms, some clotting factors are depleted and the fluid that remains is known as serum. This process of clotting is called **coagulation.**

When laboratory tubes contain an anticoagulant, blood can be separated into cells and plasma by **centrifugation.** Centrifugation is the spinning of test tubes at high speed around a central axis. When collected blood without an anticoagulant is centrifuged, it is separated into cells and serum. Recall that plasma is the liquid component of blood and serum is the liquid component of blood without clotting factors. The results of centrifugation are shown in Figure 5-15. Centrifugation will be discussed further in the chapter *Blood Specimen Handling.*

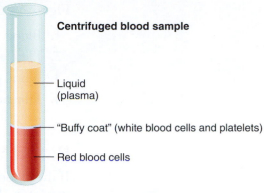

Centrifuged blood sample

Liquid (plasma)

"Buffy coat" (white blood cells and platelets)

Red blood cells

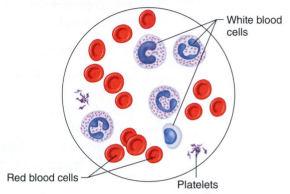

Peripheral blood smear

White blood cells

Red blood cells

Platelets

Figure 5-15 Centrifuged blood sample and peripheral blood smear showing blood components.

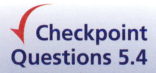

1. List the formed elements of blood and briefly describe the purpose of each.
2. What is the difference between plasma and serum?

✓ Checkpoint Questions 5.4

5.5 Hemostasis and Blood Coagulation

It is important for the phlebotomist to understand how bleeding is controlled naturally. Both venipuncture and dermal puncture create injuries to the blood vessels, and the body's natural defenses must stop the bleeding. The medical term **hemostasis** breaks down into *hemo,* meaning "blood," and *stasis,* meaning "stopping." Following an injury, there are four major events involved in stopping the flow of blood at the injured site.

Figure 5-16 illustrates the following four events:

1. Blood vessel spasm (vasoconstriction)
2. Platelet plug formation
3. Blood clotting (coagulation)
4. Fibrinolysis, or dissolving of the clot and return of the vessel to normal function

Blood Vessel Spasm

If the blood vessel is small and the injury is limited, a blood vessel spasm alone may stop the bleeding. At the time of injury, the involved blood vessel will constrict (narrow in diameter), and this decreases the amount of blood flowing through the vessel, which stops or controls the bleeding.

Platelet Plug Formation

In the event that bleeding continues in spite of the blood vessel spasms, platelets are called into action. The torn, inner lining of the blood vessels releases chemical signals, which stimulate platelets to gather at the injury site. These platelets clump together to form a platelet plug, which further decreases the flow of blood from the injured site. This process occurs within seconds after an injury and is known as *primary hemostasis*.

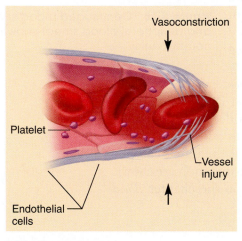

1. Blood vessel spasm

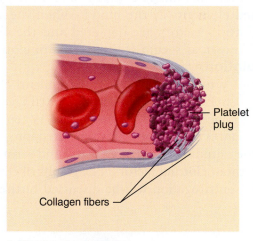

2. Platelet plug formation

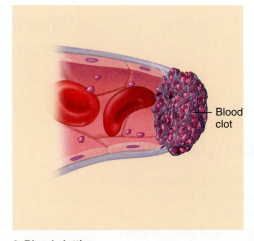

3. Blood clotting

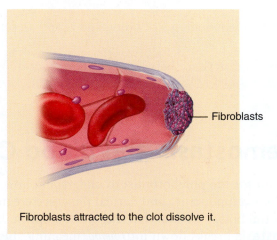

Fibroblasts attracted to the clot dissolve it.

4. Fibrinolysis

Figure 5-16 Events of hemostasis.

Blood Clotting

Extensive injury to larger blood vessels generally requires all steps in the hemostasis process. The third step is coagulation, or blood clotting, which requires the presence of specific clotting factors (Factors I, II, V, VII, VIII, IX, and X) to form a blood clot. At the time of injury to the blood vessel, certain clotting factors are called into action. These clotting factors, along with calcium ions and platelet factors, come together through a complex series of chemical reactions to produce **thrombin.** Thrombin is an enzyme used to convert the plasma protein fibrinogen into **fibrin,** which is a very strong and elastic protein. Once fibrin has been produced, the threadlike composition of fibrin forms a meshlike sac that adheres to the injury site, trapping platelets, blood cells, and other particles to form a clot. This process takes several minutes and is known as *secondary hemostasis* (see Figure 5-17).

Fibrinolysis

The clot stimulates the growth of fibroblasts and smooth muscle cells within the vessel wall. This begins the repair process, which includes the final step in hemostasis, fibrinolysis, ultimately resulting in the dissolution of the clot. The vessel finally returns to normal (see Figure 5-18).

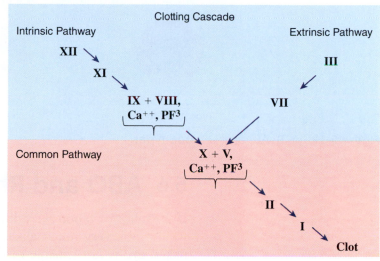

Figure 5-17 Simplified schematic of the clotting cascade, a sequence of events that result in the formation of a clot. These events occur in similar fashion to falling dominos, where one domino falling touches off a chain reaction. The clotting proteins are identified with Roman numerals. The above diagram shows the proteins involved in several pathways of clotting. The clot often forms around platelets that have adhered to the site of tissue or vessel damage as shown in Figure 5-16.

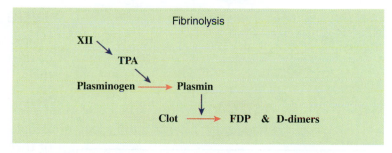

Figure 5-18 Simplified schematic of fibrinolysis. Fibrinolysis (breaking down of the clot) occurs in a similar "falling dominos" fashion to the clotting cascade. A series of reactions occurs that results in the clot being broken down into fibrin degradation products (FDPs) and D-dimers.

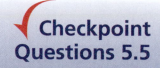

1. What is the medical term for stopping the flow of blood?
2. Explain the purpose of thrombin in the blood coagulation process.

Checkpoint Questions 5.5

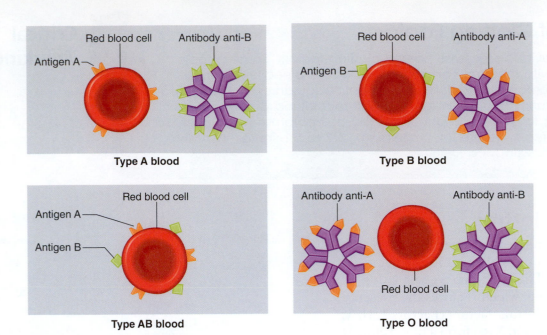

Figure 5-19 A, B, AB, and O blood types.

5.6 ABO and Rh Blood Types

If 20 tubes of blood were lined up on a counter in the laboratory, they all would look very much alike, even though they may be very different. The naked eye is not capable of detecting the inherited identifying proteins on the surface of individual red blood cells, known as **antigens.** The ABO blood group consists of four **blood types:** A, B, AB, and O. They are distinguished from each other in part by their antigens and antibodies (see Figures 5-19 and 5-20).

Medical laboratory scientists identify these blood groups by testing for **agglutination,** the clumping of red blood cells. Agglutination occurs because the antigens on the surface of red blood cells bind to antibodies in plasma.

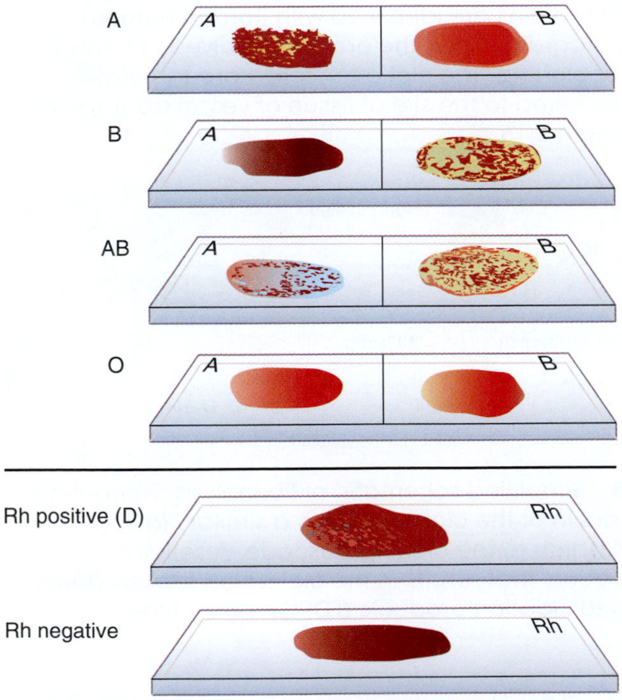

Type A

People with type A blood have antigen A on the surface of their red blood cells. They also have antibody B in their plasma. Antibody B will only bind to antigen B.

Type B

People with type B blood have antigen B on the surface of their red blood cells. They also have antibody A in their plasma.

If a person with type A blood is given type B blood, the antibody B in the recipient's blood stream will bind with the red blood cells of the donor blood because those cells have antigen B on their surfaces. The donated—in this case Type B—red blood cells are destroyed causing severe complications for the patient. This is why a person with type A blood should NEVER be given type B blood (and vice versa). It can cause complications known as transfusion reactions, which are discussed later in this chapter.

Figure 5-20 The agglutination of different ABO and Rh blood types using antisera (serum containing antibodies to either A, B, or D). A grainy appearance indicates agglutination. A smooth appearance indicates a lack of agglutination.

Type AB

People with type AB blood have both antigens A and B on the surface of their red blood cells. They have neither antibody A nor antibody B in their plasma. People with type AB blood are sometimes called universal recipients because most of them can receive all ABO blood types. They lack antibodies A and B in their plasma, so there is no reaction with antigens A and B in the donor blood.

Type O

People with type O blood have neither antigen A nor antigen B on the surface of their red blood cells. However, they do have both antibodies A and B in their plasma. People with type O blood are called sometimes universal donors because their blood can be given to most people, regardless of the recipients' blood type. Type O blood will not cause a transfusion reaction when given to other people because it does not have the antigens to bind to antibody A or antibody B.

Rh Factor

The **Rh antigen** is present on red blood cells and is classified separately from the ABO blood groups. The Rh antigen is assigned the letter D. The Rh antigen was first discovered in 1940 by Karl Landsteiner during his research with Rhesus monkeys, hence the name Rhesus factor and the abbreviation Rh.

The Rh, or D, antigen is the next most important antigen after those in the ABO blood group. Rh is tested with the same techniques as for ABO. Antibodies to the D antigen are added to a drop of patient blood and if agglutination occurs the patient is Rh-positive. No agglutination indicates Rh-negative blood (see Figure 5-20).

People who are Rh-positive have red blood cells with Rh antigens on the cell surface. People who are Rh-negative have red blood cells that do not have Rh antigens on the cell surface. A person who is Rh-negative, if given Rh-positive blood, will usually make antibodies that bind to the Rh antigens. If the Rh-negative person is given Rh-positive blood a second time, the antibodies will bind to the donor cells and agglutination will occur.

It is very important for a female to know her Rh type. If an Rh-negative female mates with an Rh-positive male, there is a 50-50 chance that her fetus will be Rh-positive. After birth, when the blood of an Rh-positive fetus mixes with the blood of a mother who is Rh-negative, the mother develops antibodies against the fetus's red blood cells. The first Rh-positive fetus usually does not suffer from these antibodies because the mother's body has not yet generated the antibodies. However, if the mother conceives another Rh-positive fetus, the fetus's blood will be attacked by the antibodies right away. The fetus then develops a condition called *erythroblastosis fetalis*, or hemolytic disease of the fetus and newborn (HDFN). The baby is born severely anemic, often needing multiple blood transfusions at birth and several times as a neonate. Without treatment, the baby may die before birth or after delivery.

Erythroblastosis fetalis is prevented by giving an Rh-negative woman drugs that suppress the production of anti-D, such as RhIg or RhoGAM®. Blood tests, such as the direct antihuman globulin test (DAT) and bilirubin, may be ordered to evaluate the newborn for any blood incompatibility between the mother and the baby.

Transfusion Reactions

A transfusion reaction occurs when a patient is transfused with blood to which he has an antibody. Initially, agglutination occurs, followed by hemolysis. Transfusion reactions can range from mild, which may produce a slight fever or hives, to severe, resulting in death. To avoid reactions, patients are given type-specific blood or blood products even in emergencies.

Phlebotomists are frequently asked to draw blood that is used to determine a patient's blood type in order to be cross-matched with appropriate blood products.

To prevent transfusion reactions, two patient identifiers must always be used. The blood and blood products must be labeled accurately. An incorrectly labeled specimen can cause a patient to die. The procedure for patient identification during blood collection for blood banks is explained in the chapter *Special Phlebotomy Procedures*.

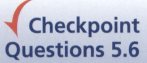
Checkpoint Questions 5.6

1. Which antigen(s) do people with O-positive blood have on their red blood cells?
2. What are the symptoms of a transfusion reaction?

Chapter Summary

Learning Outcome	Key Concepts/Examples	Related NAACLS Competency
5.1 Describe circulation and the purpose of the vascular system. Pages 106–109.	The vascular system consists of a network of vessels that, along with the heart, provides for circulation of the blood. Coronary circulation provides blood to the heart. Systemic circulation provides oxygen and nutrients to body tissues and removes waste. Pulmonary circulation replenishes oxygen in the blood and removes carbon dioxide.	3.1
5.2 Identify and describe the structures and functions of the different types of blood vessels. Pages 109–114.	Blood vessel layers include the tunica intima (innermost), tunica media (middle), and tunica adventitia (outermost). All arteries, with the exception of the pulmonary artery, carry oxygenated blood to the body. All veins, with the exception of the pulmonary vein, carry deoxygenated blood back to the heart and lungs. Arterioles are small arteries and venules are small veins. Capillaries provide a link between arterioles and venules and allow for gas exchange.	3.1, 3.6
5.3 Locate and name the veins most commonly used for phlebotomy procedures. Pages 114–116.	The three veins most commonly used for phlebotomy are located in the antecubital fossa. They include the median cubital, cephalic, and basilic veins.	3.2
5.4 Identify the major components of blood and describe the major functions of each. Pages 116–125.	The major components of blood are formed elements. Red blood cells transport oxygen and carbon dioxide. White blood cells include neutrophils for response to bacterial infections, eosinophils for response to allergies and parasitic infections, basophils for release of histamine and heparin, monocytes to fight chronic infections, and lymphocytes that assist the immune system and produce antibodies. Platelets are essential for clotting. Plasma is the liquid portion of unclotted blood. Serum is the liquid portion of blood collected in a tube without anticoagulant.	3.3

Learning Outcome	Key Concepts/Examples	Related NAACLS Competency
5.5 Define hemostasis and describe the basic coagulation process. Pages 125–127.	Hemostasis, or stopping of blood, includes four major events: blood vessel spasm, platelet plug formation, blood clotting, and fibrinolysis.	3.4, 3.5
5.6 Describe how ABO and Rh blood types are determined. Pages 128–130.	ABO and Rh blood types are determined by the type of antigen found on the red blood cells.	3.6

Chapter Review

A: Labeling

Label the arm veins commonly used for venipuncture in the following image.

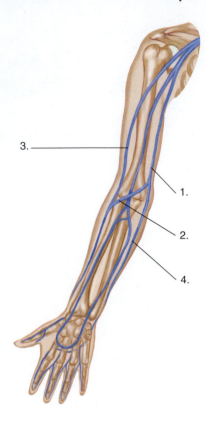

1. [LO 5.3] _____

2. [LO 5.3] _____

3. [LO 5.3] _____

4. [LO 5.3] _____

B: Matching

Match the following terms with their correct description or definition.

_____**5.** [LO 5.1] oxygenated

_____**6.** [LO 5.1] deoxygenated

_____**7.** [LO 5.2] artery

_____**8.** [LO 5.2] vein

_____**9.** [LO 5.2] venule

____**10.** [LO 5.2] arteriole

____**11.** [LO 5.1] aorta

a. carries deoxygenated blood away from the heart

b. very small vein

c. very small artery

d. blood with a high oxygen concentration

e. largest vein in the body

f. smallest blood vessel in the body

g. carries oxygenated blood to the heart

h. largest artery in the body

i. middle layer of a blood vessel

j. blood with a low oxygen concentration

___12. [LO 5.1] vena cava

___13. [LO 5.2] capillary

___14. [LO 5.2] tunica intima

___15. [LO 5.2] tunica media

___16. [LO 5.2] tunica adventitia

___17. [LO 5.4] serum

___18. [LO 5.4] plasma

___19. [LO 5.1] pulmonary artery

___20. [LO 5.1] pulmonary vein

___21. [LO 5.4] lymphocytes

___22. [LO 5.4] monocytes

___23. [LO 5.4] diapedesis

___24. [LO 5.4] eosinophils

___25. [LO 5.4] erythrocytes

___26. [LO 5.4] leukocytes

___27. [LO 5.4] neutrophils

___28. [LO 5.4] basophils

___29. [LO 5.4] platelet

k. fluid that contains fibrinogen

l. blood vessel that carries blood away from the heart

m. outer covering of a blood vessel

n. blood vessel that carries blood toward the heart

o. innermost, smooth layer of a blood vessel

p. fluid left after blood has clotted

q. perform phagocytosis to destroy pathogens

r. smallest of all the blood components and considered to be a cell fragment

s. most numerous of the WBCs

t. process by which WBCs pass through capillary walls to fight pathogens

u. least common granulocyte

v. largest of all WBCs

w. contain hemoglobin and transport oxygen and carbon dioxide

x. produce antibodies that help destroy pathogens

y. assist with inflammatory processes; level is elevated in the presence of allergies and parasites

C: Fill in the Blanks

Write in the word(s) to complete the statement or answer the question.

30. [LO 5.6] _____ are located on the surface of RBCs.

31. [LO 5.5] The liquid portion of the blood is referred to as _____ or plasma, depending on whether it contains fibrinogen and other clotting factors.

32. [LO 5.6] Women with Rh-negative blood may be given drugs to suppress the production of anti-D antibodies in order to prevent a condition called _____ in the fetus.

33. [LO 5.6] People with type _____ blood have the A antigen on the surface of their red blood cells.

34. [LO 5.6] Type _____ blood has neither A nor B antigens on the surface of the red blood cells.

D: Sequencing

As blood flows from the heart, it enters the following blood vessels in what order?

35. [LO 5.2] _____ arterioles

36. [LO 5.2] _____ arteries

37. [LO 5.2] _____ capillaries

38. [LO 5.2] _____ veins

39. [LO 5.2] _____ venules

Put the events of hemostasis (coagulation) in the correct order from 1 to 4.

40. [LO 5.5] _____ formation of the platelet plug

41. [LO 5.5] _____ blood vessel spasm

42. [LO 5.5] _____ blood clotting

43. [LO 5.5] _____ fibrinolysis

E: Case Studies/Critical Thinking

44. [LO 5.2] A phlebotomist is attempting to obtain blood from an unconscious patient. When the needle is inserted into the arm, the phlebotomist observes a bright red, pulsating flow of blood entering the syringe. What may have occurred, and what should the phlebotomist do next?

45. [LO 5.4] An immunocompromised patient requires blood to be drawn routinely, and the phlebotomist has just received a STAT page that needs to be done immediately. Should the phlebotomist proceed to the isolation room quickly and just draw this patient's blood, or should the phlebotomist go back at a later time? Give an explanation for your response.

46. [LO 5.4] A patient exposed to a parasitic infection may experience elevated WBCs. What type of WBC will increase in number during an infection of this type? Why?

47. [LO 5.4] Lymphocytes play an important role in the body's immune system. They produce antibodies and other chemicals that destroy pathogens. What are the three types of lymphocytes that play an effective role in the body's immune system?

48. [LO 5.5] You have been asked to draw blood from a patient who is known to have a low platelet count. Recall that platelets are responsible for clotting blood. When a blood vessel is damaged, the vessel's collagen fibers come in contact with the platelets. The platelets produce a sticky substance, allowing them to stick to the collagen fibers. What would happen to this patient who is experiencing a low platelet count? How would you collect blood from this patient?

F: Exam Prep

Choose the best answer for each question.

49. [LO 5.1] Circulation that is part of the cardiovascular system includes *(Choose all that apply)*

  a. coronary.

  b. pulmonary.

  c. systemic.

  d. lymphatic.

50. [LO 5.1] The heart has

  a. two chambers functioning as a single pump.

  b. two chambers functioning as a dual pump.

  c. four chambers functioning as a single pump.

  d. four chambers functioning as a dual pump.

51. [LO 5.1] Which side of the heart carries deoxygenated blood?

a. Left
b. Right
c. Both
d. Neither

52. [LO 5.1] Blood vessels are lined with the same cells as the heart's

a. endocardium.
b. epicardium.
c. myocardium.
d. pericardium.

53. [LO 5.1] The structures that keep blood flowing in the correct direction are

a. chambers.
b. septa.
c. valves.
d. vessels.

54. [LO 5.1] Blood must pass through this valve when entering the left ventricle.

a. Aortic semilunar
b. Bicuspid
c. Pulmonary semilunar
d. Tricuspid

55. [LO 5.1] The mitral valve is the same as the

a. aortic semilunar valve.
b. bicuspid valve.
c. pulmonary semilunar valve.
d. tricuspid valve.

56. [LO 5.1] Blood is kept from flowing from the aorta backward into the heart by the

a. bicuspid valve.
b. aortic semilunar valve.
c. tricuspid valve.
d. venous valve.

57. [LO 5.2] The structures that carry blood to all parts of the body are the

a. chambers.
b. endocardium.
c. ventricles.
d. vessels.

58. [LO 5.3] The vein on the back of the hand that may be used for phlebotomy procedures is the

a. basilic.
b. cephalic.
c. dorsal.
d. median cubital.

59. [LO 5.4] Which of the following white blood cells has NO phagocytic function?

a. Eosinophil
b. Lymphocyte
c. Monocyte
d. Neutrophil

60. [LO 5.4] The ability of red blood cells to pass through capillaries is due to their shape, which is

a. biconcave.
b. a flat disk.
c. spheroid.
d. uniconcave.

61. [LO 5.4] What type of blood cells have hemoglobin?

a. Erythrocytes
b. Leukocytes
c. Thrombocytes
d. All of these

62. [LO 5.4] Mononuclear leukocytes include all of these EXCEPT

a. B-cell lymphocytes.
b. monocytes.
c. neutrophils.
d. T-cell lymphocytes.

63. [LO 5.4] Various types of granulocytes exhibit these colors when stained EXCEPT

a. blue-black.
b. red-orange.
c. tan-pink.
d. yellow-green.

64. [LO 5.4] A person develops an allergy. What type of blood cells may be elevated when he is exposed to the cause of his allergy?

a. Basophils
b. Eosinophils
c. Macrophages
d. Plasma cells

65. [LO 5.4] While on vacation, a person acquires a parasitic infection. What blood cells may be elevated as a result of this infection?

    a. Basophils

    b. Eosinophils

    c. Monocytes

    d. Neutrophils

66. [LO 5.4] A function of T-cell lymphocytes is to

    a. fight bacterial infections.

    b. mediate cellular interactions.

    c. phagocytize microorganisms.

    d. produce antibodies.

67. [LO 5.4] Serum differs from plasma mainly because it contains NO

    a. electrolytes.

    b. fibrinogen.

    c. nutrients.

    d. water.

68. [LO 5.6] A woman who is pregnant is concerned that her blood type may not match that of her baby's and might harm either her or her baby. Which red blood cell antigen should be of most concern to her and her physician?

    a. A

    b. B

    c. O

    d. Rh

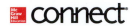

Enhance your learning by completing these exercises and more at connect.mheducation.com.

References

Harmening, D. (2009). *Clinical hematology and fundamentals of hemostasis.* Philadelphia: F. A. Davis.

Hoffman, R., Benz, E. J., Shattil, S. J., Cohen, J., & Silberstein, L. E. (1995). *Hematology: Basic principles and practice* (2nd ed.). New York: Churchill Livingstone.

Kaushansky, K., Lichtman, M., Beutler, E., Kipps, T., Prchal, J., & Seligsohn, U. (Eds.). (2010). *Williams hematology* (8th ed.). New York: McGraw-Hill.

National Accrediting Agency for Clinical Laboratory Sciences. (2012). *NAACLS entry-level phlebotomist competencies.* Rosemont, IL. NAACLS.

Owen, R. (2000). Karl Landsteiner and the first human marker locus. *Genetics, 155,* 995–998. Retrieved May 31, 2011, from www.genetics.org/content/155/3/995.full

Shier, D., Butler, J., & Lewis, R. (2010). *Hole's human anatomy and physiology* (12th ed.). New York: McGraw-Hill.

Wilson, D. (2008). *McGraw-Hill manual of laboratory and diagnostic tests.* New York: McGraw-Hill.

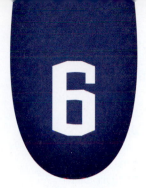

Patient and Specimen Requirements

essential terms

accession number
ambulatory
analyte
ASAP
assault
basal state
battery
bedside manner
code of ethics
confidentiality
consent
diurnal variation
edema
electronic health record (EHR)
electronic medical record (EMR)
ethics
fasting

Health Insurance Portability and Accountability Act (HIPAA)
hemoconcentration
hemodilution
interfering substances
law
lipemic
peak level
postprandial
rapport
requisition
respondeat superior
sedentary
STAT (ST)
therapeutic drug monitoring (TDM)
trough level

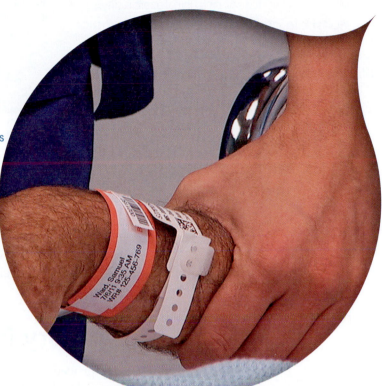

Learning Outcomes

6.1 Identify the parts and functions of a laboratory requisition.

6.2 Identify the professional communication techniques of the phlebotomist.

6.3 Comply with ethical and legal standards for professional communication.

6.4 Carry out proper patient identification.

6.5 Define the legal/ethical importance of specimen identification.

6.6 Recognize patient factors that may affect specimen quality and test results.

6.7 Explain the phlebotomist's role in maintaining accurate and secure blood collection documentation.

Related NAACLS Competencies

4.00 Demonstrate understanding of the importance of specimen collection and specimen integrity in the delivery of patient care.

4.1 Describe the legal and ethical importance of proper patient/sample identification.

4.2 Describe the types of patient specimens that are analyzed in the clinical laboratory.

4.3 Define the phlebotomist's role in collecting and/or transporting these specimens to the laboratory.

4.4 List the general criteria for suitability of a specimen for analysis, and reasons for specimen rejection or re-collection.

4.5 Explain the importance of timed, fasting, and STAT specimens, as related to specimen integrity and patient care.

7.00 Demonstrate understanding of requisitioning, specimen transport, and specimen processing.

7.1 Describe the process by which a request for a laboratory test is generated.

9.00 Communicate (verbally and nonverbally) effectively and appropriately in the workplace.

9.1 Maintain confidentiality of privileged information on individuals, according to federal regulations (e.g., HIPAA).

9.3 Interact appropriately and professionally.

9.4 Demonstrate an understanding of the major points of the American Hospital Association's Patient's Bill of Rights and the Patient's Bill of Rights from the workplace.

9.5 Comply with the American Hospital Association's Patient's Bill of Rights and the Patient's Bill of Rights from the workplace. (Patient Care Partnership)

9.8 Define and use medicolegal terms and discuss policies and protocol designed to avoid medicolegal problems.

9.10 Demonstrate ability to use computer information systems necessary to accomplish job functions. (Patient Care Partnership)

Introduction

How orders for laboratory tests are generated, the skills for professional communication with the patient, and the identification of both the patient and specimen are included in this chapter. Insights into the effect certain patient situations have on laboratory test results and how specimen collection is documented and tracked in the electronic health record are also included.

6.1 Laboratory Requisitions

The phlebotomy procedure begins when a physician or other qualified healthcare practitioner orders blood tests to be performed. The order may be entered on an inpatient's chart, **electronic medical record (EMR),** or **electronic health record (EHR),** which may interact with facility-wide computer systems (see Figure 6-1). Many inpatient facilities require that the healthcare practitioner enter laboratory test requests directly into the hospital information system (HIS) or laboratory information system (LIS). In most facilities, this is called computerized physician order entry, or CPOE.

If the patient is an outpatient, the order for laboratory tests may be written as a prescription requested on an official **requisition** form (see Figure 6-2), telephoned to the laboratory by the physician or office staff, or faxed to the laboratory from the physician's office. In addition, some laboratories have provided physician offices with access to the LIS for the purpose of ordering tests and accessing results. In this case, the physician offices are called *clients.*

In many healthcare facilities, when a laboratory test is ordered it is entered into a computer at the patient care station (part of the HIS). The computer in the laboratory (part of the LIS) receives the order and provides an **accession number** (a number assigned sequentially in the order received). This accession number is usually a Julian date (the day of the year) followed by the test number. The LIS then prints the requisition, in the form of labels, for the phlebotomist to use. Figure 6-3 shows the Julian date as the fourth day of the year (004) in the year 2011 (11-). The Julian date is followed by the number 002085, which indicates that this test is the 2,085th test ordered on that day.

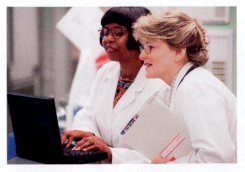

Figure 6-1 Patient information may be maintained in a hard copy file or entered into a computer system, or both.

Sample Laboratory Requisition

Patient Data (Please Print)

Last Name	First Name	Maiden Name

Address | Apt No.

City | State | Zip

SS# | Phone #

Date of Birth (Month, Day, Year) | ☐ Male ☐ Female | Date Collected | Time Collected | ☐ a.m. ☐ p.m.

Physician 1 | Physician 2

PLEASE PROVIDE MANDATORY ICD CODE BELOW

1 | 2 | 3 | 4 | 5

CALL TEST RESULTS TO: | **FAX RESULTS TO:**

Test: _____ | To: _____
To: _____ | Fax: ( ) _____
Phone: ( ) _____

☐ Veni   Tech Code _____   Tubes Received _____

Please (X) desired Panel(s) / Profile(s) / Tests. See back of requisition for profile components.

PANELS/PROFILES		INDIVIDUAL TESTS	
Hepatitis Panel, Acute	2S	ABO Group/RH	P
Basic Metabolic Panel	MT	Acid Phosphatase, Prostatic	S
Comp Metabolic Panel	MT	Albumin	MT
Electrolyte Panel (Lytes)	MT	Alkaline Phosphatase	MT
Hepatic Function Panel	MT	Amylase	MT
General Health Panel	MTL	Antinuclear Antibodies (ANA Send)	S
Lipid Panel	MT	HCG, Beta Quant	MT
Obstetric Panel AMH	P2SL	Bilirubin T / D Neonate	A
Renal Panel	MT	Bilirubin T / D Adult	MT
MICROBIOLOGY		BNP Screen	L
Source of Specimen:		BUN	MT
Culture, Anaerobe		CA-125	S
Chlamydia/GC Amp Probe		CA-125 to Dianon	S
Culture, Ear		CRP	MT
Culture, Eye		CRP Cardio	MT
Leukocytes Stool		Calcium	MT
Culture, Fungal		Carbamazepine/Tegretol	R
Culture, Genital		CBC & PLT w/o Diff	L
Culture, Herpes		CBC & PLT w Diff	L
Occult Blood Screen		Carcino Embryonic Antigen (CEA)	S
Ova & Parasites		Cholesterol Total	MT
Rapid Strep Throat		Cortisol Level	MT
Culture, Stool		Creatine Kinase, Total (CK)	MT
Culture, GROUP A BetaStrep Screen		CPK total w CKMB	MT
Culture GROUP B Screen		Creatinine Clearance	U
Culture, Throat		Creatinine	MT
Culture, Urine		D Dimer Quant	B
Culture, Wound / Abscess		DNA AB Double Strand	S
Culture, Viral		Digoxin Level	R
C. Difficile Toxin A&B AMH			

Please Indicate Bill Type Below
Attach Copy of Insurance Card

Billing Information (Please Print Clearly)

Please Bill to: ☐ Dr. Account (Client)   ☐ Patient Self Pay   ☐ Insurance Co

Responsible Party (Last, First)   Relationship to Subscriber   ☐ Self ☐ Child ☐ Spouse ☐ Other

Primary Insurance Co. Name   HMO ☐   PPO ☐

Insurance Policy #   Insurance Group #

Primary Insurance Co. Address (Street, City, State, Zip)

Insured Date of Birth   Insured SS#

INDIVIDUAL TESTS (cont.)

Drug Screen Urine	U	SGPT (ALT)	MT
Drug Screen Urine c Confirm	U	Testosterone	S
Estradiol Level	MT	Testosterone Free & Total	S
Ferritin Level	MT	TSH	MT
Fetal Fibronectin (FFN)	SWAB	Total T3	MT
Folic Acid (PROTECT)	MT	T3 Uptake	S
Follicle Stimulating Hormone	MT	Free T3	MT
GGT (Gamma Glut Trans)	MT	Free Thyroxine (FT4)	MT
Glucose	MT	Total T4	S
Glucose Fasting	MT	Free Thyroxine Index (FTI)	S
Glucose Challenge 1° Preg	MT	Thyroid Antibodies	S
Glycosylated Hemoglobin (HA1C)	L	Troponin / Quant	MT
Hepatitis B Surface AG	S	Triglycerides	MT
Hepatitis B Surface AB	S	Uric Acid	MT
Hepatitis C Antibody	S	Urinalysis	U
Herpes Simplex I & 2 IgG AB	S	Valproic Acid / Depakote	R
Herpes Simplex I & 2 IgM AB	S	Vitamin B12 (PROTECT)	MT
HIV I&II Abs	S	Vitamin D 25 Hydroxy	S
Homocysteine	L		
Iron/TIBC	MT	**ADDITIONAL ORDERS**	
Lactate Dehydrogenase (LDH)	MT		
Lipase	MT		
Lithium	R		
Luteinizing Hormone	MT		
Microalbumin Random/24 Hr.	U		
Magnesium	MT		
MONO test heterophile	S		
Phenobarbital	R		
Phenytoin/Dilantin	R		
Phosphorous	MT		
Potassium	MT		
Progesterone	S		
Prolactin	MT		
PSA Free and Total	S		
PSA Screen (Medicare)	S		
PSA Diagnostic	S		
Prothrombin Time	B		
aPTT	B		
PTH Intact	S		
Reticulocyte Count	L		
Rheumatoid Factor (RF)	MT		
RPR QUAL	S		
Rubella, IgG	S		
ESR (Sed Rate)	L		
SGOT (AST)	MT		

Figure 6-2 Physician's office staff may use a laboratory requisition form to order tests for their patients. All required patient and specimen information must be included as well as billing information.

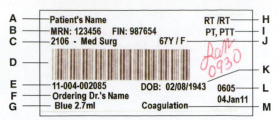

A	Patient's Name	RT /RT
B	MRN: 123456 FIN: 987654	PT, PTT
C	2106 - Med Surg 67Y / F	
D		
E	11-004-002085 DOB: 02/08/1943 0605	
F	Ordering Dr.'s Name	
G	Blue 2.7ml Coagulation 04Jan11	

Figure 6-3 A laboratory test requisition may take the form of a computer-generated label and must contain the following: (A) patient's name, (B) patient's medical record number, (C) patient's location, (D) bar code, (E) laboratory accession number, (F) requesting physician, (G) blood volume and tube type, (H) test status, (i) test to be performed, (J) patient's age and gender, (K) patient's date of birth, (l) date and time the test is to be performed, and (m) laboratory section to which the specimen should be delivered.

Some laboratories require separate requisitions for each department. These requisitions may be color-coded or numbered to identify the laboratory to which the specimen will be transported for analysis. The phlebotomist must be able to read and interpret requisition labels quickly and accurately.

Physician orders for laboratory tests will indicate the type of specimen and the time or priority of collection. Some specimens are ordered as **STAT (ST),** which means they must be collected and transported immediately. Specimens may also be referred to as **ASAP** (as soon as possible) or routine (RT), with collection times determined by the facility. Some laboratory tests require specific times for collection; these are referred to as timed tests, which will be discussed later in this chapter.

The phlebotomist is responsible for examining all requisitions carefully before leaving the laboratory to collect the specimen or before drawing blood from a patient. All requisitions must contain certain basic information to ensure that the specimen drawn and the reported test results are for the correct patient. Every requisition should contain the following information:

- Patient's name
- Patient's date of birth
- Patient's medical record number
- Patient's location (if inpatient)
- Ordering physician's name
- Type of test to be performed
- Test status (timed, fasting, STAT, ASAP)
- Date and time the test is to be performed

In special testing conditions, additional information should be included. Special testing conditions include fasting (no food or liquids except water) prior to the draw and situations in which blood must be drawn at an exact time. These requirements are also included on the requisition form.

Other information may also appear on computer-generated requisitions because they are often used as specimen labels (see Figure 6-3). Additional information may include the following:

- Computerized bar code
- Laboratory accession number
- Type of anticoagulant tube required
- Volume required
- Laboratory section performing the test

The requirements for specimen labeling are discussed later in this chapter.

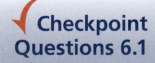

Checkpoint Questions 6.1

1. What information must requisitions for laboratory tests include?
2. Define the following: EHR, CPOE, and LIS.

6.2 Professional Communication

The phlebotomist must have a certain level of confidence before meeting a patient. Just knowing how to perform the proper technique may not be sufficient. The patient may be anxious, may be combative, or have veins that are difficult to access. In such instances, self-confidence combined with experience in dealing with all kinds of patients provides the mind-set required to successfully obtain the specimen on even the most difficult draws.

Greeting the Patient

The phlebotomist sets the tone for the venipuncture procedure when greeting the patient. Always smile and address the patient in a calm, pleasant tone of voice to gain the patient's confidence and trust. Behave as a professional. Show courtesy and respect for the patient. This is called **bedside manner** or **rapport.** Be aware of cultural differences that might make communication awkward, such as the consideration that direct eye contact may be disrespectful for individuals of certain cultures or backgrounds. Cultural diversity and professionalism are discussed further in the chapter *Practicing Professional Behavior.*

A confident manner will put the patient at ease and will help divert the patient's attention from the phlebotomy procedure. When greeting a patient, you should always identify yourself. In most cases, it is appropriate to state your first name only. A patient may become upset about treatment or become affectionate toward you and attempt to contact you outside the facility. For these reasons, many facilities recommend that phlebotomists simply identify themselves as from the lab. Check the policy of the facility where you are employed. In any case, after identifying yourself, be certain to state why you are there and what you will be doing. Remember, phlebotomists represent the laboratory profession.

Greeting the patient properly is important for both inpatients and outpatients. Outpatient situations occur in hospitals and clinics, patients' homes, long-term healthcare facilities, and physician offices, among others. In an outpatient situation, the first few seconds are even more critical than with an inpatient. If a patient is in a hospital, it is not a surprise for a phlebotomist to arrive to collect a specimen. When a patient is not in a traditional hospital or clinic setting, a person arriving to collect a blood sample may not be expected. Your arrival may cause the patient to become anxious, so conducting yourself in a professional manner is essential in an outpatient setting.

Inpatients present different circumstances (see Figure 6-4). The

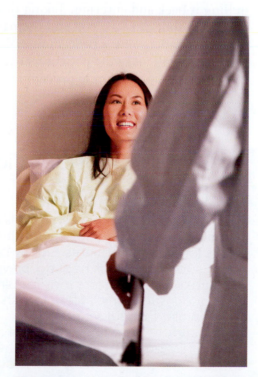

Figure 6-4 Greeting the patient in a professional manner instills confidence in the patient concerning phlebotomy skills.

Special Considerations for Children

In the healthcare field, discretion and common sense must be used at all times, but especially when dealing with children. The phlebotomy procedure usually frightens children. Never lie to patients (children or adults) by telling them, "This will not hurt." Even the most smoothly performed phlebotomy procedure will cause momentary discomfort. For children, it is best to keep them talking to distract them and then quickly proceed with the procedure. Usually, a parent is present and can assist with the phlebotomy procedure and reassure the child. For most purposes, the consent of a parent is enough informed consent to proceed with the procedure.

Because an adult usually accompanies the child in an outpatient setting, phlebotomists may approach identifying the child as they would an adult. If the child is too young or unable to respond to questions, ask the adult to verify the child's identity.

doors to most patients' rooms are usually open. Whether a patient's door is closed or open, knock and wait for a response before entering. Some patients cannot respond, especially if they are asleep, have been sedated, or have a medical appliance covering or inserted into their mouth. After waiting for a few seconds, open the door slowly and greet the patient before proceeding into the room. Even if the door is slightly ajar or open, it is still a good idea to knock lightly to make the patient aware that you are about to enter.

Sometimes the curtain is pulled around the patient's bed. Treat this situation in a similar manner. Talk to the patient through the curtain before pulling it back and entering. Taking this small extra step before entering the patient's room can save you and the patient embarrassment in the event the patient is undergoing a procedure or is using a bedpan or urinal. Following these steps will make the patient feel respected and will help create a positive setting for the phlebotomy procedure.

Special Considerations for Geriatric Patients

Just as there are certain details to keep in mind when dealing with children in the phlebotomy setting, there are also special considerations for geriatric patients. Elderly patients may exhibit sensory impairment, such as loss of hearing or vision, that requires further patient preparation. Hearing loss may require the phlebotomist to repeat questions and instructions. Phlebotomists may also encounter patients who are confused about where they are or why they are in the hospital. In an outpatient setting, a patient's loss of eyesight may require you to carefully guide the patient to the phlebotomy chair. Being patient and compassionate will make it easier to communicate with elderly patients.

Wake the Patient Gently

At any time of the day, but especially during early morning blood collections, the patient may be asleep. Gently wake the patient without startling him or her and explain why you are there (see Figure 6-5). Nudge the bed, instead of touching the patient. Talk in a soft manner and avoid turning on bright lights. Give the patient the opportunity to shield his or her eyes before turning on a light. Never attempt to collect a specimen from a sleeping patient. The patient may wake suddenly and jerk the arm. This could potently harm the patient or injure you.

Responding to Patient Questions

Patients usually want to know the purpose of the blood tests requested by the healthcare provider and how much blood will be drawn. The best response is to state that the tests are routine tests ordered by the physician. If the patient needs more information about the tests, suggest that she speak with the physician directly.

The phlebotomist should not discuss the tests with the patient. For example, if the phlebotomist were to tell a pregnant woman that a test for syphilis (a sexually transmitted disease) was to be drawn, and this was the first she had heard of it, imagine the anxiety and panic this woman might feel, not to mention the doubt created toward her husband or significant other. It is the physician's responsibility, not the phlebotomist's, to discuss this information with the patient. In such cases, the phlebotomist might respond by saying, "You will need to ask your physician about these tests or results. I am not allowed to discuss them with you."

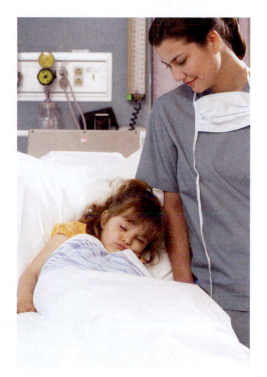

Figure 6-5 Gently waken sleeping patients of any age before beginning procedures.

Patient Interaction

Patients often do not feel well. They may be angry or scared about their medical condition, and, as a result, they may attempt to take out their frustration or anger on the phlebotomist. Regardless of what the patient says or how the patient acts, the phlebotomist must remain polite and professional. Whatever happens or whatever is said to you, do not take it personally. Being polite and as kind as possible is the easiest way to improve an unpleasant situation. However, phlebotomists should be aware of situations that are unsafe for them. For example, if a patient becomes hostile or attempts intimate physical contact, the phlebotomist should leave the room as quickly and calmly as possible.

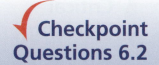

Checkpoint Questions 6.2

1. Why is it important to maintain a pleasant, professional attitude while working with patients?
2. Describe how you should let an inpatient know you are entering his or her room.

6.3 Healthcare Ethics and Law

As a phlebotomist, you need to know how law and ethics apply to your profession. This knowledge will help you

- function at the highest possible professional level
- provide competent, compassionate healthcare to patients
- avoid legal entanglements

Code of Ethics

Ethics is a moral philosophy that varies by individual, religion, social status, or heritage. A **code of ethics** is a set of written or unwritten rules, procedures, or guidelines that examine values, actions, and choices to help us determine right from wrong. Following a code of ethics is a key part of being a phlebotomist. Acting morally toward others requires putting yourself in their place. If you were a patient requiring blood tests to rule out a disease or other condition, how would you want to be treated?

Healthcare and the Law

A **law** is a rule of conduct or action prescribed or formally recognized as binding or enforced by a controlling authority. You may think of laws as rules necessary to keep society functioning. If a law is violated, a civil or criminal case may be brought to trial. In a lawsuit, there is a plaintiff (the person bringing the lawsuit) and a defendant (the person against whom the suit is brought). If the defendant is found liable and convicted, a fine, imprisonment, or revocation of (taking away) her license may be the penalty.

Respondeat superior is Latin for "Let the master answer." This doctrine states that an employer is responsible for the acts of his employees, if such acts are performed within the scope of the employees' duties.

Many lawsuits that are brought against phlebotomists involve civil law, which includes wrongful acts against a person. If a phlebotomist intentionally harms another, the plaintiff may seek remedy in a civil suit. These types of cases may involve:

- **assault**—the threat of bodily harm or "reasonable apprehension of bodily harm"
- **battery**—an action that causes bodily harm to another or bodily contact made without permission, such as drawing blood without the patient's consent

Negligence is usually the basis for professional malpractice claims. Negligence means that a professional neglects to perform in the manner expected by the profession. Four elements—known as the four *D*s—must all be present for a malpractice case:

- Duty—the professional owes a duty of care to the accuser. (The healthcare provider is expected to care for the patient. For example, a phlebotomist is expected to perform venipunctures.)

- Derelict—the professional breaches the duty of care to the patient. (The healthcare provider acts outside the standards expected of his profession. For example, if the phlebotomist repeatedly explores with the needle (probes) when drawing blood.)

- Direct cause—the breach of the duty of care to the patient is a direct cause of the patient's injury. (The care outside the standards of the profession causes the patient's injury. For example, repeated probing causes nerve damage to the patient.)

- Damages—there is a legally recognizable injury to the patient. (The injury is deemed severe enough for compensation. For example, nerve damage caused by repeated probing is severe enough to cause the patient not to be able to use her computer and her job requires 8 hours a day of computer use.)

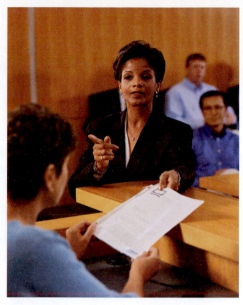

Figure 6-6 Malpractice cases are settled in a court of law.

In malpractice cases, the burden of proof is on the plaintiff (the patient, or the person who is making the case). (See Figure 6-6).

Phlebotomists can prevent malpractice cases by following these guidelines:

- *Caring*—as a phlebotomist, caring about your patients is your most important job.

- *Communication*—communicate clearly and you are more likely to earn your patient's trust.

- *Competence*—know your professional duties well, including your limitations, scope of practice, and standards of care. Participate in job-related continuing education. These parts of competence are discussed in detail in the chapter *Practicing Professional Behavior*.

Patient's Rights and Informed Consent

Patient's Rights

The issue of patient's rights is not new, and it has been clearly defined by the American Hospital Association in a document called the *Patient Care Partnership: Understanding Expectations, Rights and Responsibilities* (formerly the Patient's Bill of Rights). In addition to the right to refuse care, patients have the right to be treated with respect, to have all records and information classified as confidential, to be informed about the purpose and expected results of treatments, and to have access to their medical records.

Consent

Consent is an important legal aspect of phlebotomy. As a part of informed consent, it is the phlebotomist's responsibility to inform the patient of the pending procedure. The phlebotomist must explain to the patient in non-medical terms, using simple language, what he can expect to happen during the procedure. The phlebotomist must determine that the patient understands what is about to take place. Most people have had a blood test before, so the explanation "I'm here to draw your blood" should be sufficient.

If the patient does not understand English, the phlebotomist must use hand gestures, a demonstration of a venipuncture, or some other means to get the idea of the venipuncture procedure across to the patient. Most hospitals require a translator be present at the facility or at least a translator phone service be available. Family should not be used to translate except for extreme emergency situations because they may not correctly interpret the information to the patient, and this incorrect information may not be detected by the caregiver. Interpreting medical terminology often requires specialized study, as even someone who is fluent in a foreign language can struggle with topics as technical as medical language.

Patients generally sign a consent form for treatment during the initial admissions process before entering the hospital or before being treated by a physician in the physician office. Consents take a variety of forms, including written agreements, spoken words, implicit or unspoken/implied actions, and appointments for tests. It is important to provide quality patient education and to make sure the patient understands what is agreed upon.

Phlebotomists are also instrumental in collecting specimens for chain-of-custody, which is the documentation process for specimens of a legal nature, such as evidence. In these cases, it is essential to discuss express consent with the patient. Express consent means that the patient not only has to be informed of the procedure and its process but also must sign a consent form, agreeing to have the procedure done. Other procedures that may require written consent are drug and alcohol screens and HIV testing.

Consent must always be very clear. If a patient just puts out an arm but does not bother to stop watching TV or otherwise acknowledge the phlebotomist, this is considered implied consent. If the patient does not speak English but notices the tray and automatically extends an arm, that, too, is considered implied consent. If conflicting information is present, or if the patient doesn't understand English and seems confused about what you are there for, you *must* be very careful to verify the patient's true intent. Conflicting consent has resulted in several lawsuits.

Law & Ethics — Patient Discrimination

With few exceptions, phlebotomists are required to obtain blood specimens when ordered by the primary practitioner, regardless of the patient diagnosis. Patients with infectious diseases, such as tuberculosis, hepatitis, and AIDS, have the right to have their blood drawn just as other patients do. It is considered discrimination to refuse to draw blood from these patients and may result in disciplinary actions and/or legal liability. All patients, regardless of condition, should be treated with respect and dignity. Certain exceptions can occur, however, when a phlebotomist may not be required to draw a specimen, such as when a patient is receiving radiation treatment and the phlebotomist is pregnant or when an irate patient infected with hepatitis or AIDS might compromise the phlebotomist's safety.

Safety & Infection Control — Phlebotomist Safety

As a phlebotomist, it is important to protect yourself against harm from blood and body fluid exposure, as well as legal issues. If you feel as though there are policies and procedures that will place your safety in jeopardy, you must first alert your supervisor. If there is no resolution, take it to the next person in charge until your situation has been resolved. Phlebotomists may also purchase liability insurance through several insurance carriers that provide low-cost coverage to healthcare workers. Be sure to check with your employer to see if it carries liability coverage for employees. If so, there is no need to purchase liability insurance.

If a minor child or mentally incompetent patient is to have blood drawn, and the parent or guardian is not present, the written consent for treatment the parent signed on admission is considered adequate. There are three instances in which a patient *cannot* refuse to consent: the patient is a minor under the age of 18 and consent was obtained from the parent or guardian, the patient has a mental impairment (not able to understand), or the patient has been ordered by law to have her blood drawn.

Patient Refusal

Sometimes a patient refuses to have his or her blood drawn. When this happens, explain that the physician has ordered the test and the test results are needed to help diagnose or treat his or her medical condition. If a patient still refuses, do not attempt to draw blood; instead, politely leave the room. It is the patient's right to refuse the procedure (except in the situations listed in the previous section), and the phlebotomist should not badger or restrain the patient in order to perform the procedure. Inform the licensed practitioner (nurse or physician) of the patient's refusal and document a detailed account of the patient interaction. Be sure to document in writing—in a note on the laboratory requisition or in a comment field on the computer—that the patient refused the procedure. Make sure to include the name of the licensed practitioner whom you informed about this, along with the date, the time, and your initials. You should also inform the phlebotomy supervisor of the situation.

Patient Confidentiality

The **Health Insurance Portability and Accountability Act (HIPAA)** was established in response to information that was being transferred electronically for medical transactions. In 2003, a federal law was passed that establishes a national standard for electronic healthcare transactions and protects the privacy and **confidentiality** of patient information. Among other provisions, HIPAA states that information about a patient must not be discussed with individuals other than the patient unless the patient has given written or verbal permission for you to do so. A patient's information cannot be shared among healthcare professionals unless it is for the patient's treatment. The following is a list of other HIPAA guidelines that may apply to the care of patients during phlebotomy:

- Close patients' room doors when caring for them or discussing their health.
- Do not talk about patients in public places.
- Turn computer screens that contain patient information so that passersby cannot see the information.
- Log off computers when you are done.
- Do not walk away from patient medical records; close them when leaving.

Confidentiality

Law & Ethics

The phlebotomist may be privy to laboratory results. If you disclose results of any laboratory test to anyone other than a healthcare provider, or even access information that you do not need to know to perform your duties, you will have breached patient confidentiality and may be subject to disciplinary action, dismissal, legal action, or a monetary fine.

All information concerning the care of patients is strictly confidential and is not to be discussed. Inpatient settings may require the phlebotomist to travel throughout the facility to collect specimens, from the patient's bedside to other departments, such as the emergency room. Information obtained, no matter how seemingly insignificant, must remain confidential to protect both the patient and the facility. Fines have been set and imposed for any individual who violates the HIPAA standards.

Maintaining confidentiality sometimes involves communicating with the patient's visitors. On occasion, family members can calm the patient prior to procedures, but there are times when visitors interfere with the blood collection process. So if there are too many visitors or if the visitors appear to make the patient anxious, politely request that they leave the room for a few minutes. It is rare that visitors will resent such a request when asked politely.

✓ Checkpoint Questions 6.3

1. How would you obtain informed consent to draw blood from a 6-year-old child?
2. Describe some steps you could take to ensure you are following HIPAA guidelines.

6.4 Patient Identification

Prior to any patient procedure, proper identification of the patient is a crucial aspect and top priority of patient safety. The National Patient Safety Goals established by The Joint Commission recommends the use of at least two patient identifiers (not including the room number) before blood samples are obtained. As discussed in the chapter *The Phlebotomy and Healthcare*, The Joint Commission is the organization that sets standards for patient care in healthcare facilities.

To follow the National Patient Safety Goals and prevent an error, the phlebotomist must carefully identify every patient. Upon entering the patient area, the phlebotomist must check the patient identification. In acute care settings, patients have an armband or identification label bearing the patient's first and last names, the hospital number, the patient's date of birth, and the physician's name. Proper identification of the patient is a three-step process (see Figure 6-7).

If the three-step process is followed, correct patient identification can be established, thereby eliminating errors. The presence of doubt at any point during the three-step check calls for further investigation of the patient's

Competency Check 6-1

Patient Identification

1. Ask the patient to state his name and date of birth. Be sure that you do not call the patient by name prior to this because patients with altered mental states may simply repeat the name they hear.

2. Compare the name on the test requisition form/slip to the patient's response.

3. Confirm the patient's identity by checking the medical record number, patient armband, or some other form of identification, such as a driver's license. (See Figure 6-8.)

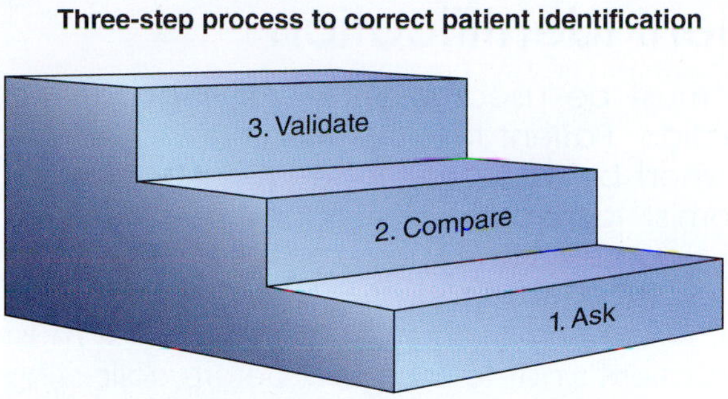

Three-step process to correct patient identification

3. Validate

2. Compare

1. Ask

Figure 6-7 Follow a three-step process for correct patient identification.

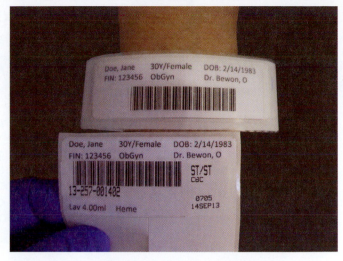

Doe, Jane   30Y/Female   DOB: 2/14/1983
FIN: 123456   ObGyn   Dr. Bewon, O

Doe, Jane   30Y/Female   DOB: 2/14/1983
FIN: 123456   ObGyn   Dr. Bewon, O

ST/ST
CBC

13-257-001402

0705
14SEP13

Lav 4.00ml   Heme

Figure 6-8 Confirm patient identification by comparing phlebotomy requisition label with inpatient armband.

identity. If the patient is unable to state his name, find another person, such as the nurse or a family member (depending on the setting), to state the name for you.

In a hospital setting, all patients must wear an identification bracelet. Most hospital policies require that a patient wear an identification bracelet in order for any procedure to be done, including phlebotomy. All laboratory specimens require a licensed healthcare provider's order; therefore, requisition labels will be available for the specimens you are to collect. Remember that all specimens require proper collection, handling, labeling, and transportation to the laboratory for testing.

Accurate patient identification and proper preparation are mandatory. It makes no difference how sophisticated or expensive the laboratory equipment is on which the specimen is tested. The results will be wrong if collected from the wrong patient. If this occurs, the effects on healthcare delivery can be disastrous. Say, for instance, that a blood specimen was collected for a cross-match because Mr. W. Buller is having surgery. Instead, the cross-match specimen is collected from a Mr. B. Buller. After Mr. W. Buller's surgery, he is given the unit of blood the doctor had requested. However, it was an incorrect cross-match, resulting in the wrong blood being administered. Mr. W. Buller can suffer serious consequences ranging from minor transfusion reactions to death as a result of this error. Because the result of identification errors can be serious or deadly, phlebotomists have been fired due to lack of proper patient identification.

Another potentially serious consequence of inaccurate patient identification occurs when specimens are needed for diagnostic testing or monitoring of treatments and medication levels. If the wrong patient's blood is drawn, the physician will receive the wrong results. The physician then adjusts the patient's treatment or medication according to incorrect information, and the patient can become ill or even die. Although these are extreme cases, such unfortunate patient identification errors have occurred and can still happen. So again, the most important step in a venipuncture procedure is proper patient identification.

Always ask the patient to state his name and date of birth. Never ask, "Are you Mr. (Name)?" A person who is on medication or is a heavy sleeper may answer yes to any question you ask. Allow the patient to answer fully, not just say yes or no. Ask for the information you have on the requisition form, such as the patient's date of birth. You can also ask an outpatient for his address, if it is supplied on the form. Remember, you must verify at least two patient identifiers before proceeding. You can also double-check the two identifiers you are using by matching information provided to you visually. For example, does the patient match the age and sex given on the requisition form?

Confirming Patient Identification

At least two identifiers must be used when identifying patients prior to specimen collection. Patient identification should not be performed hastily or cut short by using only one identifier. It is not uncommon for the phlebotomist to find a discrepancy or difference in the spelling of the patient's name on the lab requisition form when comparing it to the patient's wrist (identification) band or having the patient spell his or her name. When this occurs, the phlebotomist must find out which spelling of the patient's name is correct before collecting specimens. Make sure the correct spelling is on the requisition form, the ID band, and the specimen(s), once labeled. Most facilities have procedures in place for documenting discrepancies and taking corrective action. Be sure to follow policies and procedures at your facility.

Identification of Inpatients

As mentioned above, you must check the identification (ID) band on an inpatient's arm. This includes identification of patients in the emergency room. If the patient does not yet have an identification band, you should wait until the patient is properly banded before proceeding with blood collection unless instructed otherwise by your supervisor. Does the identification number on the armband match the one on the requisition form? Does the information on the ID band exactly match the information on the requisition? You must use at least two identifiers, such as name, birth date, and/or medical record number. Both identifiers must match the requisition. *Even if there is only one number or letter difference, you cannot proceed with the venipuncture.*

Never rely on the information on any item, such as a card, that is taped to the door, wall, or end of the bed. Patients are often transferred from room to room or out of the hospital without this information being changed. Only the information on the patient's ID band, while on the patient's wrist, should be compared. Even wristbands may be exchanged or switched. It is best to check the wristband *and* to ask the patient questions. If there is a discrepancy or contradiction, ask for assistance from the patient's nurse.

Some facilities use a bar code system of identification. The bar codes on both the requisition and the patient ID band are scanned and must match before you can proceed (see Figure 6-9). However, you must still verify the name and date of birth verbally if the patient is able to respond. Any discrepancies in patient identification must be resolved before you can proceed with specimen collection.

In some circumstances, the ID band is not on the patient's wrist. If this is the case, check if the ID band is on the patient's ankle instead. An ID band may be placed on the ankle because of burns, amputation, or **edema** (swelling) of the arm. If the patient does not have an ID bracelet, the nurse responsible for the patient must properly band the patient BEFORE any sample is collected.

If the patient is unable to speak because he is sedated, in a coma, or on a ventilator, the patient's nurse will need to come to the room to give verbal verification of the patient's identity. The phlebotomist should compare verbal information with the patient's armband and the requisition.

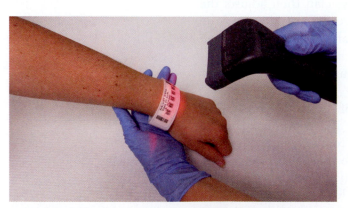

Figure 6-9 Check the identification bracelet of an inpatient. In some cases, scanners are used for proper identification.

Sometimes you will be expected to collect a specimen from an unconscious or nonresponsive patient. You must still identify yourself and inform the patient of the procedure you are about to perform. Unconscious patients may still be able to hear what is being said to them; they just cannot respond. Also, an unconscious patient may be able to feel pain, so you should be prepared for the patient to move once you have inserted the needle. You may need to have someone assist you in holding the arm steady. In addition, the phlebotomist must apply pressure until the site has stopped bleeding after the venipuncture for these patients because the patient is not able to apply adequate pressure.

If the patient is not in the assigned room, proceed to the nurses' station to find out where the patient is and when the patient is expected back. This is especially important if the specimen to be collected is a STAT (immediate) or timed specimen. Make every attempt to locate the patient because sometimes the patient is only walking in the hallway or undergoing a procedure in another part of the hospital. If you cannot locate the patient or the patient has not returned within a reasonable length of time, inform the appropriate healthcare provider at the nurses' station that the specimen was not collected. On the request slip, document the time and the name of the person you spoke with at the nurses' station. Ask that the laboratory be informed when the patient returns and be sure to tell the laboratory supervisor that the patient specimen was not collected, in case the laboratory is called for results.

Identification of Outpatients

An outpatient normally does not have an armband or identification band. Outpatients arrive in the laboratory area with a physician order form or prescription form—or an electronic order is sent to your lab—listing the requested laboratory tests.

Patient Identification

Critical Thinking

In the event of two spellings for the same last name, such as *Stevenson* and *Stephenson,* the phlebotomist must determine the correct spelling before obtaining the blood specimen. Also check at least one other identifier, such as date of birth and/or medical record number. Consider what you would do if a requisition form indicated that the patient's name was John M. Smith but, when you checked the identification band, it showed "John N. Smyth."

Outpatients must be correctly identified BEFORE they are registered and tests are ordered. This is done by asking for some sort of identification card and requesting that the patient state his or her full name and date of birth. After the receptionist has verified the patient's identification, registered the patient, and entered the test request into the computer, the phlebotomist must verify the patient's identification. The patient must be asked to state his or her full name and date of birth. Before any specimen is collected, a three-way match must be made between the written or electronic order from the physician, the information on the labels, and the patient's statement of name and date of birth. If there is any doubt about the patient's identity, additional information that may help to establish correct identity includes the physician's name, the patient's ID number (if it appears on the laboratory requisition form), or the patient's home address or telephone number. This does not have to be a prolonged identification process; usually, two or three verification items are sufficient to ensure proper identification.

Life Span Considerations

Identification of Children

If the patient is an infant or child under 18 years of age, the parent or legal guardian with the child must state the child's full name and date of birth. In addition, the parent or legal guardian must provide valid photo identification with the physician's written order (if not already ordered electronically).

Patient Education & Communication

Special Considerations for Psychiatric Patients

The challenges presented by patients with a mental illness may test both your technical skills and your interpersonal skills. These patients may have a hard time remaining calm and still during the procedure. They can be combative, scared, or anxious due to fear of the unknown. Or they may simply not understand the procedure that is taking place because of their frame of mind or medication. Patients with a mental illness can have a difficult time grasping an idea or a concept, thus making your job as a phlebotomist more difficult. For example, patients may intentionally provide incorrect information. Evaluate the patient carefully for any signs that the process of blood collection might be difficult. If you have a concern, ask another phlebotomist or staff member to assist you when obtaining specimens from patients who have a mental illness.

✓ Checkpoint Questions 6.4

1. A phlebotomist enters a patient's hospital room and says, "Mr. Wilson, I am from the lab and I am here to draw some blood." What error did the phlebotomist make and what should she have said?
2. How should you ensure proper identification of a child under 18?

6.5 Specimen Identification

Proper specimen identification goes hand in hand with proper patient identification. Specimen identification must follow facility policies and procedures to ensure patient safety and quality patient care. Occasionally, unlabeled specimens are sent to the laboratory. There is no way of positively knowing whom the specimen is from, even if this information is included on paperwork that accompanies the specimen.

Unlabeled specimens are rejected according to laboratory policy and must be re-collected. This causes delays in testing and reporting of results. Mislabeled specimens are especially dangerous. Laboratory personnel may have no idea that a specimen is labeled with the wrong patient's information. Tragic consequences can result from mislabeling a patient specimen in the event that the results from that specimen are used to diagnose and/or treat the wrong patient.

Labeling the Specimen

All specimens must be labeled properly before leaving the patient's room or the blood collection area. Label all specimens immediately, using computer-generated labels or writing the necessary information directly on the tubes with a permanent marker (see Figure 6-10). In an effort to standardize labeling procedures and reduce labeling errors, the Clinical Laboratory Standards Institute (CLSI) developed standards for specimen labeling. Five elements must appear on each patient specimen label:

- Patient's name
- Patient's date of birth
- Unique patient identifier (medical record number or other number used by the facility)
- Specimen collection time and date (printed or recorded on the label after collection)
- Collector's identification (name, initials, or operator identification, recorded after collection)

In addition, the label may include other information required by the laboratory, such as the following:

- Patient location
- Ordering physician
- Computer accession number (unique number in a sequence)
- Specimen requirements (test ordered, tube type, special handling)
- Other comments or special instructions

Figure 6-10 Specimen labels include, at a minimum, the patient's name and date of birth, a unique identification number, the time and date of collection, and the initials or identification code of the person performing the specimen collection.

Make sure you write the time of collection on the computer-generated labels and initial them. Your initials or code number must be present, in case there is a question about the specimen, so that laboratory personnel will know whom to ask. The actual time of collection is critical for fasting specimens and the monitoring of therapeutic drug levels. Some bar code readers are equipped with a label printer that will print the time of draw on the label; they may be programmable to include phlebotomist information as well.

Always label the blood tubes AFTER drawing the blood. This is done for several reasons. A tube may have lost its vacuum, in which case the label is wasted because it is difficult to transfer most computer labels. You may not be able to obtain a sample and an unused tube then has the wrong phlebotomist's name on the label. This tube might accidentally be used to draw blood from another patient. At an inpatient facility, sometimes blood tests are canceled or the patient has been discharged by the time the phlebotomist reaches the floor. Having tubes pre-labeled creates a potential for mistakes and wasted supplies.

Another reason to avoid pre-labeling tubes is that you may be interrupted by a STAT request while away from the laboratory, drawing blood. This request requires that you respond immediately and postpone drawing another patient's blood until you have collected the STAT blood specimen. The only safe way to collect specimens is to label them at the time of collection, after obtaining the blood but before leaving the patient.

Mislabeled specimens can lead to serious patient complications. Imagine that a potassium level is drawn on a patient who has a very low level, yet the specimen

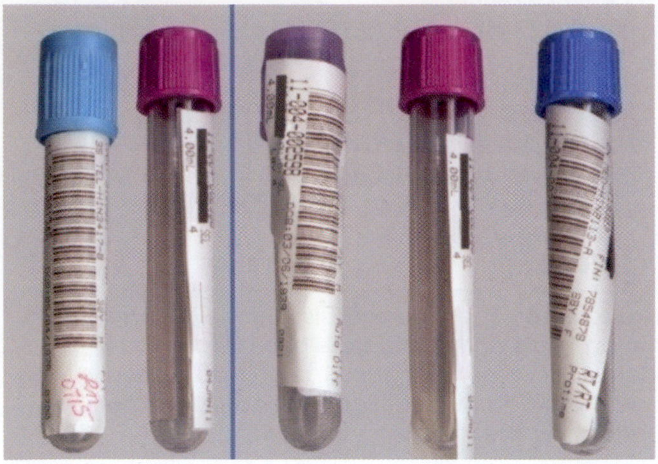

Correct | Incorrect

A   B   C   D

Figure 6-11 Specimen collection tubes: (A) properly labeled, (B) label over the cap, (C) label hanging off the bottom, (D) label not straight on the tube.

bears the label of another patient. The patient whose blood has been drawn may then receive unnecessary potassium supplements, whereas the other patient may not get the needed potassium replacement therapy. Both patients' medical care would be greatly compromised, and the mix-up may even result in death. Thus, proper labeling is a matter of life or death.

Labels must be placed on tubes as shown in Figure 6-11(A). Information on the left end of the label should be placed near the cap end of the tube. The label should be straight, smooth, and not overlapping the cap. The label should be placed so that the tube contents can easily be viewed. Improper label placement, as shown in Figure 6-11(B)–(D), may cause problems with performing laboratory tests. A label over the cap may cause problems with opening the tube or loss of information when the cap is removed; a label hanging over the bottom will cause tubes to get stuck in instrumentation, such as blood cell counters and chemistry analyzers, or loss of information may occur when this part of the label is cut off so as not to jam in the instrument. Crooked bar codes do not scan properly by instrumentation. Remember, improperly labeled tubes cause delays in testing and reporting of results.

Critical Thinking

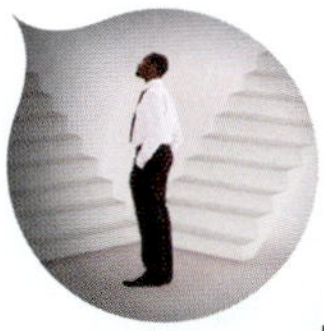

Specimen Identification

Imagine the following scenario involving specimen identification. Blood for a platelet count was collected from two patients occupying the same room. The platelet count on the patient who had entered the hospital to have his low platelet count monitored was now normal and he was sent home. The blood draw for the other patient was his first since being admitted, and his platelet count was critically low. This patient is scheduled for consult with a hematologist about possible bone marrow analysis procedures. Later in the week, the patient who was discharged returns because of a bleeding problem. Upon investigation, it was discovered that the platelet count samples for these two patients had been switched. How could this have occurred? How could this mistake have been avoided? What could have been the outcome for these patients? What may have happened to the phlebotomist because of this mistake?

Phlebotomists may also be confronted with issues involving team members. Serving as a member of a team is a challenge because all the "players" affect the outcome. The team concept implies working together to achieve common goals. The ultimate goal is to provide quality care to consumers accessing your healthcare facility. All blood specimen tubes must be properly labeled at the patient's bedside. If you find specimen tubes without a label, bring it to the attention of other team members. Do not label specimens that you did not collect. If you label a specimen as requested by a team member, you become accountable for the accuracy of that specimen. Unless you saw your team member obtain the specimen, you cannot be sure that the blood specimen belongs to that patient. Just imagine the potential implications of placing the wrong patient label on a specimen: a patient with a potentially abnormal test result may not receive needed treatment and a patient not needing that treatment may receive it. Both of these situations can compromise patient safety and lead to disciplinary actions, so never label specimens for which you should not assume responsibility.

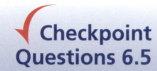

Checkpoint Questions 6.5

1. When should a specimen tube be labeled, and why?
2. What are the five elements that must appear on each patient specimen label?

6.6 Factors Affecting Specimen Quality and Test Results

Phlebotomists have an essential role in ensuring the quality of the specimens collected. Laboratory test results depend not only on proper specimen collection but also on patient status. Various factors affect laboratory results. The factors that occur prior to performing laboratory tests, such as patient identification and specimen labeling, are called pre-examination variables. Some pre-examination variables depend on the patient, whereas others are controllable by the phlebotomist.

Patient Factors

Healthcare professionals should have a basic understanding of patient factors that can affect laboratory results. The phlebotomist must also understand why patient preparation before collection and the timing of the collection can be critical to a patient's care and well-being. Phlebotomists often have little to no control over the effects of patient status on laboratory tests. Table 6-1 lists some patient variables that affect laboratory results. Pre-examination variables due to the order of draw, complications of specimen collection, and specimen processing, over which phlebotomists may have control, are discussed in more detail in the chapters *Blood Collection Equipment*, *Venipuncture*, *Capillary Puncture*, and *Blood Specimen Handling*.

Normal ranges, also called *reference ranges*, for some laboratory **analytes** (chemicals and other substances being measured) vary with patients' age and gender. All laboratories have established reference ranges for their patient population. These ranges are reported with patient test results. Examples of laboratory results that vary by age and/or gender are RBC count, hemoglobin, white blood cell differential, and nutrient levels.

Environmental Factors

Altitude

Normal, or reference, ranges for laboratory analytes are typically determined on populations living at sea level. Laboratories at higher elevations must determine normal ranges for their patient populations residing at these higher elevations (see Figure 6-12). Analytes that show a significant increase at higher elevations

TABLE 6-1 Some Patient Variables That Affect Laboratory Tests

Variable	Tests Affected
Nonfasting	Glucose Lipid profile • Total cholesterol • HDL • LDL • VLDL • Triglycerides
Stress	Adrenal hormones Fatty acids Lactate White blood cells
Posture	Albumin Bilirubin Calcium Enzymes Lipids Total protein Red blood cells White blood cells
Exercise	Aldolase Creatinine Fatty acids Lactate Sex hormones AST CK LD White blood cells
Diurnal variations	Cortisol Serum iron White blood cells
Alcohol	Lactate Triglycerides Uric acid GGT HDL
Tobacco	Catecholamines Cortisol Hemoglobin White blood cells

include RBC count and hemoglobin. This is because there is less oxygen at higher elevation, so the body needs more RBCs and hemoglobin to provide greater oxygen-carrying capacity. Certain enzymes involved in oxygen exchange are also increased at higher altitudes. For example, urates (by-product of protein degradation) may increase due to the increased turnover of red blood cells.

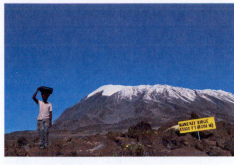

Figure 6-12 People living at high altitude may normally have blood results that are far different from people living at sea level.

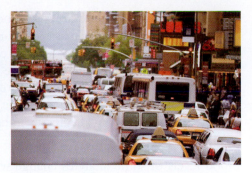

Figure 6-13 In areas of high automobile traffic, a patient may have higher levels of lead and carboxyhemoglobin in his or her blood.

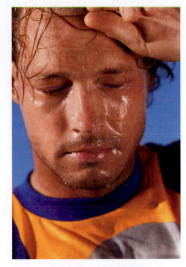

Figure 6-14 Exposure to extreme temperatures can cause a shift in fluid balance that may affect blood test results.

Geographic Location

The environment in which people live can affect the composition of their blood. For example, people residing in areas of high automobile traffic may have higher levels of lead and carboxyhemoglobin (carbon monoxide attaching to hemoglobin) in their blood (see Figure 6-13). Trace elements, such as lead and zinc, may be found at higher concentrations in those living near smelting plants, and people living in areas where the water is "hard" may have higher lipid and magnesium levels.

Changing Altitudes

People who visit areas of higher elevation for a length of time may show a transient, or temporary, rise in their red blood cells, hemoglobin, and related test results. If they are tested immediately after returning to lower elevations, their results may be interpreted as abnormal. Understanding the effects of such travels on laboratory values is important when discrepancies with patients' previous results arise.

Critical Thinking

Temperature

Changes in environmental temperature affect the distribution of water between the tissues and the blood. If more water enters the blood vessels, some analytes may decrease; conversely, as water leaves the blood vessels, some analytes may increase. Plasma protein levels can drop slightly during acute or severe exposure to heat. Electrolytes can be out of balance during profuse sweating (see Figure 6-14).

Hydration

Water is essential to maintaining a balance among the cells and chemicals in the bloodstream and tissue fluids (see Figure 6-15). Disruptions in this balance may lead to health problems, and they create difficulties in interpreting laboratory results. When patients are dehydrated (decreased plasma water), the effective concentration or percentage of many substances in the blood increases. This phenomenon is called **hemoconcentration.** Dehydration leading to hemoconcentration may occur due to persistent vomiting, diarrhea, diabetic acidosis, or inadequate fluid intake.

The opposite imbalance in hydration is **hemodilution.** Hemodilution is an increase in plasma water, which may result in decreased concentrations of substances in the blood. The physical levels (presence/amounts) are not actually affected in this case, but their concentration is diluted

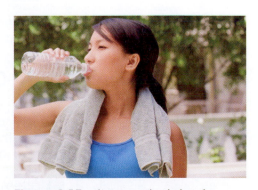

Figure 6-15 A person's state of hydration can affect blood test results by causing hemoconcentration or hemodilution.

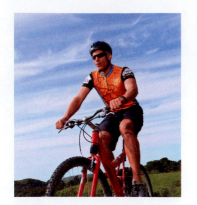

Figure 6-16 Strenuous exercise can cause imbalances in many cellular and chemical components of blood.

by the excess fluid. Hemodilution can occur in water intoxication, salt retention syndromes, and infusion of massive amounts of intravenous fluids. Imagine a cup half full of water that has a drop of food coloring added. Now imagine the change in the intensity of the color when more water is added to the cup, lowering the concentration of the dye. Similarly, more water in blood will result in lower concentrations of cells and chemicals in the blood. Blood cell counts and chemistry tests are most commonly affected by imbalances in hydration.

Posture, Exercise, and Stress

Blood levels of some analytes change when a patient's posture changes or as a result of changes in activity from **ambulatory** (walking about) to **sedentary** (no physical activity). The lack of activity causes the body's tissues to allow more water to enter the circulation, which increases the plasma volume. Some analytes, such as total calcium, may be diluted ("watered down") more than normal and appear decreased in bedridden patients. Strenuous exercise (see Figure 6-16) can cause an elevated white blood cell count, alterations in the coagulation system, and fluctuations in various enzyme and other chemical levels. Stress, such as anxiety, fear, or nervousness, can also affect laboratory tests in a way similar to exercise.

Timing of Specimen Collection

Many laboratory tests can be drawn at any time throughout the day because eating and exercise have little effect on the results. However, certain laboratory tests require special patient preparation and timing. The phlebotomist must understand why preparation of the patient before the collection and timing of the collection can be critical to a patient's care and well-being.

Patient Basal State   A patient who is at rest and has been **fasting** (nothing to eat or drink, except plain water) for at least 12 hours is said to be in **basal state.** A patient who arises in the morning and immediately exercises is not in a basal state, even if he is fasting, because the exercise alters the body's metabolic processes. Specimens collected during basal state, early in the morning, provide the most accurate assessment of some blood constituents (substances) like electrolytes, glucose, lipids, and proteins.

Diurnal Variation   **Diurnal variation,** also called diurnal rhythm, is the variation in an analyte at different times throughout the day. Certain hormones, such as testosterone, decrease during the afternoon, whereas others, such as thyroid-stimulating hormone, increase in the evening. The levels of some types of white blood cells may rise during the day. Some analytes may show a drop in blood levels and a rise in urine levels at the same time. Thus, specimens for hormones and other tests are often required to be drawn at the time of day corresponding to the diurnal variation of a particular analyte.

Timing for Drug Levels   Frequently, laboratory requisitions note the time a blood sample should be drawn. As mentioned previously, some specimens need

Life Span Considerations

Crying Infants

Similar to strenuous exercise, excessive crying by an infant can cause his leukocyte count to be elevated. It takes 60 minutes for the leukocyte count to return to normal. Thus, if an infant has just had a procedure (e.g., circumcision or vaccination) that has resulted in excessive crying (see Figure 6-17), you should wait 60 minutes before attempting blood collection. If you are asked to collect the specimen anyway, include a note on the requisition or in the comment section on computerized documentation that the infant was crying excessively.

to be collected when the patient is in basal state; others must be collected **postprandial** (after eating). Another reason for specimens to be drawn at a specified time is **therapeutic drug monitoring (TDM).** TDM is monitoring the amount of a therapeutic drug in the blood. The healthcare provider needs to know if the dose of a medication is at the appropriate level to ensure that it is effective. A drug peak level may be requested. A **peak level** is a specimen collected when the serum drug level is at its highest, shortly after a medication is given. The laboratory results for the peak level determine the amount of medicine the physician orders for the patient's next dose. For therapeutic drug monitoring, both peak and **trough levels** may need to be collected. Trough levels are collected when the drug level in the blood is at its lowest, usually immediately before the next scheduled dose. Figure 6-18 displays a graph that helps to determine when specimens for peak and trough levels should be collected.

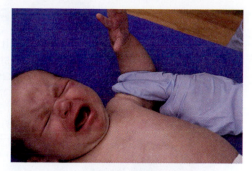

Figure 6-17 Infants who have been violently crying will have altered blood test results. It is best to return to collect the specimen after the child has been calm for at least one hour. If a specimen must be collected while the child is crying, note it on the requisition or enter this information into the laboratory information system.

Timing Not Followed

Critical Thinking

Phlebotomists should become familiar with the tests that are most likely to require specific collection times. These tests include measuring the level of antibiotics, such as gentamicin. Consider the consequences of blood for therapeutic drug monitoring (TDM) being collected several hours before or after the requested time. What is the phlebotomist's responsibility in TDM collections?

Dietary Restrictions

After properly identifying the patient and obtaining patient consent for the phlebotomy procedure, you must verify any special dietary restrictions or instructions. These restrictions include fasting and the avoidance of certain foods. Laboratory tests can be affected by what a patient eats or doesn't eat, or even by whether the patient has smoked within a designated time. To verify that a patient has followed the instructions given when the test was ordered, simply ask, "When was the last time you had anything to eat, drink, or smoke?" The most common dietary restriction that affects specimen collection is fasting. This restriction requires the specimen to be drawn after the patient has not ingested foods or liquids for a specified period of time. Routinely, the fast is for 12 hours. In some instances, the licensed practitioner may request a fast of 4, 8, 10, or 16 hours.

Some laboratory tests require special diet instructions. The patient may be instructed to eat or not eat certain foods for a specified number of days or hours before the specimen is taken. A common test request is for a 2-hour postprandial glucose test. This laboratory specimen must be drawn 2 hours after the patient has started eating a meal, usually breakfast. If a restriction or special diet is required and the patient has followed this requirement, make a notation on the requisition

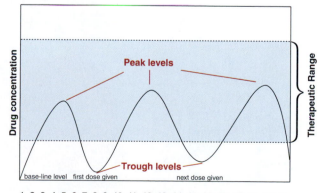

Figure 6-18 Blood for therapeutic drug monitoring is collected when concentrations are at their highest levels for the dose (peak) and lowest levels (trough), just before the next dose.

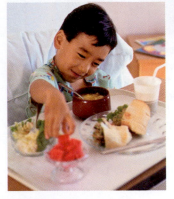

Fasting

It is important for the licensed practitioner, nurse, or laboratory staff to inform patients about fasting prior to blood collection. Fasting means having nothing to eat or drink (except for minimal amounts of water) for 8 to 12, or even 16, hours before blood is to be collected. However, drinking water is allowed and even encouraged, as abstaining from water can result in dehydration, which can cause inaccurate laboratory results. Written instructions with detailed explanations should be provided to all patients.

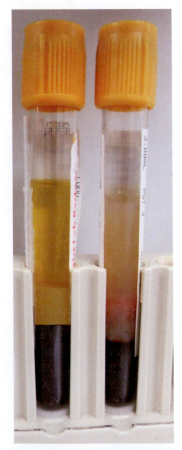

Figure 6-19 Ensure that the patient has not eaten if he is supposed to have a fasting specimen collected.

slip. Also note the last time the patient had anything to eat, drink, or smoke, and note if special dietary instructions were followed or not.

Sometimes patients forget or are not informed of the dietary restrictions necessary before blood is drawn (see Figure 6-19). Ensure that the patient has not eaten if he is supposed to have a fasting specimen collected. In these circumstances, you will need to ask the licensed practitioner if a nonfasting specimen will be adequate. In some instances, this will be allowed. The normal values of some laboratory tests, such as cell counts, are not markedly different if the patient was nonfasting before the specimen was drawn. However, for some tests—especially glucose and lipid profiles—the specimen has to be fasting. If the licensed practitioner approves collecting the nonfasting specimen, note "nonfasting" on both the tube and the laboratory requisition. Additionally, make a notation on the laboratory requisition of the name of the person who approved taking the specimen from a nonfasting patient. It is good practice to notify the laboratory section performing the test that the licensed practitioner approved the nonfasting sample. Some laboratories will not report results if proper patient procedures (such as fasting) were not followed unless approval is noted.

If blood is drawn shortly after a meal, the serum may appear cloudy, or **lipemic.** Lipemia is due to the large amount of fatty compounds in blood after a meal and it interferes with many laboratory tests. Severely lipemic specimens have an appearance similar to milk instead of the normal serum appearance of clear yellow fluid. See Figure 6-20.

Medications as Interfering Substances

Interfering substances are substances that can alter laboratory test results. Substances the phlebotomist has no control over include medications or other drugs the patient is taking (see Figure 6-21). Some medications contribute an abnormal color to blood and/or body fluids, which can interfere with test procedures. For example, some antibiotics (such as erythromycin) and vitamins (such as B_{12}) add orange and yellow coloring

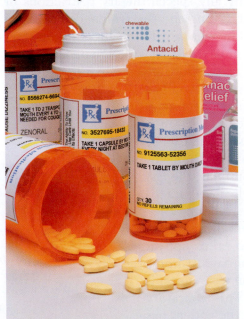

Figure 6-21 Some medications can have an effect on laboratory test results.

Figure 6-20 The lipemic serum sample on the right is very milky compared with the normal (clear) serum on the left.

(respectively) to blood and urine. These abnormal colors may interfere with tests that require the detection of a color change during testing. Medications can also have an effect on various body systems and may alter the level of chemicals, such as enzymes, that they produce. For example, statins (drugs used to lower cholesterol) may affect liver function and thereby cause an elevation in liver enzymes in the blood. Interfering substances that are under the control of the phlebotomist are those contained in collection tubes (additives) and are discussed in the chapter *Blood Collection Equipment*.

Specimen Transporting and Processing

Laboratory test results can be greatly affected by the way specimens are handled. Thus, the phlebotomist's role is crucial, as she is responsible for ensuring that specimens are handled properly. Specimens must be transported to the laboratory in a timely manner and under test-specific conditions.

Some laboratory tests, especially STAT tests, must be performed within 1 hour of collection. Other laboratory tests must be centrifuged, or separated, within a specified amount of time. The phlebotomist must be aware of the tests that require special handling and apply facility policies concerning the specimens for these tests. Special handling applies to specimens that are to be kept warm or cold, protected from light, centrifuged, or even separated. Specimen processing and transport is covered in further detail in the chapter *Blood Specimen Handling*.

1. Name at least five factors that can interfere with laboratory test results.
2. You enter the room of a crying infant to draw his or her blood. What should you do?

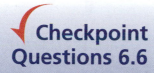

Checkpoint Questions 6.6

6.7 Documenting Specimen Collection

Electronic Health Records

Because research shows that health information technology helps save lives and lower healthcare costs, the Health Information Technology for Economic and Clinical Health Act (HITECH) was passed in 2010. This bill encourages the use of electronic health records (EHRs) and hopes to cause 90% of doctors and 70% of hospitals to use comprehensive EHRs by the end of the decade. The act helps establish standards for EHRs that will allow nationwide exchange of patient health information. Given this, phlebotomists must be knowledgeable and able to work with electronic health records as part of their day-to-day responsibilities.

An electronic health record is an electronically stored record of patient health information. This information is generated over one or multiple encounters and includes information about patient demographics, progress notes, problems, medications, vital signs, past medical history, immunizations, laboratory data, and radiology reports. The purpose of EHRs is to provide secure, real-time access to patient-centered information, thereby reducing delays in planning, treatment, reporting, quality management, and billing. In the hospital setting, laboratory information found in the EHR includes not only laboratory test results but also collection dates and times, as well as who collected the specimen, who received the specimen in the lab, and who performed or verified the laboratory test results. All comments that were entered during collection verification also appear in this record.

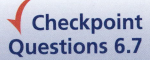

Critical Thinking

EHR versus EMR?

Although some people use the terms EHR (electronic health record) and EMR (electronic medical records) interchangeably, they are different. EMR came first and was only for medical records used by doctors for diagnosis and treatment. EHRs are health records that cover more information, encompassing the total health of the patient. EMRs and EHRs both track data over time; easily identify which patients are due for preventive screenings or checkups, such as blood pressure readings or vaccinations; and help monitor and improve the quality of care within the practice. The difference lies in the ability of EHR systems to travel from facility to facility and from one healthcare provider to another in a secure way. EHRs are used by laboratories and other specialists and allow all members of the healthcare team to access the latest patient information, providing for coordinated patient-centered care.

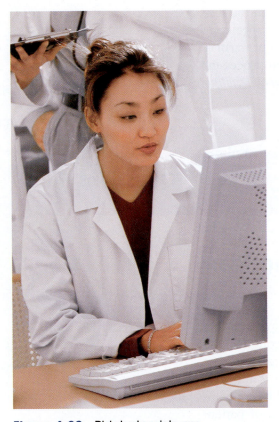

Figure 6-22 Phlebotomists are responsible for recording collection data and entering them into the laboratory information system.

Specimen Tracking

The phlebotomist's responsibility for documentation includes recording his identification on requisitions and specimen labels and entering collection information and comments into the laboratory log book or into the patient's EHR using the laboratory information system (LIS). See Figure 6-22. Bar code systems with an LIS interface can be used to download time of draw and phlebotomist information from the bar code reader. The entry of these data allows for specimen tracking. Having collection information is helpful when specimen quality concerns arise or when the laboratory staff receives inquiries as to the status of laboratory test collections and anticipated completion times.

In many hospitals, the LIS communicates with the hospital information system (HIS), providing nursing and other staff direct access to this information in the patient's EHR. The LIS may also connect to laboratory analyzers, which expedites the entry of test data and reduces transcription errors. Laboratories may choose to provide remote locations, such as physician offices, with access to the LIS. The interconnectedness of computer systems often means that all patient data, orders, results, and charges may be viewed by anyone connected to the system.

In order to help safeguard the patient's privacy and personal information, phlebotomists must be aware of their responsibility to appropriately access only the information needed to perform their specific job-related duties.

✓ Checkpoint Questions 6.7

1. Briefly describe the phlebotomist's responsibilities regarding documentation of laboratory specimens.
2. Why are electronic health records useful?

Chapter Summary

Learning Outcome	Key Concepts/Examples	Related NAACLS Competency
6.1 Identify the parts and functions of a laboratory requisition. Pages 138–140.	Laboratory requisitions must include doctor's name; patient's name, age, date of birth, and identification number; tests to be performed; and date and time for specimen collection.	7.00, 7.1
6.2 Identify the professional communication techniques of the phlebotomist. Pages 141–144.	Communicating with patients in a professional manner helps instill patient confidence in the phlebotomist.	9.00, 9.3
6.3 Comply with ethical and legal standards for professional communication. Pages 144–148.	Following a code of ethics during patient interactions helps prevent accusations of malpractice. Patients must give consent to and have the right to refuse any procedures.	9.4, 9.5, 9.8
6.4 Carry out proper patient identification. Pages 148–152.	Patients must be identified using a minimum of two unique patient identifiers.	4.1
6.5 Define the legal/ethical importance of specimen identification. Pages 152–155.	Specimen labels must include the patient's name, date of birth, and unique patient identifier (medical record number); the actual specimen collection time and date; and the collector's identification. Improperly labeled specimens can cause errors in treatment, which in turn can result in malpractice.	4.1
6.6 Recognize patient factors that may affect specimen quality and test results. Pages 155–161.	Phlebotomists must document patient situations that can compromise the quality of the specimen. Patient factors that may affect laboratory results include deviation from basal state, age and gender, dietary restrictions, hydration, activity, and health status. Proper specimen handling includes appropriate collection and transport for each type of specimen collected and timely delivery to laboratory sections.	4.00, 4.2, 4.3, 4.4, 4.5
6.7 Explain the phlebotomist's role in maintaining accurate and secure blood collection documentation. Pages 161–162.	Proper documentation ensures that tests are performed on the correct patient's specimen and allows for test status tracking; it often requires the use of hospital and/or laboratory computer systems. Patient information is stored in hospital and laboratory computers as part of the patient's electronic health record (EHR). Phlebotomists have access to patient information and must maintain utmost confidentiality.	9.10

Chapter Review

A: Labeling

Identify each item on this test requisition label.

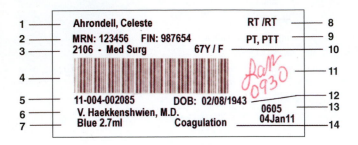

1. [LO 6.1] _____

2. [LO 6.1] _____

3. [LO 6.1] _____

4. [LO 6.1] _____

5. [LO 6.1] _____

6. [LO 6.1] _____

7. [LO 6.1] _____

8. [LO 6.1] _____

9. [LO 6.1] _____

10. [LO 6.1] _____

11. [LO 6.1] _____

12. [LO 6.1] _____

13. [LO 6.1] _____

B: Matching

Match the terms and abbreviations on the left with their meanings.

___14. [LO 6.1] accession number

___15. [LO 6.6] analyte

___16. [LO 6.6] basal state

___17. [LO 6.6] diurnal variation

___18. [LO 6.6] fasting

___19. [LO 6.6] HIS

___20. [LO 6.6] lipemic

___21. [LO 6.6] LIS

___22. [LO 6.6] peak

___23. [LO 6.6] postprandial

___24. [LO 6.6] trough

a. highest blood concentration of a drug level

b. after a meal

c. increased fats in the blood

d. lowest blood concentration of a drug level

e. nothing to eat or drink except water for a specified amount of time

f. 12-hour period without intake of food and exercise

g. normal daily changes in lab values

h. substance undergoing analysis

i. reflects the sequence in which the laboratory receives an order

j. facility-wide computer system

k. computer system for the laboratory

C: Fill in the Blanks

Write in the word(s) to complete the statement or answer the question.

25. [LO 6.2] Displaying a professional manner that includes behavior, appearance, courtesy, and respect toward patients is called _____.

26. [LO 6.3] A rule of conduct or an action prescribed or formally recognized as binding or enforced by a controlling authority is a(n) _____.

27. [LO 6.3] A(n) _____ is a set of written rules, procedures, or guidelines that examines values, actions, and choices to help determine right from wrong.

28. [LO 6.3] _____ results in patient injury caused by a breach in the duty of care to the patient.

29. [LO 6.1] A test for which a specimen must be collected immediately is a(n) _____ test.

30. [LO 6.6] When a chemical in the blood is normally higher at one time of the day and lower at another, it is showing a(n) _____.

D: Sequencing

Place the following in the correct order of performance. Write the correct number to the left of each statement.

31. [LO 6.4] _____ Collect blood specimens.

32. [LO 6.4] _____ Deliver specimens to the laboratory.

33. [LO 6.4] _____ Examine the requisitions.

34. [LO 6.4] _____ Label specimen collection tubes.

35. [LO 6.4] _____ Proceed to next patient if not a STAT order.

36. [LO 6.4] _____ Verify patient identification.

E: Case Studies/Critical Thinking

37. [LO 6.6] You are sent to the newborn nursery to collect blood from a newborn. When you arrive, the infant is just being brought back from a circumcision and has been crying. What should you do?

38. [LO 6.3] Your patient, Mr. Tykodi, is not in his hospital room and you happen to see him in the family waiting area with his grandson. In the waiting area are several other patients with their families, several with young children. You approach Mr. Tykodi and tell him you are here to draw his blood. He says, "Why not do it here in the sunshine?" What are your concerns about this situation? What would you do?

39. [LO 6.2] You are on the pediatric floor, and Jennifer Burnham, a 5-year-old girl, needs to have her blood drawn for a blood test. You enter her room and notice she is alone. You inform Jennifer you are there to take a blood test. She starts to cry and says, "Please, no more needles!" What would you do?

40. [LO 6.4] You are on your morning rounds on the fifth floor of the hospital. John Stallings in room 250 is scheduled to have blood drawn. When you enter the patient's room, he identifies himself as James Stallings, but the armband says John Stallings. What is your next step?

41. [LO 6.5] You are going back to the laboratory to drop off your first set of specimens. As you begin to log the samples into the computer system, you find that you are missing a label on one of the specimens. What do you do?

F: Exam Prep

Choose the best answer for each question.

42. [LO 6.1] Which of the following does not necessarily need to be on a laboratory requisition?

   a. Laboratory accession number
   b. Ordering physician information
   c. Patient's name and date of birth
   d. Type of test to be performed

43. [LO 6.1] Which of the following pieces of information found on a specimen label is NOT optional?

   a. Computerized bar code
   b. Laboratory accession number
   c. Volume and type of anticoagulant tube required
   d. Time the specimen was collected

44. [LO 6.5] Specimen tubes should be labeled in this order:

   a. after obtaining the requisition, before leaving the laboratory.
   b. after entering the patient's room, before collecting the specimen.
   c. after collecting the specimen, before leaving the patient's room.
   d. after performing all collections, on arriving back in the laboratory.

45. [LO 6.2] Which of the following behaviors will NOT help calm an anxious patient?

   a. Talking quickly and being direct
   b. Showing respect and concern
   c. Using a pleasant tone of voice
   d. Dressing and acting professionally

46. [LO 6.3] Appropriate behavior for maintaining your own privacy includes

   a. not identifying yourself; patients know what you want.
   b. providing business cards with your contact information.
   c. not displaying your name badge when entering patient rooms.
   d. stating only your first name when introducing yourself.

47. [LO 6.2] What is the most appropriate way to enter an inpatient room?

   a. Walk in and ask if the patient is here, using her first and/or last name.
   b. Walk in, introduce yourself, and proceed to check the patient's wristband.
   c. Knock, walk in, introduce yourself, and ask for the patient by name.
   d. Knock while asking permission to enter, introduce yourself, and ask the patient her name.

48. [LO 6.5] Which of the following specimens will NOT be accepted by the laboratory and must be re-collected? *(Choose all that apply.)*

   a. A specimen without a label that the person who collected it can identify

   b. A specimen with its label upside down

   c. A specimen with a computer label for "John Smith" affixed over handwriting on the tube that reads "Jonathan Smith"

   d. A specimen that has a handwritten label for "Mary Jones" but is not yet labeled with the computer label for "Mary Jones"

49. [LO 6.4] How should a patient be identified who cannot speak for himself? *(Choose all that apply.)*

   a. Check the name on the door.

   b. Check the name on the wristband.

   c. Check the name above the bed.

   d. Check the name with the unit nurse.

50. [LO 6.3] How should you respond when patients ask about their lab tests?

   a. Tell them that they don't need to know anything at this time.

   b. Inform them that you are not allowed to tell them anything.

   c. Tell them what it says on the requisition, but no more.

   d. Ask them to ask their doctor to explain the tests to them.

51. [LO 6.3] Why should you NOT collect blood from a sleeping patient? *(Choose all that apply.)*

   a. She might get startled.

   b. She might not consent to the procedure.

   c. She might jerk her arm unexpectedly.

   d. She cannot help during the procedure.

52. [LO 6.3] If you collect a blood specimen on a patient who has not given consent, he might bring a civil lawsuit for

   a. assault.

   b. battery.

   c. direct injury.

   d. negligence.

53. [LO 6.3] If a patient feels threatened by the phlebotomist, she may bring suit under civil law for

   a. assault.

   b. battery.

   c. direct injury.

   d. negligence.

54. [LO 6.3] Which of the following is NOT acceptable for patient consent concerns?

   a. Patients give consent by simply being admitted to the hospital.

   b. The phlebotomist explains the procedure and asks permission to proceed.

   c. An interpreter explains the procedure to non-English-speaking patients.

   d. Parents give consent for procedures on their child.

55. [LO 6.6] How much time without food or drink is considered fasting?

   a. 4 to 6 hours

   b. 2 to 4 hours

   c. 6 to 7 hours

   d. 8 to 12 hours

56. [LO 6.5] Which of the following actions by the patient will least likely affect fasting-level test results?

   a. Chewing sugarless gum

   b. Drinking tea or coffee without sugar

   c. Smoking cigarettes

   d. Drinking water

57. [LO 6.6] The serum of a specimen appears slightly cloudy after centrifugation. This is a clue that

   a. the patient is in a basal state.

   b. the patient is smoking cigarettes.

   c. the patient was not fasting.

   d. the centrifuge is malfunctioning.

58. [LO 6.6] Which of the following tests most often needs a fasting specimen?

   a. Complete blood count

   b. Triglycerides and other lipids

   c. Therapeutic drug monitoring

   d. Vitamin levels

59. [LO 6.6] A postprandial specimen collection should occur

    a. after a blood transfusion.

    b. before the next dose of medication.

    c. early in the morning.

    d. at a specific time after eating.

60. [LO 6.6] What specimens are most likely to be collected only early in the morning? *(Choose all that apply.)*

    a. Basal state

    b. Diurnal analytes

    c. Fasting

    d. Postprandial

61. [LO 6.6] What specimens are most likely to be collected for therapeutic drug monitoring? *(Choose all that apply.)*

    a. Fasting

    b. Peak

    c. Postprandial

    d. Trough

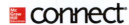

Enhance your learning by completing these exercises and more at connect.mheducation.com

References

American Hospital Association. (2003). *The patient care partnership.* Chicago, IL.

American Medical Association. (2013). *HIPAA violations and enforcement.* Retrieved July 20, 2013, from www.ama-assn.org/ama/pub/physician-resources/solutions-managing-your-practice/coding-billing-insurance/hipaahealth-insurance-portability-accountability-act/hipaa-violations-enforcement.page

Burtis, C. A., Ashwood, E. R., & Bruns, D. E. (Eds.). (2005). *Tietz textbook of clinical chemistry and molecular diagnostics* (4th ed.). Philadelphia: W. B. Saunders.

Clinical and Laboratory Standards Institute. (2010). *Accuracy in patient and sample identification; approved guideline.* Wayne, PA: CLSI.

Clinical and Laboratory Standards Institute. (2007). *Procedures for the collection of diagnostic blood specimens by venipuncture; approved standard—sixth edition.* Wayne, PA: CLSI.

Clinical and Laboratory Standards Institute. (2010). *Specimen label: Content and location, font and label orientation.* Wayne, PA: CLSI.

Healthcare Information and Management Systems. (2011). *Electronic health records.* Retrieved March 22, 2011, from www.himss.org/ASP/topics_ehr.asp

Judson, K., & Harrison, C. (2010). *Law and ethics for medical careers* (5th ed.). New York: McGraw-Hill.

Saltin, B. (1996). Exercise and the environment: Focus on altitude. *Research Quarterly for Exercise and Sport. 67,* 3: S1-S10.

Wilson, D. D. (2008). *McGraw-Hill manual of laboratory and diagnostic tests.* New York: McGraw-Hill.

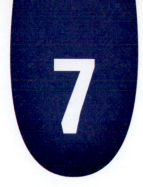

7

Blood Collection Equipment

essential terms

ACD
additive
aerosol
aliquot
antiglycolytic
antiseptic
bacteriostatic
bevel
capillary action
citrate
clot activator
dermal
EDTA
evacuated collection tube

evacuated tube holder
gauge
heel warmer
heparin
lancet
microcollection
sharps container
sterile
thixotropic separator gel
tourniquet
venipuncture
winged infusion set

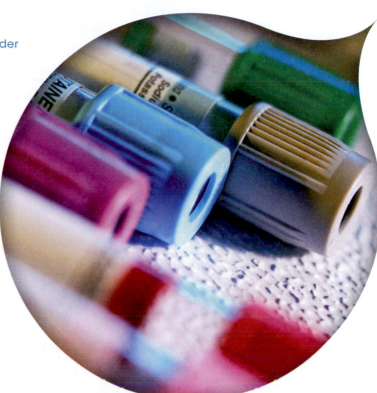

Learning Outcomes

7.1 Select equipment used for both venipuncture and capillary puncture.

7.2 Select equipment specific for venipuncture procedures.

7.3 Select equipment specific for dermal/capillary puncture procedures.

7.4 Identify the various types of additives and color-coding used in blood collection and explain the reasons for their use.

7.5 Implement the correct order of draw for venipuncture and capillary puncture procedures.

7.6 Compare blood collection equipment from various manufacturers

Related NAACLS Competencies

5.00 Demonstrate knowledge of collection equipment, various types of additives used, special precautions necessary, and substances that can interfere in clinical analysis of blood constituents.

5.1 Identify the various types of additives used in blood collection, and explain the reasons for their use.

5.2 Identify the evacuated tube color codes associated with the additives.

5.3 Describe the proper order of draw for specimen collections.

5.4 Describe substances that can interfere in clinical analysis of blood constituents and ways in which the phlebotomist can help to avoid these occurrences.

5.5 List and select the types of equipment needed to collect blood by venipuncture and capillary (dermal) puncture.

5.6 Identify special precautions necessary during blood collections by venipuncture and capillary (dermal) puncture.

Introduction

Phlebotomists must become familiar with the equipment used at their facilities and any facility modification to the order of draw. The various types of equipment used in the collection of blood samples are presented in this chapter. In addition, a commonly accepted sequence for collecting multiple samples is discussed, as well as the tubes used for specimen collection in the same order of draw. Further equipment unique to special procedures is discussed in the chapter *Special Phlebotomy Procedures*.

7.1 Common Blood Collection Equipment

For any blood test, collecting a blood specimen—by **venipuncture** (puncture of a vein) or capillary/**dermal** (skin) puncture—is the first step. This process is often referred to as "drawing blood." The phlebotomist must become familiar with each item used in the collection of blood by venipuncture and dermal puncture (Figure 7-1). Proper handling of phlebotomy equipment is of the utmost importance for the safety of both the phlebotomist and the patient. Equipment used by the phlebotomist is universal but may vary in appearance depending on its manufacturer. Although much of the equipment is used during both venipuncture and **microcollection** procedures (capillary/dermal puncture), there are some items that are used only for specific types of collection. Table 7-1 lists each type of blood collection equipment and when it is used.

Phlebotomy Tray or Cart

Phlebotomists use a tray or cart to store and transport blood collection equipment (Figure 7-2). Trays and carts should be clean, orderly, and well stocked with sufficient equipment for the number and types of tests ordered, as well as the types of patient situations that may be encountered. A phlebotomist should take the time to restock the phlebotomy tray or cart as needed on a regular basis.

Gloves

OSHA regulations require that gloves be worn during the phlebotomy procedure and changed after each patient. Nonsterile gloves are acceptable for blood collection because, unlike surgery, blood collection is not a sterile procedure. Gloves are used to prevent the spread of infection, but pathogens are not completely eliminated as they would be during a sterile procedure. Because the powder in gloves can contaminate the specimen during blood collection, powder-free gloves are recommended.

Gloves are available in a variety of materials and in many sizes and styles. Nitrile, vitrile, synthetic vinyl, or other nonlatex gloves are frequently used (Figure 7-3). Although latex gloves were widely used in the past, most healthcare facilities have discontinued stocking them to protect employees and patients who may have latex allergies. Even when permitted by the healthcare facility, latex gloves should not be used when a patient has latex allergies.

Glove liners are available, but these are only for long-term glove use, such as specimen processing.

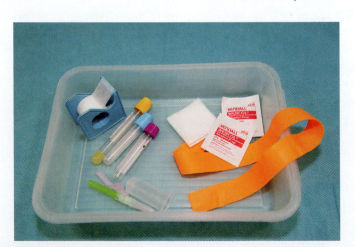

Figure 7-1 A variety of equipment is needed to perform routine blood collection.

They can make it difficult to palpate veins during blood collection. Thus, wearing well-fitting, nonlatex gloves is the best policy for the phlebotomist.

TABLE 7-1 Blood Collection Equipment

Equipment	Routine Venipuncture	Difficult Venipuncture	Capillary Puncture
Phlebotomy tray or cart	Yes	Yes	Yes
Gloves	Yes	Yes	Yes
Hand sanitizer	Yes	Yes	Yes
Alcohol prep pads	Yes	Yes	Yes
Gauze pads	Yes	Yes	Yes
Adhesive bandage or tape	Yes	Yes	Yes
Sharps (needle disposal) container	Yes	Yes	Yes
Permanent fine-tipped marking pen	Yes	Yes	Yes
Labels (preprinted)	Yes	Yes	Yes
Specimen transport bags	Yes	Yes	Yes
Evacuated tube holder or syringe	Yes	Yes	No
Evacuated tubes	Yes	Yes	No
Tourniquet	Yes	Yes	No
Needles	Yes	Yes	No
Winged infusion set	No	Yes	No
Syringe	No	Yes	No
Lancets	No	No	Yes
Capillary tubes and sealant	No	No	Yes
Microcollection tubes	No	No	Yes

Hand Sanitizers

Phlebotomists must wash their hands after removing their used gloves and prior to donning new gloves for procedures with the next patient. If soap and running water are not available, a suitable alcohol-based hand sanitizer may be used to cleanse hands between patients (Figure 7-4). However, if your hands

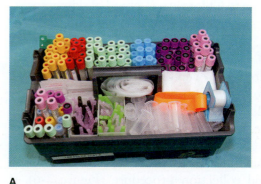
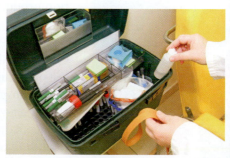
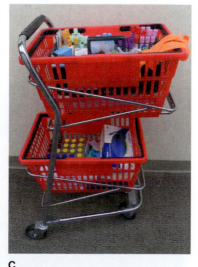

Figure 7-2 (A) Blood collection tray. (B) Some trays are available with covers that are used for storage and during transport between departments. (C) Blood collection carts on wheels provide an ergonomic way for phlebotomists to transport all the equipment they may need during blood collection rounds.

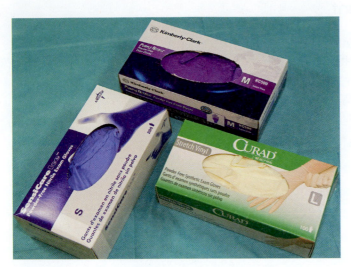

Figure 7-3 Several sizes and types of gloves.

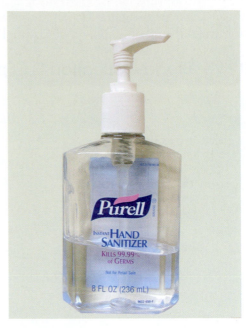

Figure 7-4 Alcohol-based hand sanitizer.

show any type of visible contamination or soilage, you should wash your hands rather than use an alcohol-based hand sanitizer.

Alcohol Prep Pads

To prevent infection, the blood collection site must be cleaned using an **antiseptic**—a germicidal solution—before the blood specimen is collected. *Alcohol prep pads* are a frequently used type of antiseptic. These sterile pads are saturated with 70% isopropyl alcohol (Figure 7-5). Seventy percent isopropyl alcohol is a **bacteriostatic** antiseptic, meaning that it inhibits the growth of bacteria. This prevents contamination by normal skin bacteria during a venipuncture procedure.

However, alcohol preps are not recommended for the collection of blood alcohol levels, in order to eliminate any concerns over alcohol contamination. This is especially important if the alcohol test results are to be submitted as evidence in a court of law. Follow your facility's policy when collecting specimens for legal purposes.

Stronger antiseptics may be used depending on the site or collection procedure. A blood culture collection or an arterial puncture requires additional sterility. For these procedures, antiseptics such as Betadine®, iodine, or chlorhexidine gluconate (the ingredient contained in the Chloraprep is a brand. Change to ChloraPrep® brand of skin preparation products) are used to clean the puncture site.

Gauze Pads

Gauze is a loosely woven cotton fabric used to cover the puncture site when applying pressure immediately upon completion of the procedure. In some facilities, sterile gauze is used to dry the puncture site after it is cleaned. Gauze pads are available in several sizes, including the 2-inch by 2-inch squares normally used after a blood collection procedure (Figure 7-6). If needed, gauze can be folded into quarters and taped to the patient's skin to serve as a pressure bandage, which will maintain a firm amount of pressure to

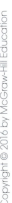

Figure 7-5 Alcohol prep pads.

the site. Note that cotton balls are not recommended for post-procedure care of a blood collection site because the cotton may adhere to the site and cause the site to reopen when the cotton ball is removed.

Adhesive Bandages

An adhesive bandage or gauze held by paper tape is placed over the puncture site to stop the bleeding. Adhesive bandages should not be used on patients with fragile skin, such as the elderly. In some facilities, paper tape may be used on patients with fragile skin. However, applying bandages of any type is not advisable for infants and small children because they may remove and place the bandage in their mouth and possibly aspirate and choke on it. Patients may be asked to hold pressure on the gauze while the phlebotomist is finishing the collection procedure. However, it is the phlebotomist's responsibility to ensure bleeding has stopped before releasing the patient. The patient should be advised to watch the site and remove the bandage in 15 to 30 minutes. In

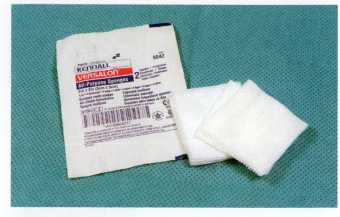

Figure 7-6 Gauze pads.

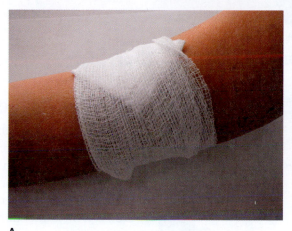

A

B

Figure 7-7 (A) Roller gauze dressing. (B) Coban® bandage.

many cases, a roller gauze is wrapped entirely around the arm, so tape is not placed on the skin. A Coban® bandage can also be used to apply pressure (Figure 7-7). Acute care facilities may not use Coban® since certain patients may be unable to remove the bandage after 15 to 20 minutes. Leaving a Coban® or other pressure dressing in place too long can cause constriction of the tissues and possible circulation issues. The patient should also be instructed to avoid lifting and frequent bending of the elbow to prevent the return of bleeding. Select a bandage size appropriate to the type of puncture performed and the patient's situation (Figure 7-8).

Sharps Container

Needle disposal containers, also known as **sharps containers,** are designed to protect healthcare personnel from accidental needle-sticks by contaminated needles (Figure 7-9). Sharps containers are rigid, leak-proof, puncture resistant, and clearly marked with the biohazard symbol. These containers are usually red and are available in a variety of shapes and sizes. Used needles, lancets, and other sharp items must be disposed of immediately in these special containers. To prevent possible needlesticks, the needle should not be removed from the holder. Dispose of the needle holder in the sharps container as well. Never reach into, tamper with, or attempt to pry open a sealed sharps container. These disposal units are marked with a biohazard label and are to be disposed of according to the biohazard guidelines established by OSHA.

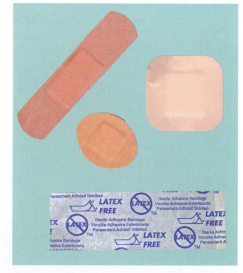

Figure 7-8 A variety of adhesive bandages.

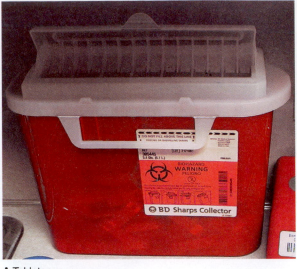
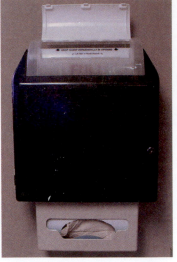

A Tabletop   B Wall-mounted

Figure 7-9 Biohazard sharps containers.

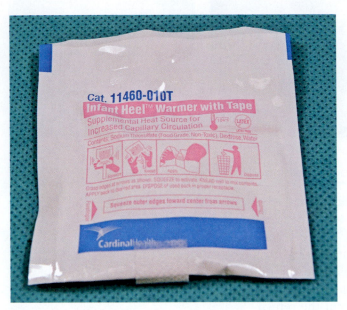

Figure 7-10 Heel warmer.

Tissue Warmers

Tissue warmers, such as a warm towel, cloth, or chemical warmer packet, are used to increase the blood flow to the intended puncture site. A **heel warmer** packet (Figure 7-10) is commonly used for dermal puncture on infants. Larger tissue warmers are used on adults during venipuncture.

Computer Label/Permanent Marking Pen

Each evacuated tube must be labeled at the time of specimen collection, immediately after drawing each patient's blood. Tubes must be labeled before the phlebotomist leaves the patient's side but never before the specimen is drawn. Tubes may be labeled with a computer-generated label or with a permanent marker or pen. A computer-generated label usually includes a bar code that provides specimen information to laboratory information systems within the EHR (Figure 7-11). Place the computer-generated label over the original tube label, not over the clear area of the tube. This will allow the amount and condition of the blood to be viewed during testing. Any label, whether computer generated or handwritten, should contain the patient's full name, a unique patient identifier, the patient's date of

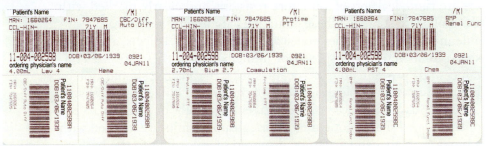

Figure 7-11 Computer labels.

birth, the specimen collection time and date, and the collector's identification (initials, signature, or code).

When using a computer label, the phlebotomist must initial and date the label and affix it to the tube after collection. If computer labels are not provided, the same required patient identification information and collection information must be written on specimen labels of all tubes collected. Specimens for the blood bank (such as type and cross-match) may have other special requirements, including patient banding procedures. Identification of specimens for the blood bank's transfusion service is explained in the chapter *Special Phlebotomy Procedures*.

Specimen Transport Bags

Specimen transport bags are plastic, ziplocked bags that display a biohazard symbol and include a separate outer pocket in which paperwork is placed (Figure 7-12). These bags not only identify the contents as being a biohazard but also help contain specimen spills if the collection container breaks. A specimen bag must be used to transport blood from the collection location to the testing location. The specific type of transport bag varies, depending on your place of employment. For transport between facilities, adding an absorbent pad in the specimen containment portion of the transport bag will provide extra safety from spills and breakage.

The specimen bag protects the person handling the specimens from biohazard exposure. Blood and other laboratory specimens may contain disease-producing organisms, and preventing exposure is part of Standard Precautions. Once a specimen is placed in the bag, handle it gently and keep it vertical, with the tube cap or closure on top. For blood samples, this will prevent *hemolysis* (destruction of red blood cells) caused by excessive agitation.

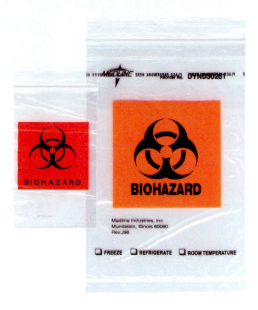

Figure 7-12 Specimen transport bags (biohazard bags).

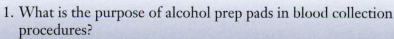

1. What is the purpose of alcohol prep pads in blood collection procedures?
2. What items should be placed in a sharps container?

Checkpoint Questions 7.1

7.2 Equipment Unique to Venipuncture

Blood collection involving various venipuncture procedures requires equipment designed specifically for these procedures. This section describes the equipment used in venipuncture procedures. The actual procedures are discussed in the chapter *Venipuncture*.

Tourniquets

A **tourniquet** is a length of rubber tubing or strapping that is wrapped around the arm to slow the flow of venous blood (blood in the veins), causing a backup of blood and increased pressure. Tourniquets are used during venipuncture to make it easier to locate a patient's veins. A tourniquet is applied 3 to 4 inches above the puncture site, tightly enough to slow the blood flow but not stop it.

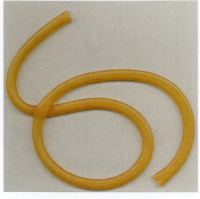
A Tubing-type tourniquet

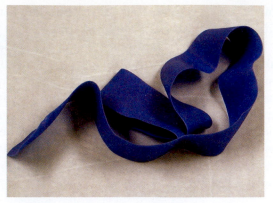
B Flat latex-free band-type tourniquet

Figure 7-13 Tourniquet examples.

As a result, the veins become enlarged, making them easier to find and penetrate with a needle. Several styles of tourniquets are available, and each phlebotomist must decide his or her preference. The most commonly used is soft and pliable, measuring 1 inch wide by 18 inches long. Common types are rubber tubes, thin rubber bands, and strips of elastic fabric (Figure 7-13). The Clinical and Laboratory Standards Institute (CLSI) and The Joint Commission (TJC) require that a new tourniquet be used on each patient. Non-latex tourniquets are preferred to avoid any chance of a latex allergic reaction.

Whatever type of tourniquet is used, it must be disposed of after the procedure or used again ONLY on the same patient and only if it is not visibly contaminated. For example, when a patient at an inpatient facility requires multiple blood collections, a tourniquet may be kept at the bedside and reused only if it is not visibly contaminated. Tourniquets should *not* be cleaned and reused.

The tourniquet should not be left on the arm longer than 1 minute at a time. Leaving the tourniquet on too long can change the results of certain blood tests. If it takes longer than 1 minute to complete the procedure, loosen the tourniquet for at least 2 minutes; then reapply the tourniquet.

Sometimes a blood pressure cuff is used to help locate an appropriate site for venipuncture in people with veins that are difficult to palpate. When using a blood pressure cuff, the cuff should be inflated to a pressure between the systolic and diastolic pressures. Do not leave the cuff inflated for more than 1 minute.

Needles

The needle is composed of the hub, or plastic section; the shaft; and the **bevel,** or slanted tip at the point. The bevel should always be facing upward (you should be able to see the bevel when looking down) before the needle is inserted into the skin to puncture the vein (Figure 7-14A). **Sterile** needles (those free of microorganisms) are available in peel-apart packages or plastic cases. The tip of the needle should be checked for damage and for burrs, which are small imperfections or rough edges on the end of the needle. These burrs will cause unnecessary pain for the patient. Also, a blunt or bent tip can be harmful to the patient and interfere with collecting a blood sample. It is rare that disposable needles display these defects; however, you may occasionally encounter a "bad" needle. If you find a damaged needle, discard it in the sharps container and get a new one.

The double-pointed needle has a rubber sleeve over one end with a screw hub in the center: one end is designed for the venipuncture and the other is used to puncture the evacuated collection tube's rubber stopper (Figure 7-14B). This rubber sleeve makes it easier to draw multiple tubes because the sleeve covers the needle inside the tube holder (adapter), preventing blood from dripping into the holder before another tube is inserted.

Because of the large number of documented needlestick injuries, the Needlestick Safety and Prevention Act was put into place in 2001. This act states that needles used in phlebotomy should have safety features, known as *engineering devices,* to protect the phlebotomist from accidental puncture with a contaminated needle. In most cases, the user must actively engage the safety feature. The safety device is attached to either the needle or the holder (Figure 7-14C). These safety features should

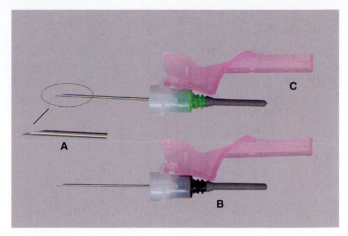

Figure 7-14 Needles showing (A) enlarged bevel, (B) rubber sleeve, and (C) safety device.

be activated as soon as the procedure is completed. Some safety devices are designed to be activated just before the needle is removed from the collection site, whereas others are designed to be activated immediately on removing the needle from the site. In either case, the entire assembly is disposed of in one piece as a safety measure. Use a one-handed technique when activating the safety device. Do not attempt to activate the device with your other hand. Always keep your fingers away from the point of the needle. An audible click or color change will occur to indicate that the safety feature is engaged. Table 7-2 provides examples of safe needle devices for phlebotomy.

A phlebotomist generally uses three types of needles: (1) a multiple-sample needle, used as part of an evacuated collection system (a double-pointed needle and collection tube that contains a vacuum); (2) a hypodermic needle, used with a *syringe;* and (3) a **winged infusion set** (*butterfly needle*) that can be used with either syringe or evacuated tube systems.

Needles vary in length from ¾ to 1½ inches. The bore size, lumen, or **gauge** of the needle also varies from large, 16-gauge needles used to collect units of blood to smaller, 23-gauge needles used for very small veins. The smaller the number assigned to the gauge, the larger the lumen size, or inside diameter, of the needle. As a safety precaution, the caps of the needles are usually color-coded to aid in quick identification of the needle's gauge (Figure 7-15A). The most commonly used sizes and coded colors of needles for venipuncture on adults are 20-gauge (yellow), 21-gauge (green), and 22-gauge (black) in 1- to 1½-inch lengths.

Needles have a manufacturer's label, which identifies the needle's gauge and seals the caps of both ends. On assembly, if the needle already has a broken seal, you should assume that the needle is not sterile and discard it (Figure 7-15B). In addition, an expiration date is printed either on the label or on the smaller needle cap, as shown in Figure 7-15C. Expiration dates indicate the date at which time needle sterility cannot be ensured. Never use needles with questionable sterility on patients.

Winged Infusion Set

Winged infusion sets, also called butterfly needles, are used for blood collection from infants, from small children, and in other situations when routine equipment might be difficult to use. These situations are discussed in detail in the *Venipuncture* chapter.

The butterfly needle has plastic wings attached to the needle and includes two types of systems. The needle gauge is 21 to 23 with plastic tubing attached

TABLE 7-2 Safe Needle Devices

Feature	Example	Activation
Self-blunting needle	Blunt-tip blood-drawing needle / Blood collection tube / Sharp point / Blunt point	After the blood is drawn, a push on the collection tube moves the blunt needle forward through the outer shell and past the needle point. The blunt point can be activated before it is removed from the vein or artery.
Self-blunting butterfly needle		After collection and before the removal of the needle, the wing is flipped to the other side, blunting the needle.
Hinged cap		Using the thumb, a protective hinged cap is flipped over the needle and locks into place.
Protective shield		The user slides a plastic cover over the needle and locks it in place. Syringes also have this device.
Retractable needle		The needle is spring-loaded and retracts into the barrel when a button is pushed to activate.

to the needle. The difference between the two systems is at the end of the plastic tubing. There is a hub end, designed to attach to a syringe, or a rubber sleeve end, designed to insert into a holder just like the evacuated needles. The butterfly needle has a safety device attached to the plastic wing end. When disposing of the butterfly assembly, the best way to avoid a needlestick injury is to place the needle end into the sharps container first and then let the rest of the assembly drop into the sharps container.

The "wings" of the butterfly needle are used to hold the needle during insertion into the vein (Figure 7-16). Butterfly needles are typically ¾" inch long and have a protective shield that slides in place on completion of the procedure. The butterfly set is not used as extensively as the evacuated blood collection system. Winged sets can be used with an evacuated tube holder or a syringe. One of the main reasons for butterfly sets is to have more control with non-stable patients.

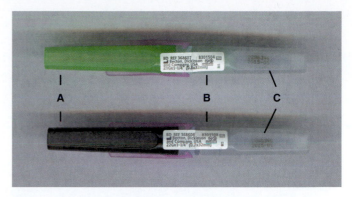

Figure 7-15 Needles showing (A) gauge-related color-coded caps, (B) a needle safety label, and (C) a needle sterility expiration date.

Syringe

A syringe consists of a barrel and a plunger. The barrel is usually graduated in milliliters or fractions of a milliliter. Two types of hypodermic needles are available for attachment to syringes, the "slip tip" and the "luer lock." Luer locks are preferred because there is no danger of the syringe slipping off during the procedure. Some syringes come with a pre-attached needle (Figure 17-17A). Syringes may also be used with butterfly needles; the hub at the end of the butterfly tubing slips over the tip of the syringe (Figure 17-17B).

Transfer Adapters

Transfer adapters provide a safe and easy way to transfer blood from a syringe to evacuated tubes. Transfer adapters can also be used when collecting samples using butterfly needles. Transfer adapters are available with female or male connectors, allowing for coupling with equipment that has the opposite gender connector. Figure 7-18 shows various types of couplings using these connectors. Some transfer adapters are designed to accommodate evacuated tubes as well as blood culture bottles, which are explained in the *Special Phlebotomy Procedures* chapter. See Figure 7-19.

Evacuated Tube Holder

An **evacuated tube holder,** called a *barrel* or an *adapter,* is a specialized plastic adapter that holds both a needle and a tube for blood collection (Figure 7-18). Needles are designed so that they can be screwed onto one end of the holder. An evacuated tube is inserted into the other end after the needle has been inserted into the patient's vein. The evacuated tube holder, often made of clear, rigid plastic, has a flange at the end where the tube is inserted. This flange area is helpful during the venipuncture procedure. The evacuated needles that attach to the holder are designed with or without a safety engineering device. If the needle does not have a safety device, you must use a holder that has a built-in safety device, such as a holder that snaps a cover over the needle. These holders are to be discarded after use. If a safety needle is used, it is activated immediately after the needle is removed from

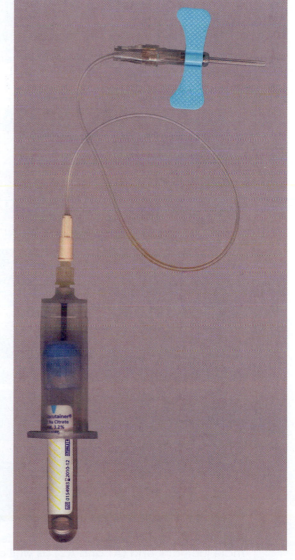

Figure 7-16 Winged infusion, or butterfly, assembly.

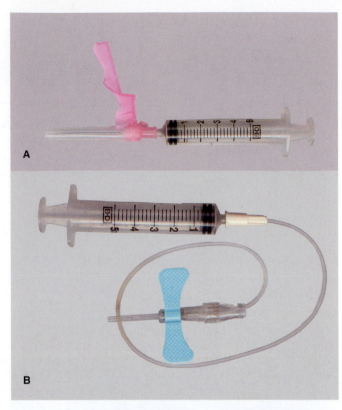

Figure 7-17 Syringe with (A) a hypodermic needle and (B) a butterfly needle.

the skin. After use, this entire assembly is disposed of in one piece as a safety measure. Safety holders come in two sizes: one for the standard-size collection tube and a smaller version for a small-diameter tube. A tube adapter is available that allows the use of small-diameter tubes with an adult-size holder (Figure 7-21). Updated engineering devices for both holders and needles are constantly being developed to protect the phlebotomist from an accidental needlestick.

Evacuated Tubes

Evacuated collection tubes contain a premeasured vacuum and are the most widely used system for blood collecting. Some evacuated tubes contain **additives** (substances that either inhibit or promote clotting). These tubes are sterile inside to prevent contamination of the specimen and the patient. The tubes also have an expiration date, which indicates that, at the end of the month of the expiration date, the tube should no longer be used because the additives and vacuum are not guaranteed to perform as intended. Tubes are available in a variety of sizes and colors and are

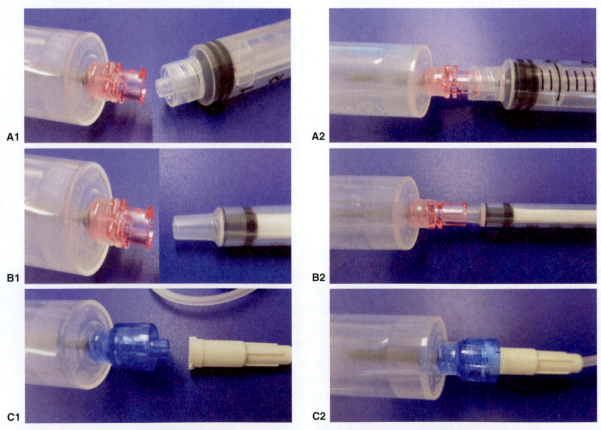

Figure 7-18 A transfer adapter with a female connector can couple with a syringe that has a male luer-lock end (A1 and A2) as well as a syringe with a plain male end (B1 and B2). A transfer adapter with a male connector can couple with a butterfly needle that has a female-ended tubing (C1 and C2).

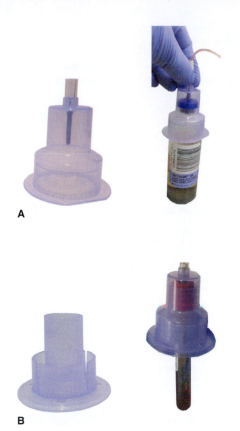

A

B

Figure 7-19 Specialized transfer adapter: (A) Adapter as used with blood culture bottles. (B) The adapter sleeve fits into the blood culture bottle adapter and allows for collection of evacuated tubes.

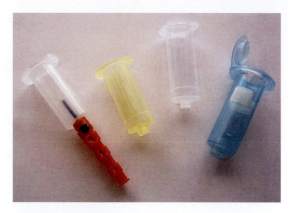

A Evacuated tube holders

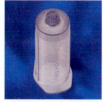

B Vacutainer® holder

Figure 7-20 Various types of tube holders.

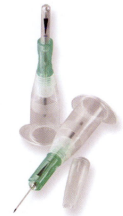

C BD Vacutainer®

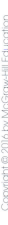

made of glass or plastic. Sizes range from 2 to 15 milliliters (Figure 7-22). The colors of the stoppers vary based on the additives inside the tube and the type of test to be completed. Plastic tubes have less chance of breakage, which helps prevent spillage and possible exposure to bloodborne pathogens. In the closed system of evacuated tubes, the patient's blood goes directly from the vein into a rubber-stoppered tube without being exposed to the air (Figure 7-23). The evacuated tube system allows many tubes to be collected with just one venipuncture.

Evacuated tubes fill automatically with blood because a vacuum exists inside the tube. The vacuum inside the collection tube helps "draw" the blood out of the patient's vein. The amount of vacuum is adequate for the tube to fill to the required amount for testing. Some evacuated collection tubes have a plastic splashguard that covers the sides of the tube. This splashguard is a safety device that helps reduce the **aerosol** mist (particles suspended in the air) that may be generated when the tube's stopper is removed from the evacuated tube during specimen processing.

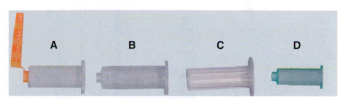

Figure 7-21 Various tube holders and adapter types.

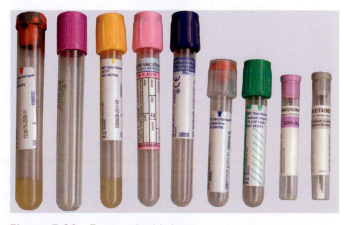

Figure 7-22 Evacuated tubes.

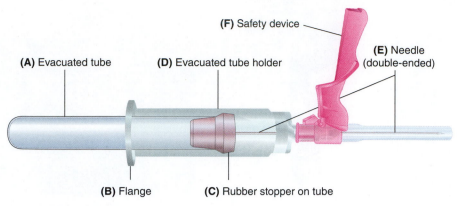

(F) Safety device

(A) Evacuated tube   **(D)** Evacuated tube holder   **(E)** Needle (double-ended)

(B) Flange   **(C)** Rubber stopper on tube

Figure 7-23   Evacuated collection tube assembly.

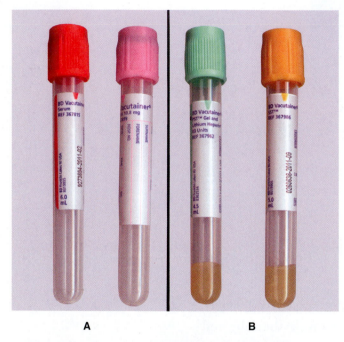

A   B

Figure 7-24   Evacuated tubes: (A) no separator gel, (B) with separator gel.

Serum—the liquid portion of blood that has been allowed to clot or coagulate—will form when blood is collected in a tube with no anticoagulant. When plastic tubes are used for a serum sample, a clot activator is added to the tube during the manufacturing process because blood takes longer to clot in a plastic tube. The clotted cells and serum will separate when centrifuged.

Plasma is the result of blood collected in a tube that contains an anticoagulant. Some tubes contain a **thixotropic separator gel** to separate serum and plasma from cells (Figure 7-24). When the specimen tube is centrifuged, this gel will create a barrier between cells and either plasma or serum. Cells, which are heavier than the gel, descend to the bottom of the tube, while the liquid portion of the blood (plasma or serum) remains above the gel.

The anticoagulant in the evacuated tube prevents the specimen from clotting by neutralizing

Safety & Infection Control

Check the Expiration Dates

Manufacturers print an expiration date on each tube label. As tubes age, the vacuum may be lost and the effectiveness of the additives deteriorates. Do not use tubes past their expiration date. Using an expired tube with loss of vacuum interferes with the collection. If the tube has loss of vacuum or the tube additive has deteriorated, then any specimen collected in the tube will be unacceptable and could result in error in patient treatment.

or removing one of the essential factors necessary for the clotting or coagulation process. Tubes containing an anticoagulant should be mixed or inverted gently several times (usually 8 to 10 times) immediately after drawing blood to ensure uniform mixing of the specimen with the anticoagulant. Check the manufacturer's directions for the proper number of inversions to perform.

7.3 Equipment Unique to Microcollection

Although venipuncture is the most frequently performed phlebotomy procedure, current laboratory instruments and procedures enable phlebotomists to use smaller and smaller amounts of blood. Thus, obtaining microsamples by capillary/dermal puncture is also popular. This section describes the equipment used specifically for microcollection procedures. The actual microcollection procedures are discussed in the chapter *Dermal/Capillary Puncture*.

Lancets

Lancets are small cutting instruments designed to control the depth of the dermal puncture. Lancets come in several depths: low blood flow, 1.5 mm; medium blood flow, 1.8 mm; and high blood flow, 2.0 mm. Lancets with depths greater than 2.0 mm should not be used, to avoid injuring the underlying bone. Phlebotomists must select the appropriate lancet based on the amount of blood needed and the location of the puncture site. Safety lancets with retracting blades should be used to prevent sharps injuries. To produce adequate blood flow, the depth of the puncture is actually less important than the width of the incision. This is because the major vascular area of the skin is located near the skin's surface, usually within 2 mm of the surface. A variety of dermal puncture devices are available (Figure 7-25).

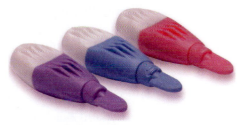

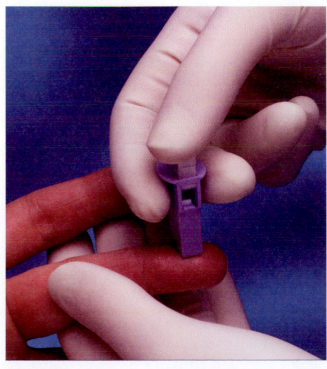

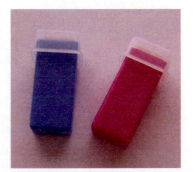

Figure 7-25 Dermal puncture devices.

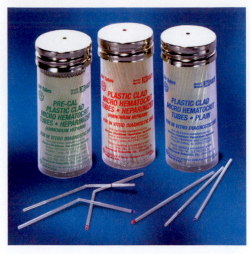

Figure 7-26 Bottles of capillary tubes.

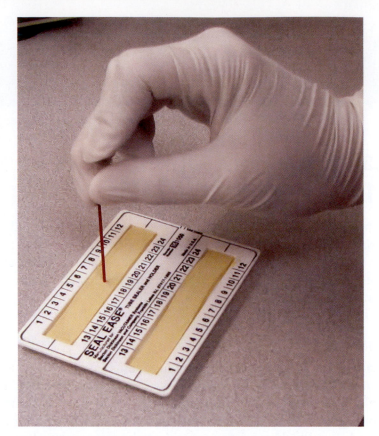

Figure 7-27 Sealing a capillary tube.

Capillary Tubes and Sealant

Capillary tubes, also called *microhematocrit tubes*, may be used to collect blood from a dermal puncture when only a small amount of blood is required (Figure 7-26). Capillary tubes are small plastic or glass tubes with a thin Mylar filament wrapping (a clear, nonstick coating). Mylar, wrapped glass and plastic tubes are used to avoid easy breakage. Capillary tubes use **capillary action,** which is the physical process of a fluid flowing, or being pulled, into a very thin tube. Capillary action eliminates the need to tip the tube downward, thus reducing the risk of getting air bubbles in the sample.

Three types of capillary tubes are available: red-tipped tubes, blue-tipped tubes, and black-tipped tubes. Red-tipped capillary tubes have an anticoagulant (heparin) coating on the inside to prevent specimen clotting and are used to measure the hematocrit. When the phlebotomist has collected sufficient blood in the red-tipped capillary tube, one end of this tube can then be closed by embedding it in a clay sealant (Figure 7-27). Also available are self-sealing capillary tubes that require no clay sealant after collection; however, care must be taken to collect from the opposite end of the sealant. Blue-tipped capillary tubes have no anticoagulant coating on the inside, so specimens will clot in these tubes. Blue-tipped capillary tubes are used when no anticoagulant is required. Black-tipped tubes have a smaller diameter in order to collect a smaller amount of blood.

Microcollection Tubes

Microcollection containers are usually plastic tubes that provide a larger collection volume than capillary tubes (Figure 7-28). Some containers are designed for a specific test, whereas others are used for multiple purposes. For example, some containers have a capillary tube end, whereas others have a scoop or a wide-mouth opening to collect drops of blood. Microtainers®, manufactured by Becton Dickinson, are one such type of collection device.

Microcollection containers or devices come with the same variety of anticoagulants as do evacuated tubes, including separator gels. The same color-coding system is used for microcollection containers as is used for commonly used evacuated tubes (Figure 7-28).

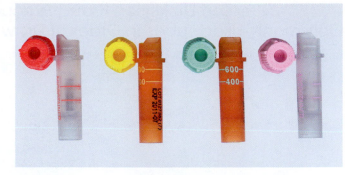

Figure 7-28 Microcollection containers.

Equipment Selection

The volume of blood normally drawn on pediatric and geriatric patients with fragile veins is less than the volume normally drawn on adult patients. Selecting the appropriate method of collection is crucial to the successful collection of a quality specimen. Microcollection techniques and equipment are most often used when collecting blood from infants and young children. Routine venipuncture procedures and equipment are used for uncomplicated blood collection from older children and adults. Special equipment, such as the butterfly assembly, may be required for venipuncture procedures on any patient with difficult veins.

Life Span Considerations

The mixing process for microcollection devices is the same as for evacuated tubes, although the number of inversions times may vary. Immediate and proper mixing is very important with the microcollection devices because the coagulation system is initiated during dermal puncture. Without proper mixing of the anticoagulant and specimen for tests requiring whole blood, the specimen will clot. A clotted specimen *cannot* be used for laboratory testing.

Checkpoint Questions 7.3

1. What is the difference between a capillary tube and a microcollection tube?
2. What depth of lancet would be used to have high, medium, and low blood flow when performing a capillary/dermal puncture?

7.4 Additives and Color-Coding

A variety of colors are used for the rubber stoppers that function as closures for evacuated blood collection tubes. Each color indicates the presence of a specific additive contained in the tube. An additive is any substance in a blood collection tube that acts as an anticoagulant, a clot activator, or a preservative. A tube stopper color-coding system helps ensure that the correct additive is used during blood collection for specific laboratory tests. Although the colors used are fairly universal among manufacturers, the shades of these colors may vary. For the purposes of this color-code discussion, common Becton Dickinson brand colors are explained in Tables 7-3 and 7-4. Table 7-3 shows frequently used evacuated tube stoppers and additives. Table 7-4 shows evacuated tube

Stopper Image		Tube Color	Additive/ Action	Laboratory Section
Standard Stopper	Splashguard Stopper (Adult/Pediatric)			
		Red/gray or clear/red	None (plastic tube)	Coagulation (may be required to purge air from butterfly tubing.)
		Light blue	Sodium citrate/ binds calcium	Coagulation
		Red	None (may use as discard) or clot activator	Chemistry Immunology
		Red/black or gold	Separator gel/ forms barrier and clot activator	Chemistry
		Green	Heparin (sodium, lithium, or ammonium)/ inhibits thrombin	Chemistry Hematology Flow cytometry
		Green/gray or light green	Heparin (as above) plus separator gel	Chemistry
		Lavender	EDTA/chelates calcium	Hematology Chemistry
		Pink	EDTA spray/same as lavender plus special labeling requirements	Blood bank
		Gray	Sodium fluoride/ glycolysis inhibitor and potassium oxalate/binds calcium	Chemistry

stoppers and additives for special tubes. Phlebotomists should be familiar with the specific evacuated tube types and additives used at the facility where they are employed.

Evacuated tubes that draw a full volume have a solid-color top. Evacuated tubes with translucent splashguard tops contain less vacuum and draw less volume. Volumes are indicated on the tube label. The tubes that draw less volume are often used for pediatric blood collection. Older-style tubes for pediatric blood collection are physically smaller with a colored rubber stopper.

Stopper Image		Tube Color	Additive/ Action	Laboratory Section
Standard Stopper	Splashguard Stopper			
		Yellow	Sodium polyanethol sulfonate/ neutralizes antibiotics	Microbiology/Blood cultures
		Yellow	Acid citrate dextrose/ maintains cell viability	Blood bank HLA lab
		Royal blue	Clot activator or EDTA specially formulated cap certified trace element free	Chemistry/Trace elements
		Tan	EDTA specially formulated cap certified lead free	Chemistry/Lead levels
		White	EDTA with separator gel	Molecular diagnostics
		Orange or Gray/ Yellow	Thrombin/ accelerates clotting	Chemistry/STAT tests

Because of the possibility of additive carryover from one tube to another, the Clinical and Laboratory Standards Institute (CLSI) has suggested a specific order of draw for the types of blood collection procedures. The order of draw discussed in this section follows the color code for the order suggested for routine venipuncture. Phlebotomists must adhere to the policies and procedures for order of draw as outlined by their employers. Some laboratories may have determined an alternate order of draw for procedures specific to their needs.

Tubes with additives should *always* be inverted several times immediately after collection to ensure proper mixing of these additives with the sample.

Tube Selection

When drawing blood, you notice that the tubes are only filling half-way. To determine why this is happening, you should first ensure that you have selected the appropriate type of tube. If using BD brand splashguard tubes, you should use tubes with solid-color caps. Check the draw volume indicated on the label. Tubes with solid-color caps draw a larger volume of blood than those with translucent caps. In addition, check the expiration date on the label. Expired tubes may have lost some or all of their vacuum.

Critical Thinking

Best practice includes mixing all tubes, regardless of additive status, so that you don't forget to mix a tube containing an additive. Follow the manufacturer's instructions for the minimum number of tube inversions for proper mixing.

Routinely Used Tubes

Discard Tubes

Red-topped tubes that *do not* contain a **clot activator** may be used as discard tubes when needed. More often, the plastic red-stoppered tube with a clear splashguard cap is used for discard purposes. Another tube designed for discard draws is topped with a red and light gray rubber stopper. A discard tube is recommended when using a winged infusion set and evacuated tubes to remove the air from the tubing. This allows subsequent tubes to fill adequately. According to protocols at some facilities, a discard tube must precede tubes drawn for coagulation (light blue). Always follow your facility's protocols for order of draw.

Light-Blue-Topped Tubes

Light-blue-topped tubes are used primarily in the coagulation section of the laboratory. The primary additive or anticoagulant in the light-blue-topped tube is sodium **citrate.** Sodium citrate binds calcium, thus preventing coagulation. In order to have accurate laboratory results, this tube must be filled to its draw capacity and all vacuum must be exhausted. In most cases, a line is found on the tube to designate the proper fill level. Anything less than full could change the results of the blood test ordered, possibly changing the patient's treatment. Light-blue-topped tubes have a relatively large amount of additive, a 9:1 ratio of blood to sodium citrate. This ratio of blood to additive is more important than in other tubes with additives. The tube should be inverted several times immediately after collection to prevent clotting. Commonly performed coagulation tests include prothrombin time (PT), activated partial thromboplastin time (APTT) or partial thromboplastin time (PTT), fibrinogen, and D-dimers. Collecting the light-blue tube in the incorrect order of draw may alter the results of these tests.

Red-Topped Tubes

Red-topped tubes, which may be glass or plastic, are used primarily in the chemistry section of the laboratory. Glass red-topped tubes may be used for serum testing and do not contain any additives or gel. The glass tube allows for access to the clot, should these cells be required for testing. Plastic red-topped tubes may contain a clot activator. The clot activator, which consists of very small silica particles (sandlike granules), speeds up the coagulation process, causing the sample to clot faster.

Serum Separator Tubes

Serum separator tubes (SSTs) are used in the laboratory's chemistry section. Rubber-stopper SSTs have a speckled look, with black mixed into the red portion of the top. Plastic splashguard SSTs are gold-topped. SSTs contain a clot activator and a thixotropic separator gel. The gel separates the serum from the blood cells by getting between the clot and the serum during centrifugation. This separation process helps prevent chemical changes caused by cellular metabolism and fibrinolysis (dissolving of the clot). Even after leaving the body, cells continue to consume glucose and create waste products. The changes in these substances over time would invalidate test results if the gel were not present to keep the cells away from the serum or plasma. The gel separator makes it easier for laboratory personnel to obtain the serum for testing; with the gel in place, the cells will not mix with the serum, making it easier to **aliquot** the liquid for testing. Aliquoting is the process of removing small samples from the original specimen and placing them in another container. Tests commonly performed in chemistry that may require blood collection in an SST include those involving electrolytes, enzymes, glucose, hormones, lipids, and proteins.

Green-Topped Tubes

Green-topped tubes are used by several laboratory sections. They contain the anticoagulant sodium **heparin,** lithium heparin, or ammonium heparin. Heparin stops the coagulation process mainly by inactivating thrombin, thereby preventing clot formation.

Plasma Separator Tubes

Light-green-topped tubes, or green-gray-stoppered tubes, have lithium heparin and a thixotropic gel. Similar to serum separator tubes (SST), plasma separator tubes (PST) are used to form a barrier between blood cells and plasma. Many facilities use light-green-topped tubes for STAT chemistry tests.

Lavender-Topped Tubes

Lavender-topped tubes are used frequently in the hematology section of the laboratory. Most lavender-topped tubes contain liquid **EDTA** (ethylenediaminetetraacetic acid). EDTA prevents blood from clotting by binding with calcium, which is essential for clot formation. EDTA is the anticoagulant of choice for hematology because it maintains the cells' shape and size better than other anticoagulants. Other anticoagulants may distort the size and shape of cells, causing them to mimic the appearance of a disease process. EDTA also inhibits platelet clumping and does not interfere with routine staining procedures in hematology. Commonly performed hematology tests performed are the CBC (complete blood cell count), a differential (percentage of each type of white cell), reticulocyte counts (percentage of early red blood cells), and erythrocyte sedimentation rates (the distance in millimeters that red blood cells settle in 1 hour).

Pink-Topped Tubes

The pink EDTA tube is the preferred tube type for use in blood collection in the blood bank (immunohematology) section of the laboratory. Pink-topped tubes are evenly coated with a sprayed-on, powdered EDTA. In addition, the label on the pink-topped tube contains lines for additional information required by the American Association of Blood Banks (AABB). Tests commonly performed by the blood bank are blood typing, donor blood testing, crossmatching blood, and preparation of blood and blood products for transfusion.

Gray-Topped Tubes

Gray-topped tubes are most often used by the laboratory's chemistry section. These tubes contain potassium oxalate (an anticoagulant), which stops the coagulation process by binding with calcium. Gray-topped tubes also contain an **antiglycolytic** agent, or glucose preservative, such as sodium fluoride. An antiglycolytic, also known as a *glycolytic inhibitor,* prevents the red blood cells from using glucose and changing it to lactic acid. The gray-topped tube is preferred for glucose levels over red or gold because a blood sample drawn in a tube without a glycolytic inhibitor will produce a lower glucose result. In addition to glucose, gray-topped tubes are used for lactic acid analysis and may be used for blood alcohol levels, depending on the analysis method used by the laboratory.

Specialty Tubes

Yellow-Topped Tubes

Yellow-topped tubes are specialized tubes that are available with two different additives. Although the tubes look identical, one contains sodium polyanethol sulfonate (SPS) and is used for blood culture collections. The SPS acts as an anticoagulant and neutralizes the effect of bacterial growth inhibitors, such as antibiotics. The SPS yellow-topped tube is sterile and must be drawn first before any other tube is collected. When a blood culture is ordered along with coagulation tests, this tube replaces the discard tube in the order of draw. Many facilities no longer use SPS tubes. These facilities use specialized blood culture collection bottles, which are discussed in the chapter *Special Phlebotomy Procedures*.

The other yellow-topped tube available contains acid citrate dextrose (**ACD**), which is an additive that maintains red cell viability or growth and is used for cellular studies in blood banks or human leukocyte antigen (HLA) typing. Discretion must be used when selecting a yellow-topped tube to ensure that it contains the correct additive for the laboratory test ordered.

Royal-Blue-Topped Tubes

Royal-blue-topped tubes are specialized tubes that are available with different additives. These tubes display additive-specific color-coding on the label: a red bar on the label indicates a clot activator, a lavender bar on the label indicates EDTA, and a green bar on the label indicates heparin. The royal blue stoppers are certified to have very low levels of trace elements, such as aluminum, lead, mercury, zinc, and other metals, making these tubes a requirement for trace element studies, toxicology, and nutritional chemistry tests. Care must be used when selecting a royal-blue-topped tube to ensure that the correct additive is present in the tube for the specific laboratory test ordered.

Tan-Topped Tubes

Tan-topped tubes are specialized tubes that contain EDTA. The tan top is certified to have very low levels of lead, making these tubes a requirement when an accurate blood lead level is needed.

White-Topped Tubes

White-topped tubes are specialized tubes that contain EDTA and a plasma separator gel. The white-topped tubes may be required by laboratories performing molecular diagnostic tests that involve DNA-based methods.

Orange-Topped Tubes

Orange-topped tubes are specialized tubes that contain *thrombin*. Thrombin is a powerful clotting factor that promotes quick clot formation. This tube is used for specimen collections needing immediate testing (STAT) for tests where serum is required.

Miscellaneous Tubes

Phlebotomists may need to use other tubes that are designed for inclusion with a specific test kit. One such test is for fibrin degradation products (FDP), also known as fibrin split products (FSP). FDPs are formed when blood clots break down. The tube that accompanies the FDP test kit may have either a light blue top (similar to the citrate tube) or a black top. This tube displays a label that identifies it as being specific for FDP. The FDP tube contains two

Tube Selection

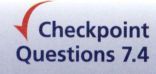
Blood collection equipment color codes are fairly standard and most blood collection product manufacturers attempt to color-code additive tubes and needle gauges with similar colors. However, due to patent rights, different shades of standard colors will be used. Phlebotomists must become familiar with equipment and test requirements specific to their places of employment. Checking with procedure manuals, supervisors, and laboratory section staff will help ensure that the correct equipment is used in the collection of specimens.

additives: thrombin to quickly clot the specimen, and a fibrinolytic inhibitor, so that the clot does not break down. The FDP tube is usually kept refrigerated until needed.

Another type of black-topped tube is used with some test kits for erythrocyte sedimentation rate (ESR). These black-topped tubes contain a specific amount of citrate anticoagulant, which provides the correct ratio of additive to perform the ESR directly in this tube.

Microcollection Container Colors

Although the previously described colors and additives are the same for evacuated tubes and microcollection containers, there are two varying characteristics for microcollection containers. Microcollection containers are not evacuated tubes. There is no light blue (citrated) microcollection container, which is used for coagulation tests, because the coagulation system is activated during the dermal puncture. In addition, the gold-stoppered serum separator and light green plasma separator microcollection containers are available in an amber-colored plastic. The amber color tube protects the specimen from light and is used primarily for bilirubin testing.

1. What is the purpose of color-coding the tops of blood collection tubes?
2. Explain why coagulation tests cannot be run on blood obtained by dermal puncture.

✓ **Checkpoint Questions 7.4**

7.5 Order of Draw

Routine Venipuncture

Routine venipuncture usually does not include a blood culture, for which special tubes are required to be drawn first. The CLSI recommends that uncomplicated blood draws use the following order:

1. Nonadditive (red or clear discard tube, if required by your facility)
2. Citrate (light blue)
3. Serum tube (clot activator tube: red, royal, or orange)
4. Serum separator (gold or red/black speckled)
5. Plasma separator (light green or green/black speckled)

6. Heparin (green)

7. EDTA (lavender, pink, royal, tan, or white)

8. Sodium fluoride (gray)

Sterile Venipuncture

When a blood culture is included with orders for other blood draws, the tubes for the blood culture must be drawn first. These tubes may be SPS yellow-topped tubes or blood culture bottles. The CLSI recommends the following order of draw when sterile procedures are included with routine blood draws:

1. Sterile tubes (SPS yellow or blood culture bottles)

2. Citrate (light blue)

3. Serum tube (clot activator tube: red, royal, or orange)

4. Serum separator (gold or red/black speckled)

5. Plasma separator (light green or green/black speckled)

6. Heparin (green)

7. EDTA (lavender, pink, royal, tan, or white)

8. Sodium fluoride (gray)

The common mnemonic used to help phlebotomists remember the order of draw for venipuncture includes the sterile tube and is outlined in Table 7-5.

TABLE 7-5 Order of Draw Mnemonic

Tube Cap	Acronym	Mnemonic meaning
	STOP	Sterile specimens for blood culture
	LIGHT	Light blue citrate tubes
	RED	Red-topped clot activator tubes
	STAY	Serum separator tubes
	PUT	Plasma separator tubes
	GREEN	Green-topped heparin tubes
	LIGHT	Lavender-topped EDTA tubes
	PLEASE	Pink-topped EDTA tubes
	GO	Gray-topped potassium oxalate/sodium fluoride tubes

This mnemonic has evolved over the years as newer evacuated tubes are added or discoveries are made that alter the order of draw. Unnecessary tubes are skipped, but the tubes that are collected should follow the same order.

Butterfly Venipuncture

When a winged infusion set is used to collect blood with evacuated blood collection tubes, the order of draw remains the same as for routine venipuncture or sterile blood draws. However, because the assembly tubing contains air, a discard tube must be drawn even for sterile blood draws. Using a discard tube for butterfly draws will ensure that the other tubes will fill with the proper amount of blood.

When using the butterfly assembly with a syringe, or using a syringe and hypodermic needle for blood collection, the blood must be transferred to the evacuated tubes. Using a syringe transfer device (Figure 7-29) lessens the chances for needlestick injury. The order of filling tubes in this manner is the same as for sterile blood draws. The CLSI has determined that using an alternate order of draw (filling of tubes) is not necessary for syringe draws.

Capillary/Dermal Puncture

During capillary/dermal puncture, the first drop of blood is *not* collected. Microcollection tubes are filled in the following order:

1. EDTA (lavender or pink)
2. Heparin (green, light green)
3. Sodium flouride (gray)
4. Nonadditive (red) or serum separator (gold)

Avoiding Interfering Substances

An *interfering substance* is one that produces incorrect laboratory test results. These substances can enter the test system during the pre-examination phase (during specimen collection and handling). Improper patient preparation (discussed in the chapters *Patient and Specimen Requirements*, *Venipuncture*, and *Dermal/Capillary Puncture*) may contribute to the presence of an interfering

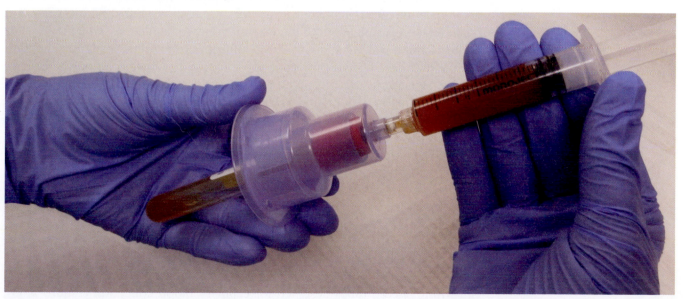

Figure 7-29 Syringe transfer device.

substance. However, interfering substances can also be introduced into the sample if the phlebotomist uses an incorrect draw order.

The order in which blood is collected using evacuated tube systems is critical to avoid introducing contaminants into the specimens. When the skin is punctured, it releases tissue thromboplastin, which may be present in the first tube collected. A citrate tube (light blue) should not be the first tube collected because the thromboplastin will activate the clotting system and render any results obtained invalid. Some facilities require a discard tube be collected first, then the citrate tube.

It is also possible to contaminate tubes with anticoagulants from other tubes. Anticoagulants or clot activators may adhere to the tube end of the double-ended needle and may be introduced into the next tube. Therefore, the light-blue-topped tube is best drawn before any other tube containing an additive because other additives may become interfering substances, altering coagulation test results. Always follow the policies and procedures established by your facility.

✔ Checkpoint Questions 7.5

1. What is the difference in the order of draw between routine blood collection and blood collection that includes a specimen for a blood culture?
2. Why is it important to use a discard tube when collecting blood with a winged infusion set directly into evacuated tubes?

7.6 Blood Collection Equipment Manufacturers

There are many blood collection equipment manufacturers. This section will discuss three common ones: Becton Dickinson, Greiner Bio-One, and Sarstedt. As a phlebotomist, you should always be familiar with the equipment that you will be using.

Becton Dickinson

Becton Dickinson (BD) manufactures equipment for blood and urine collection, including the Vacutainer® and Microtainer® systems. These tubes are available with various anticoagulants and are color-coded, as explained earlier in this chapter. BD Vacutainer® tubes, appropriate for venous blood collection from adults, have a solid cap, while those used for pediatric venous blood collection have a translucent cap. See Figure 7-30 for a comparison of adult and pediatric tube caps. Vacutainer® tubes containing a separator gel have a unique color to code them. For example, the cap on a Vacutainer® tube containing a clot activator is red, but the cap on a Vacutainer® tube containing a clot activator and separator gel is gold. Likewise, the cap on a Vacutainer® tube containing heparin is green, while the cap on a Vacutainer® tube containing heparin and a separator gel is light green. See Figure 7-31 for a comparison of these cap colors.

Greiner Bio-One

Greiner Bio-One manufactures equipment for blood and urine collection, including VACUETTE® tubes designed for venous blood collection (Figure 7-32) and MiniCollect® tubes designed for capillary blood collection (Figure 7-33). These tubes are available with various anticoagulants and are color-coded with

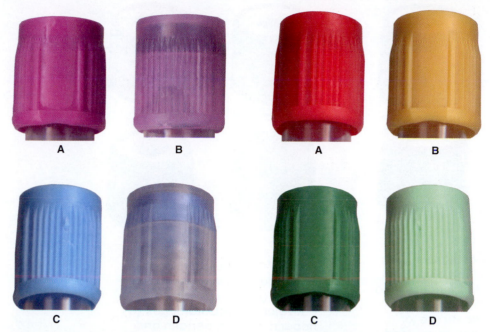

Figure 7-30 Becton Dickinson uses (A and C) solid colored caps to indicate use for adult venous blood collections and (B and D) translucent caps to indicate use for pediatric or difficult venous blood collections.

Figure 7-31 Becton Dickinson tube caps indicate the presence of (A) clot activator, (B) clot activator and separator gel, (C) heparin, and (D) heparin and separator gel.

similar colors as the BD brand tubes. VACUETTE® tubes have solid-colored tops regardless of amount of vacuum. Tubes appropriate for adult blood collection have a black ring on the cap top. Tubes appropriate for pediatric blood collection have a white ring on the cap top (Figure 7-34). VACUETTE® tubes with a separator gel use the same additive color code as the tubes without a separator gel but have a yellow ring on the cap top (Figure 7-35).

Sarstedt

Sarstedt manufactures diagnostic specimen collection equipment including the S-Monovette®, Microvette®, and Multivette® collection systems. S-Monovette® is a closed blood collection system that allows the user to collect venous

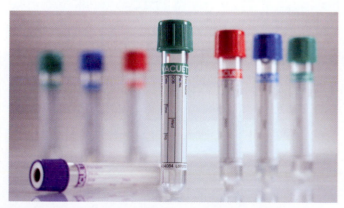

Figure 7-32 VACUETTE® tubes are part of the evacuated tube system that is manufactured by Greiner Bio-One.

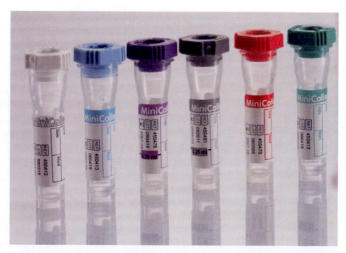

Figure 7-33 MiniCollect® tubes are microcollection containers manufactured by Greiner Bio-One.

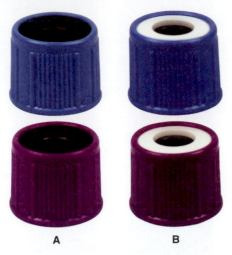

Figure 7-34 Greiner Bio-One uses (A) a black ring in tube caps to indicate use for adult venous blood collections and (B) a white ring in tube caps to indicate use for pediatric or difficult venous blood collections.

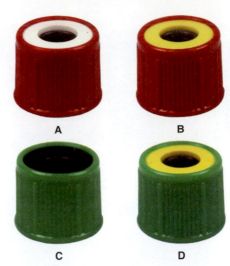

Figure 7-35 These Greiner Bio-One tube caps indicate the presence of (A) clot activator, (B) clot activator and separator gel, (C) heparin, and (D) heparin and separator gel.

blood by either syringe aspiration or the vacuum principle (Figure 7-36). S-Monovette® devices can be used like a syringe to better control vacuum pull or used like an evacuated tube if the plunger is pulled back and removed before blood collection. The S-Monovette® is color-coded to indicate the additive present. The color codes are similar to BD brand tubes. However, the cap on serum separator tubes is brown. The Microvette® enables blood sampling using either the capillary action principle or the gravity-flow principle, using the special rim (Figure 7-37). The Multivette® allows for the collection of both venous and capillary blood. For venous blood collection, a luer needle is connected to the capillary tube of the Multivette®, which automatically fills by normal venous pressure. Capillary blood is collected using the capillary tube (Figure 7-38).

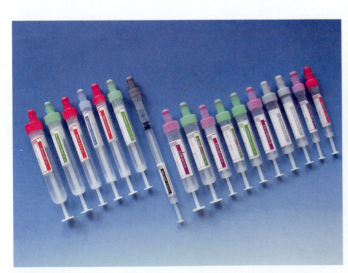

Figure 7-36 Sarstedt S-Monovette® closed blood collection system.

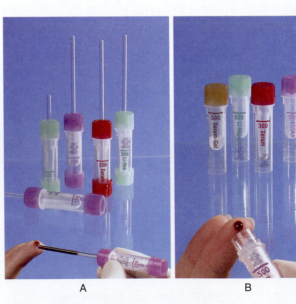

Figure 7-37 Sarstedt Microvette® tubes can be filled by (A) capillary action or (B) gravity fill.

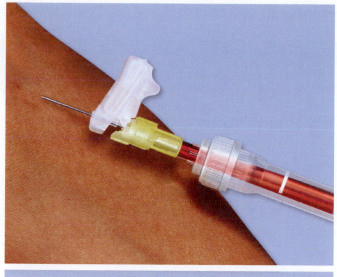
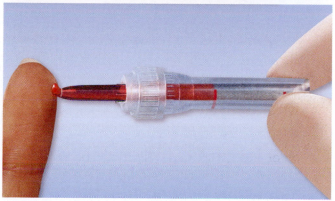

Figure 7-38 Sarstedt Multivette® can be used for small samples of venous blood or capillary blood.

1. How does Becton Dickinson indicate the difference between full volume (adult) evacuated tubes and small volume (pediatric) evacuated tubes? What about the presence of a separator gel in an evacuated tube?

2. How does Greiner Bio-One indicate the difference between full volume (adult) evacuated tubes and small volume (pediatric) evacuated tubes? What about the presence of a separator gel in an evacuated tube?

3. What is unique about the venous blood collection system manufactured by Sarstedt?

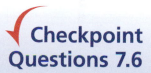 **Checkpoint Questions 7.6**

Chapter Summary

Learning Outcome	Key Concepts/Examples	Related NAACLS Competency
7.1 Select equipment used for both venipuncture and capillary puncture. Pages 170–175.	Common equipment and supplies needed for phlebotomy include gloves; alcohol prep pads; gauze pads; tissue warmers; adhesive bandages or tape; sharps container; permanent marker, pen, or computer labels; specimen transport bags; and evacuated tubes. Equipment is stored and transported on a tray or cart.	5.00, 5.5, 5.6
7.2 Select equipment specific for venipuncture procedures. Pages 175–183.	Phlebotomy equipment specific to venipuncture procedures includes tourniquets, needles or butterfly assemblies, evacuated tube holders or syringes, and evacuated tubes. The winged infusion set (butterfly assembly) includes a needle that has butterfly wings; short, thin tubing; and a place to attach a syringe or an evacuated tube holder for blood collection. The syringe set includes a needle and syringe, plus a transfer device for adding blood to the evacuated blood tubes. Evacuated tubes are a closed system of collection that allows for multiple tubes to be collected with one venipuncture. Evacuated tubes come with tops of different colors and with different additives and are designated for different tests based on their additives. Phlebotomists should be familiar with the tube color-coding system used at their facility.	5.5, 5.6
7.3 Select equipment specific for dermal/capillary puncture procedures. Pages 183–185.	Phlebotomy equipment specific to capillary/dermal puncture includes a lancet or puncture device and special microcollection tubes.	5.5
7.4 Identify the various types of additives and color-coding used in blood collection and explain the reasons for their use. Pages 185–191.	Additives used in blood collection containers are indicated by the color used in the tube closure. Commonly used additives and colors are nonadditive (white or clear with red center, depending on brand), citrate (blue), clot activator and gel (gold or red with yellow ring, depending on brand), heparin (green), EDTA (lavender), and potassium oxalate with fluoride (gray).	5.00, 5.1, 5.2
7.5 Implement the correct order of draw for venipuncture and capillary puncture procedures. Pages 191–194.	The order of the draw using the routine venipuncture procedure is dependent upon the facility's policies. An accepted order of draw may include a non-additive discard tube being collected first, followed by citrate tube, SST serum separator tube, heparin and heparinized plasma separator tubes, EDTA tube, and lastly sodium fluoride/potassium oxalate tube. Specimens requiring sterile blood collection procedures (blood cultures) must be drawn first, regardless of order of draw. Sterile tubes replace the discard tube in the order of draw using the evacuated tube system. The order in which blood is collected using evacuated tube systems is critical for avoiding contamination with interfering substances.	5.3, 5.4, 5.6
7.6 Compare blood collection equipment from various manufacturers. Pages 194–197.	Several companies manufacture blood collection equipment. The coding used to indicate additives and draw volumes vary among manufacturers. Phlebotomists must become familiar with the equipment used at their facilities.	5.2

Chapter Review

A: Labeling

Label the parts of this evacuated tube assembly.

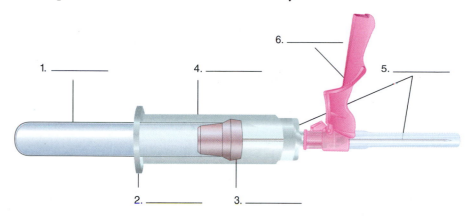

1. [LO 7.2] _____

2. [LO 7.2] _____

3. [LO 7.2] _____

4. [LO 7.2] _____

5. [LO 7.2] _____

6. [LO 7.2] _____

B: Matching

Match the items on the left with their descriptions.

____**7.** [LO 7.2] anticoagulant

____**8.** [LO 7.2] gauge

____**9.** [LO 7.2] winged infusion set

____**10.** [LO 7.2] evacuated tube

____**11.** [LO 7.2] evacuated tube holder

____**12.** [LO 7.2] safe needle device

a. covers the needle after specimen collection
b. plastic holder for both the needle and the blood collection tube
c. closed collection tube containing a premeasured vacuum
d. agent that prevents blood from clotting
e. also known as a butterfly needle
f. needle diameter or bore

C: Fill in the Blanks

Next to each additive listed on the left, write the colors of the tubes containing that additive on the right.

13. [LO 7.4] none _____

14. [LO 7.4] EDTA _____

15. [LO 7.4] sodium citrate _____

16. [LO 7.4] sodium fluoride/potassium oxalate _____

17. [LO 7.4] heparin (either sodium, lithium, or ammonium) _____

18. [LO 7.4] clot activator _____

19. [LO 7.4] thixotropic gel _____

D: Sequencing

For the following types of tubes to be drawn, indicate the correct order of draw (1 = first; 2 = second; and so on).

20. [LO 7.5] _____ light blue (coagulation)

21. [LO 7.5] _____ sterile specimens (blood cultures or yellow SPS tube)

22. [LO 7.5] _____ pink or lavender (EDTA)

23. [LO 7.5] _____ gold or red/black (SST)

24. [LO 7.5] _____ red plastic or glass (serum)

25. [LO 7.5] _____ green (heparin)

26. [LO 7.5] _____ gray (fluoride)

E: Case Studies/Critical Thinking

27. [LO 7.4] Your supervisor asks you to collect an EDTA sample on a patient waiting in the outpatient drawing room. Which tubes contain EDTA? How will you determine which tube to collect?

28. [LO 7.3] You are going to collect blood from an elderly person with fragile veins. What are your options for blood collection equipment in this case? What other things do you need to consider for your selection of equipment?

29. [LO 7.2, 7.3] A young child needs blood drawn for coagulation studies prior to going to surgery. What are your options for blood collection equipment? What are the concerns for order of draw?

30. [LO 7.4] While you are drawing blood on a patient, he asks why there are so many different colors of tubes. How would you respond to this question?

F: Exam Prep

Choose the best answer for each question.

31. [LO 7.1] The term *evacuated tube* refers to a venipuncture collection tube that

    a. does not contain a vacuum.

    b. contains a vacuum.

    c. does not contain an anticoagulant.

    d. contains an anticoagulant.

32. [LO 7.4] The purpose of an anticoagulant in a blood collection container is to

    a. decrease the chance of hemolysis.

    b. preserve the life span of red blood cells.

    c. prevent blood from clotting.

    d. produce serum for testing.

33. [LO 7.1] Needles used with evacuated tube systems have a (Choose all that apply)

   a. single point.
   b. double end.
   c. continuous shaft.
   d. rubber sleeve.

34. [LO 7.2] Syringes are used with which type of needle? (Choose all that apply.)

   a. Butterfly
   b. Double-ended
   c. Hypodermic
   d. Surgical

35. [LO 7.2] When performing a venipuncture on a patient with small veins, the best size of needle to use is

   a. 19-gauge.
   b. 20-gauge.
   c. 21-gauge.
   d. 22-gauge.

36. [LO 7.1] Gloves are *not* required while

   a. transporting specimens to the lab.
   b. performing a venipuncture.
   c. performing a capillary puncture.
   d. cleaning the venipuncture site.

37. [LO 7.3] The depth of a dermal puncture device is controlled during capillary collection in order to

   a. puncture an artery.
   b. control excessive clotting.
   c. avoid puncturing a bone.
   d. avoid bacterial contamination.

38. [LO 7.1] An alcohol prep pad is

   a. not an appropriate antiseptic to use in blood collection.
   b. a bacteriostatic preventing contamination of the puncture.
   c. saturated with a 70% iodine solution.
   d. used after the venipuncture to stop bleeding at the site.

39. [LO 7.4] A plastic red-topped tube contains

   a. an anticoagulant.
   b. an antiglycolytic agent.
   c. a clot activator.
   d. no additives.

40. [LO 7.4] A gray-topped tube contains

   a. an antiglycolytic agent.
   b. a clot activator.
   c. no additives.
   d. separator gel.

41. [LO 7.4] Blood specimens for coagulation testing are collected in _____ tubes.

   a. citrate
   b. EDTA
   c. fluoride
   d. heparin

42. [LO 7.4] EDTA is the anticoagulant found in _____ topped tubes. (Choose all that apply.)

   a. lavender
   b. pink
   c. tan
   d. white

43. [LO 7.4] Gel separation barriers are included in which tubes? (Choose all that apply.)

   a. Gold
   b. Light blue
   c. Light green
   d. Tan

44. [LO 7.4] Tubes with a gel separation barrier may also contain (Choose all that apply)

   a. heparin.
   b. EDTA.
   c. clot activator.
   d. citrate.

45. [LO 7.5] When collecting blood using a butterfly assembly, which tubes must have a discard tube drawn prior to their filling? (Choose all that apply.)

   a. Gray
   b. Lavender
   c. Royal blue
   d. Light blue

46. [LO 7.5] If gray, green, and lavender tubes are needed, the correct order of draw is

   a. green, lavender, gray.
   b. gray, lavender, green.
   c. lavender, gray, green.
   d. gray, green, lavender.

47. [LO 7.5] An erroneous coagulation test result was obtained on a specimen. What may have happened in the pre-examination phase of testing to cause this?

   a. The blue-topped tube was filled to capacity.

   b. A nonadditive tube was drawn before the blue-topped tube.

   c. The blue-topped tube was underfilled.

   d. The blue-topped tube was drawn before the lavender-topped tube.

48. [LO 7.5] To avoid contamination of sterile specimens,

   a. sterile tubes should be collected first.

   b. sterile tubes should be collected last.

   c. discard tubes should be collected before sterile tubes.

   d. blue-topped tubes should be collected before sterile tubes.

49. [LO 7.5] Interfering substances that may contaminate specimens for coagulation testing may be introduced into specimens EXCEPT when

   a. nonadditive tubes are collected first.

   b. fluoride tubes are collected first.

   c. heparin tubes are collected first.

   d. clot activator tubes are collected first.

50. [LO 7.6] Which tube would you use to collect a pediatric coagulation study?

   a. Translucent, lavender-topped tube

   b. Solid, light-green-topped tube

   c. Solid, blue-topped tube

   d. Translucent, blue-topped tube

51. [LO 7.6] You have to complete a difficult microcollection draw. Which of the following tubes would you most likely use?

   a. Greiner Bio-One black ring tube cap

   b. Becton Dickinson solid, blue-topped tube

   c. Greiner Bio-One white ring tube cap

   d. Sarstedt closed blood collection system

connect

Enhance your learning by completing these exercises and more at connect.mcgraw-hill.com.

References

Becton Dickinson. (2005). Components of the BC Vacutainer® SST tube. *Tech Talk*, 4(2). Retrieved January 15, 2011, from www.bd.com/vacutainer/pdfs/techtalk/TechTalk_November2005_VS7436.pdf

Becton Dickinson. (2007). Proper handling of BD Vacutainer® Plus citrate tubes. *Tech Talk*, 5(1). Retrieved January 15, 2011, from www.bd.com/vacutainer/pdfs/techtalk/BDVS-TechTalk-9947_D2.pdf

Becton Dickinson. (2008). *BC Vacutainer® venous blood collection tube guide.* Retrieved January 15, 2011, from www.bd.com/vacutainer/pdfs/plus_plastic_tubes_wallchart_tubeguide_VS5229.pdf

Clinical and Laboratory Standards Institute. (2007). *Procedures for the collection of diagnostic blood specimens by venipuncture; approved standard* (6th ed.). Wayne, PA. CLSI H3-A6. 27(26).

Emst. D. J., and Calam, R. C. (2004, May). *NACCLS simplifies the order of draw: a brief history.* MLO. 26–27.

Greiner Bio-One GmbH. (n.d.). *Vacuette® Preanalytics Manual.* Greiner Bio-One North America Inc.

Greiner Bio-One GmbH. (2012). *Vacuette® Preanalystics Catalog.* Retrieved July 21, 2013, from http://us.gbo.com/preanalytics/documents/?page=documents

National Accrediting Agency for Clinical Laboratory Sciences. (2010). *NAACLS entry-level phlebotomist competencies.* Rosemont, IL. NAACLS.

Sarstedt. (n.d.). *S-Monovette®: The enclosed blood collection system.* Sarstedt, Inc., North Carolina.

Wilson, D. D. (2008). *McGraw-Hill manual of laboratory and diagnostic tests.* New York: McGraw-Hill.

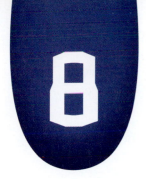

8

essential terms

antecubital
anticoagulant
aseptic
collapsed vein
concentric circles
ecchymosis
edematous
exsanguination
hematoma

hemoconcentration
iatrogenic anemia
lymphostasis
palpate
petechiae
sclerosis
syncope
venous reflux

Venipuncture

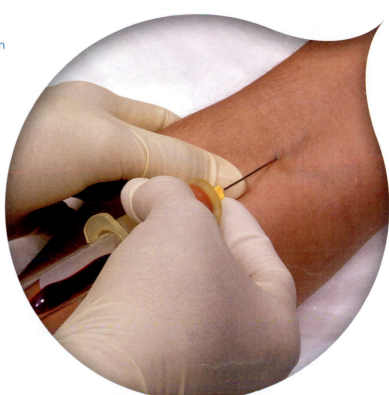

Learning Outcomes

8.1 Summarize the steps necessary to perform a competent/effective venipuncture.

8.2 Describe special procedures needed for venipuncture on difficult-to-draw veins.

8.3 Describe signs and symptoms of venipuncture complications.

Related NAACLS Competencies

5.00 Demonstrate knowledge of collection equipment, various types of additives used, special precautions necessary, and substances that can interfere in clinical analysis of blood constituents.

5.5 List and select the types of equipment needed to collect blood by venipuncture and capillary (dermal) puncture.

5.6 Identify special precautions necessary during blood collections by venipuncture and capillary (dermal) puncture.

6.00 Follow standard operating procedures to collect specimens.

6.1 Identify potential sites for venipuncture and capillary (dermal) puncture.

6.2 Differentiate between sterile and antiseptic techniques.

6.3 Describe and demonstrate the steps in the preparation of a puncture site.

6.4 List the effects of tourniquet, hand squeezing, and heating pads on specimens collected by venipuncture and capillary (dermal) puncture.

6.5 Recognize proper needle insertion and withdrawal techniques, including direction, angle, depth, and aspiration, for venipuncture.

6.7 Describe the limitations and precautions of alternate collection sites for venipuncture and capillary (dermal) puncture.

6.8 Explain the causes of phlebotomy complications.

6.9 Describe signs and symptoms of physical problems that may occur during blood collection.

6.10 List the steps necessary to perform a venipuncture and a capillary (dermal) puncture in order.

6.11 Demonstrate a successful venipuncture following standard operating procedures.

Introduction

Routine and difficult venipunctures are essential tasks for the phlebotomist. This chapter outlines the procedures for routine and difficult venipunctures as well as the complications that may occur during these procedures.

8.1 Venipuncture

Venipuncture is the most common technique for obtaining blood specimens. The routine venipuncture procedure consists of a series of detailed steps that must be performed safely and accurately. Follow the steps in Competency Check 8-1 when performing venipuncture.

Competency Check 8-1

Basic Blood Collection
1. Greet and properly identify the patient (chapter *Patient and Specimen Requirements*).
2. Select and assemble the appropriate equipment (chapter *Blood Collection Equipment*).
3. Use aseptic technique and Standard Precautions during venipuncture and blood specimen collection (chapter *Infection Control and Safety*).
4. Provide proper post-puncture patient care.
5. Adhere to specimen labeling requirements (chapter *Patient and Specimen Requirements*).
6. Correctly handle and transport specimens (chapter *Blood Specimen Handling.*

Assembling the Venipuncture Equipment

After you greet and properly identify the patient but before beginning a venipuncture, you must gather and assemble the equipment and supplies you need for the procedure (see Figure 8-1). As outlined in the chapter *Blood Collection Equipment*, a routine venipuncture requires the following items:

- Gloves
- Tourniquet
- Alcohol prep pads
- Gauze pads

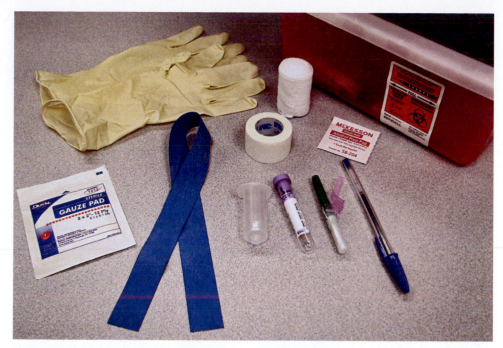

Figure 8-1 Assemble the equipment for venipuncture.

- Needle
- Evacuated tube holder or syringe
- Appropriate evacuated tubes
- Needle disposal (sharps) container
- Adhesive bandage or tape
- Permanent marker, pen, or computer labels

Line up the venipuncture equipment needed for the procedure near the patient, by having the phlebotomy cart or tray placed next to the patient's bed. Attach the needle into the tube adapter and make sure that the needle-tube adapter assembly is secure. As many different manufacturers make venipuncture equipment, check to see if the tube adapter and needle are compatible. Sometimes needles and tube adapters that are made by different companies are not interchangeable. Using holders and needles from different manufacturers may cause the needle to fall out of the holder.

Make sure that the needle is screwed all the way up to the tube adapter. DO NOT remove the needle cap at this time. The first tube to be collected may be placed loosely into the tube holder/adapter. Push the tube up to the adapter guideline or indentation in the tube adapter, but DO NOT push the tube all the way onto the needle because this will result in a loss of vacuum in the tube (see Figure 8-2). Always check the directions of the equipment you are using and follow your facility's guidelines and standard operating procedures.

Keep the Needle Sterile

The needle must not touch anything. If you touch or lay the unsheathed needle down for any reason, it becomes contaminated and a new needle must be used in its place. In addition, you must ensure that the needle safety label was not broken and that the expiration date on the label has not passed. Never use needles that have uncertain sterility.

Safety & Infection Control

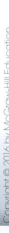

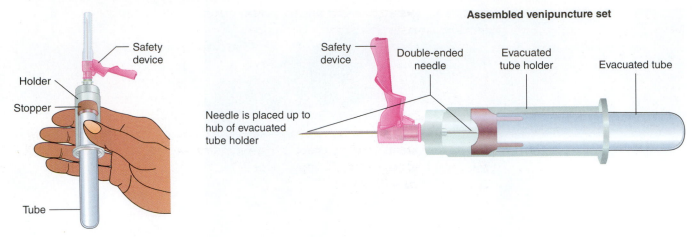

Assembled venipuncture set

Safety device

Holder

Stopper

Tube

Safety device

Double-ended needle

Evacuated tube holder

Evacuated tube

Needle is placed up to hub of evacuated tube holder

Figure 8-2 Complete venipuncture assembly.

Patient Positioning

The patient's position is another critical factor for a successful venipuncture. The patient should be either lying down or sitting in a special phlebotomy chair designed for outpatients. Most phlebotomy chairs have a movable arm support that helps in positioning the patient's arm (see Figure 8-3). Never attempt a phlebotomy procedure with a patient standing. This is not only uncomfortable for the patient but also dangerous if he or she should become dizzy or faint and be injured in a fall. A stool is not acceptable either because it is too unstable.

Not all phlebotomy locations have a specially designed phlebotomy chair. If a phlebotomy chair is not available, a phlebotomy procedure can still be performed. A straight chair with an arm is preferable to a chair without arms. The arm of the chair will help support the patient's arm during the procedure. If only an armless chair is available, the patient will need to place his or her arm on the thigh for proper support during the procedure. If an armless chair is used, the phlebotomist should position the chair against a wall or some other stable object. If the patient were to faint, the phlebotomist could then push the patient against the wall to keep him or her from falling out of the chair. If necessary, a pillow or rolled up towel placed under the patient's arm can be used to position the arm. When the patient is seated, the arm needs to be supported and should extend downward in a straight line from the shoulder to the wrist. The arm should not be bent at the elbow.

Inpatients, on the other hand, are usually in their hospital beds for the phlebotomy procedure. The supine position, with the patient lying on the back, face upward, is the most common for phlebotomy. The patient's arm should be extended in a straight line from the shoulder and not bent. A rolled towel or pillow can be used to support the arm and aid in positioning it in a downward fashion. Hyperextending the elbow slightly can help the phlebotomist locate a vein.

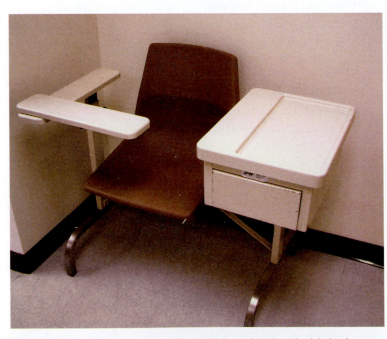

Figure 8-3 The arm supports on this outpatient phlebotomy chair are designed for the comfort and correct positioning of the patient during outpatient phlebotomy procedures.

Hospital Bedrails

Bedrails are a major concern when performing venipuncture in a hospital situation. If you lower the bedrail for a procedure, you must raise it before leaving the room. Leaving a bedrail down increases the risk of a patient falling out of bed.

Areas Not Designed for Blood Collection

In most cases, you will be drawing blood in outpatient and inpatient facilities that are designed for blood collection, and the necessary materials will be at hand. In some cases, phlebotomists are asked to draw blood in a location not typically used for blood collection, such as a person's home. Organization is key to safety in these environments. Consider using the 1-2-3-2-1 method to ensure you are set for the procedure:

1—pair of gloves

2—tourniquet and alcohol swab

3—needle, holder, and tubes (in the order to be drawn)

2—gauze/cotton swab and bandage

1—sharps container

Making sure you have each of these pieces of equipment in this order will ensure that you are prepared. Also, be certain to have additional tubes and needles available and close by in case you need them during the procedure.

Applying the Tourniquet

Placing a tourniquet on the arm makes the veins more visible and will help you decide which vein to use. When a tourniquet is applied, the flow of venous blood is slowed, which increases pressure in the veins, making them more visible and palpable (noticeable by touch). Application of a tourniquet makes it easier to feel, or **palpate,** the vein for possible venipuncture.

A tourniquet is applied to the arm 3 to 4 inches above the venipuncture site, which is usually inside the elbow in the antecubital fossa (around the crease of the elbow). The tourniquet should not pinch the patient's skin, but it should feel slightly tight. However, it should not be so tight that the arm goes numb or turns colors. To maintain the best possible comfort level for the patient, avoid twisting the tourniquet. A twisted tourniquet will pinch and feel as if it is digging into the patient's arm, causing unnecessary discomfort and pain. Thus, the tourniquet should be kept flat against the arm (see Figure 8-4). If a patient has delicate or sensitive skin, place the tourniquet over his or her sleeve. If a patient with fragile skin is wearing a shirt without sleeves, place a hand towel or washcloth over the skin; then place the tourniquet over the towel to reduce the risk of tearing the skin or creating any damage to the patient's arm. Proper application of the tourniquet—as

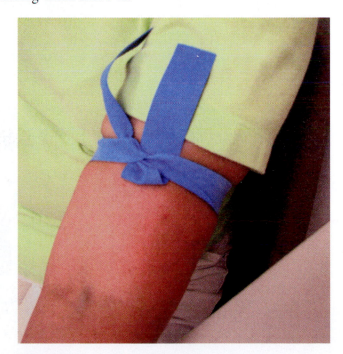

Figure 8-4 Tourniquet on arm.

seen in Competency Check 8-2—will help ensure success and prevent complications during venipuncture. Left-handed phlebotomists may prefer to switch the "left and right" positions in this sequence.

Tourniquet Application

1. Position the tourniquet under the arm while grasping the ends above the arm and venipuncture area.

2. Cross the left end over the right end and apply a small amount of tension to the tourniquet by pulling on each half of the tourniquet.

3. Grasp both ends of the tourniquet close to the patient's arm between the thumb and forefinger of the left hand.

4. Using the right middle finger or index finger, tuck the left end under the right end. The loose end of the tourniquet will be pointing toward the shoulder and the loop will be pointed toward the hand (see Figure 8-5).

5. When tugged after the venipuncture procedure, the loose end will easily release the tourniquet from the arm.

Selecting the Venipuncture Site

The most common area to perform a venipuncture is the inside of the elbow, or **antecubital** area of the arm (see Figure 8-6). This is the area on the inside bend of the elbow where the median cubital, cephalic, and basilic veins lie close to the surface of the arm (see the figure of *commonly used arm veins* in the chapter *The Cardiovascular System*). Locate the median cubital vein, which is usually the largest and best-anchored vein, near the center of the antecubital area. This vein is usually preferred for venipuncture. The cephalic vein or basilic vein may also be used for venipuncture. Always examine the antecubital area first because the easiest veins to collect from are located in this area of the arm. Patients generally have more prominent veins on their dominant arm. For example, if the patient is left-handed, look for a vein in the left arm first. You should check and palpate both arms before deciding on the venipuncture site.

To help you locate veins, position the arm at a downward angle, using the force of gravity as an aid in making the veins more prominent. In addition, instruct the patient to make a fist, but NOT to pump the fist because this can cause **hemoconcentration** (temporary increase in cells and chemicals

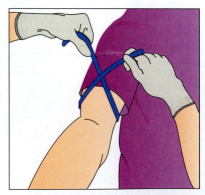

A Position the tourniquet under the arm while grasping the ends above the arm and venipuncture area. The tourniquet should be 3 to 4 inches above the site.

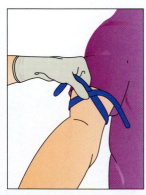

B Cross the left end over the right end and apply a small amount of tension to the tourniquet.

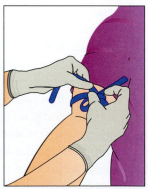

C Using the right middle finger or index finger, tuck the left end under the right end.

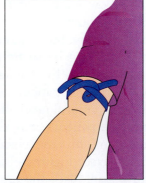

D A loose end of the tourniquet will be pointing toward the shoulder and the loop will be pointed toward the hand.

Figure 8-5 Follow these steps for proper tourniquet application.

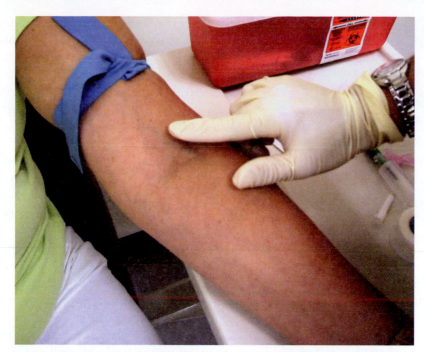

Figure 8-6 The antecubital area of the arm is the most common site to perform venipuncture.

in the blood). If increasing the vein size is necessary to make the venipuncture easier, apply heat by using a moist compress at or near body temperature (37° C) for 3 to 5 minutes (Figure 8-7). A tissue warmer may also be used for warming a venipuncture site because it reaches a temperature of 40° C when activated. Warming the venipuncture site will dilate the veins and increase the blood flow and can be used only when necessary.

Keeping the Arm Still

Patient Education & Communication

If the patient moves during the venipuncture procedure, the needle can "tear" the vein and muscle, causing pain and damage to the venipuncture site. If a patient moves during phlebotomy, the phlebotomist could miss the venipuncture site and fail to collect the blood specimen. While you are selecting the venipuncture site, explain to the patient the importance of holding the arm very still, but do not alarm the patient by telling him or her too many details. Tell the patient that holding the arm still will reduce the discomfort of the venipuncture. If the patient has anxiety over having blood drawn, help him or her relax by focusing the conversation on calming topics and get assistance to hold the arm if necessary.

Palpating the antecubital area will help you determine the vein's size, depth, and direction. Palpate the vein using the tip of the index finger. Select a vein that is large and does not roll from side to side or move easily. The larger the vein, the easier the blood collection. It is common to feel for the bulge of the vein, but try feeling for the valley instead of the bulge. Try closing your eyes if you have trouble feeling a vein, as this will enhance your sense of touch. An appropriate vein for venipuncture will bounce and have resilience to it. A vein that exhibits **sclerosis,** or feels hard and cordlike (i.e., lacks resilience), should be avoided. A vein that feels hard tends to roll easily and should not be used for venipuncture. In addition, paralyzed limbs and sites with shunts and fistulas should be avoided.

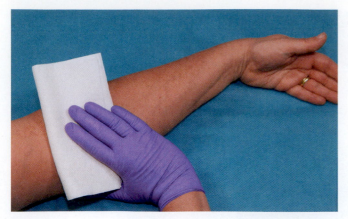

Figure 8-7 Warming the site is the preferred way to increase blood flow and make the venipuncture easier.

Carefully select the vein to be used for venipuncture. Try to mentally visualize the location of this vein and note the position of the vein in reference to hair, skin creases, scars, or a mole. Once a vein has been selected, release the tourniquet to lessen the chance of causing hemoconcentration in the venipuncture area during the cleansing procedure. Mentally visualizing the vein will help you locate the vein after releasing the tourniquet. You must clean the skin before venipuncture, and having a landmark will help you locate the selected site again. An experienced phlebotomist, who is able to identify the venipuncture site quickly and easily, may choose to apply the tourniquet, clean the area, and perform the venipuncture all in one step. This is only done if the venipuncture site is dry before the blood is collected and the tourniquet stays on the arm less than 1 minute. Meeting these two conditions is difficult, especially for the new phlebotomist.

As you may recall from the chapter *The Cardiovascular System*, arteries should never be selected for a routine venipuncture procedure. Because arteries are usually located much deeper than veins, you probably will not encounter them. However, you need to be aware of the differences between an artery and a vein. Arteries are more elastic and have thicker walls than veins. In addition, arteries will pulsate when palpated.

Tendons can also be mistaken for veins, although tendons do not have the elastic feel of veins and are hard and stringy to the touch. To differentiate between a vein and a tendon, have the patient rotate his or her wrist. The tendon will move with the muscle movement, but the vein should still be in nearly the same place and remain easy to feel.

If no acceptable vein is available in the antecubital area of both arms, remove the tourniquet and check the dorsal side of the wrist or hand for acceptable venipuncture sites (see the figure of *veins in the back of the hand* in the chapter *The Cardiovascular System*). Dorsal veins in the back of the hand may be used only if necessary. Veins on the anterior side of the wrist and hand are never used for venipuncture because of their close proximity to nerves and the risk of causing nerve damage. Ankle veins are not used for venipuncture by the phlebotomist.

Critical Thinking

Special Considerations When Selecting a Venipuncture Site

The venipuncture site should be free of lesions, abrasions, and scar tissue. Never select an arm that is **edematous,** or swollen. Because of the fluid buildup in the tissue, the vein will not be prominent. If you apply a tourniquet, it will not be effective in showing the vein and it will leave an indentation on the arm. If the patient has an IV in place, perform the venipuncture procedure on the other arm. Venipuncture should never be performed above the IV site. If a specimen is collected above an IV, the fluid given through the IV will affect the laboratory results. However, if no other site is available, drawing a blood sample below an IV site is acceptable. The arm on the side of a mastectomy (breast removal) should also be avoided because of the potential harm to the patient due to lymphostasis. **Lymphostasis,** or lack of fluid drainage in the lymphatic system, commonly occurs in patients who have had lymph nodes removed, such as during a mastectomy.

Special Considerations for Children

Just as adults can become anxious during a phlebotomy procedure, so can children—perhaps even more so. When greeting the child, phlebotomists can squat down to the child's height to reduce any intimidation the child is feeling. Never lie to children. If they ask if the procedure will hurt, respond that it will hurt a little but can hurt less if they hold absolutely still.

A good practice is to ask the child's caregiver to help with the procedure. Sometimes the parent has brought a small toy that the child can hold. This will help take the child's mind off the procedure and make the phlebotomy process easier for you. Special restraining chairs and arm boards are available to help immobilize children. If specimens from children are routinely collected, it is a good idea to have special bandages or stickers available as rewards for good helpers. Being honest and direct with the child is best; however, the child should be allowed to view the needle for as short a period as possible to help reduce anxiety.

A winged infusion set or butterfly with pediatric tubes may be used for dorsal venipuncture. Hand veins are delicate and small, so the smaller vacuum tubes, such as those for pediatric use, may be best for this procedure. The air in the tubing of the butterfly set can decrease the amount of blood obtained, so a smaller needle and adapter are preferred over the butterfly set.

Veins in the hand tend to move, or "roll." To avoid this, ask the patient to help by positioning the hand downward to hold the vein taut. Then place the thumb of the nonsticking hand about 1 to 2 inches below the insertion site. Apply pressure on the vein and pull slightly downward.

Standard Precautions

As emphasized in the *Infection Control and Safety* chapter, phlebotomists must be aware that any patient may be a carrier of an infectious disease. Always adhere to Standard Precautions when collecting blood by venipuncture, dermal puncture, or venous access devices. Your attention to detail can prevent the transfer of an infectious disease from patient to patient or from the patient to yourself.

Special Geriatric Considerations

The process of aging presents physical problems that can be challenging for the phlebotomist. Physical conditions such as arthritis and diseases that cause tremors require the phlebotomist to take extra time with the patient. Because the skin of an elderly person is thinner, the venipuncture can be more difficult. The phlebotomist must hold the skin down taut, so that the vein does not move or roll. Also, as people age, the muscles become smaller, so the angle of venipuncture should be shallow during needle insertion.

Cleansing the Venipuncture Site

After the venipuncture site is identified, the tourniquet is released and the site is cleansed using **aseptic** technique (a procedure for minimizing contamination by pathogens). Cleaning the venipuncture site with an antiseptic (alcohol pad) helps prevent microbial contamination of the specimen and the patient's venipuncture site. However, it will not sterilize or remove all the microorganisms from the site. *Sterile* puncture is discussed in the *Special Phlebotomy Procedures* chapter.

For routine puncture, the recommended antiseptic is 70% isopropyl alcohol—the kind used in alcohol pads. Cleanse the site by using **concentric circles**. Start the circular motion at the center of the selected site and move outward in an ever-widening circle. See Figure 8-8. To remove surface dirt, you must apply sufficient pressure. If the site is especially dirty, repeat the procedure (with a new alcohol pad) to ensure that the site is thoroughly clean. Allow the alcohol to dry completely. The drying action of the alcohol dries out the cells of bacteria. Never blow on the site or fan it to hasten the drying process.

Safety & Infection Control

Concentric Circles

Rubbing an antiseptic back and forth over a puncture site may bring bacteria from areas distal to (away from) the site and deposit them on the site of blood collection. Drawing concentric circles with the antiseptic, from the center-point outward, pushes microorganisms farther and farther away from the puncture site.

Law & Ethics

Use of Alcohol

If the venipuncture is attempted before the alcohol dries, it can result in a burning sensation for the patient when the needle enters the skin. The patient may perceive this as an injury incurred by the procedure. In addition, if alcohol enters the needle and becomes mixed with the specimen, the specimen will be hemolyzed and the laboratory results will be affected. In this case the patient will be subjected to another blood collection unnecessarily.

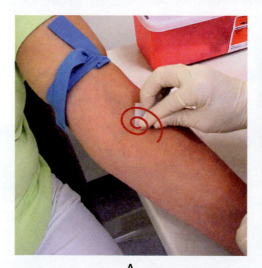
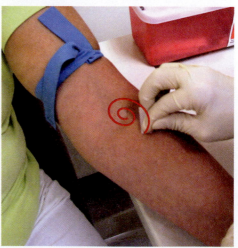

A   B

Figure 8-8 When cleaning the venipuncture site, (A) use an alcohol prep pad with firm pressure and (B) move outward in concentric circles.

Performing the Venipuncture

Verifying the Venipuncture Site

After reapplying the tourniquet, have the patient make a fist again to help with visualization of the vein. Using the dominant hand, pick up the venipuncture assembly with the thumb on the top of the tube adapter and the fingers underneath. Remove the needle cover and visually inspect the needle tip. Look for obstructions, imperfections, or barbs along the needle shaft and needle tip. If you notice abnormalities, the needle must be replaced with a new sterile needle. While inspecting the needle, note the bevel area (slanted opening at the tip of the needle) and position the bevel up. Positioning the needle bevel upward will make it easier to insert the needle into the skin and will cause less pain to the patient. In addition, if you position the bevel down, skin cells at the puncture site can only enter the needle, thus increasing the chance of contamination of the specimen. Hold the adapter assembly so that the needle is at a 30-degree angle to the vein. This angle may be less for veins lying close to the surface.

Inserting the Needle

Use the thumb of your nondominant hand (the one not holding the assembly) to pull the skin taut 1 to 2 inches below the needle insertion site while gently grasping the patient's arm. Holding the patient's arm will help anchor the arm and the vein. Pulling the skin taut will also help anchor the vein, keeping it from rolling or moving during insertion of the needle. For a successful venipuncture, line up the needle with the vein, so that the needle's position is the same as the vein's position (see Figure 8-9). Make sure the bevel of the needle is facing you, upward, while pointing in the same direction as the vein. To avoid startling the patient, warn the patient when the puncture is about to occur. Reminding the patient to remain very still and saying something like "You may feel a pinch now" will allow the patient to get ready.

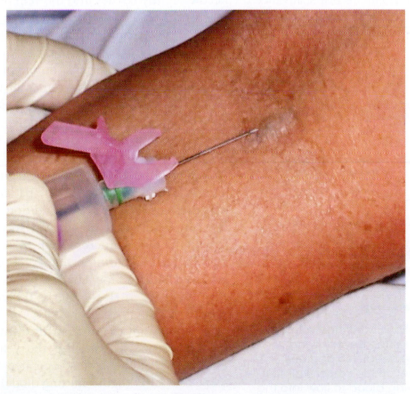

Figure 8-9 Align the needle with the chosen vein. Make sure the bevel is facing up.

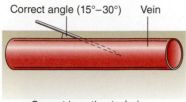

Correct angle (15°–30°)　　Vein

Correct insertion technique
(Blood flows freely into needle)

Figure 8-10 Insert the needle at a 15- to 30-degree angle.

Using one smooth motion, insert the needle into the skin at a 15- to 30-degree angle (see Figure 8-10). You will feel a decrease in resistance or a slight "pop" when the needle enters the vein. Fully engage the evacuated tube by pushing on it, causing the needle to puncture the tube's stopper. The first sign of a successful venipuncture is blood in the evacuated tube, after the tube is completely inserted.

If the Venipuncture Is Not Successful

In some cases, the venipuncture is not successful. However, failure to obtain a blood specimen can be remedied by various techniques. It is important to note that insufficient vacuum in the tube can cause blood collection failure. Because there is no way to check tube vacuum before a venipuncture, always keep an extra tube close at hand. If the needle position appears correct, a loss of tube vacuum is the most likely reason for the failure of blood to appear in the tube. Replace the defective tube with another tube.

Law & Ethics

Number of Attempts

Each healthcare facility has its own policy regarding the number of times a phlebotomist may attempt to get a blood specimen. Generally, two is the maximum number of times venipuncture should be attempted. If you are unsuccessful after two tries, you need to ask for assistance. Repeated, unnecessary needlesticks can cause damage to the patient. You can be held personally liable if you fail to follow your institution's policies and patient injury occurs as a result.

If you still cannot obtain a blood specimen, reposition the needle by pulling back slightly. The bevel may be against the wall of the vein, stopping the blood flow. If no blood flows, advance the needle slightly farther into the vein because the needle may not have penetrated the vein wall. If the needle is over halfway into the patient's arm, pull the needle back slowly until it is positioned inside the vein and blood begins to enter the tube. The needle can penetrate too far into the vein and exit beyond the vein wall to the other side. Problematic needle positions are shown in Figure 8-11. Applying the tourniquet too tightly can also stop blood flow, so try releasing the tourniquet slightly.

Never probe the site with the needle. This is extremely painful to the patient and may cause tissue damage. In addition, probing may result in a hemolyzed specimen. Probing is much different than repositioning the needle. During probing, the needle is moved back and forth or side to side in an effort to hit a vein. It is better to try another site rather than probe.

You may want to use an instrument, such as a venoscope, to visualize the vein (see Figure 8-12). The battery-operated venoscope uses LED (light-emitting diode) lights to illuminate the subcutaneous tissue and highlight the veins that absorb the light.

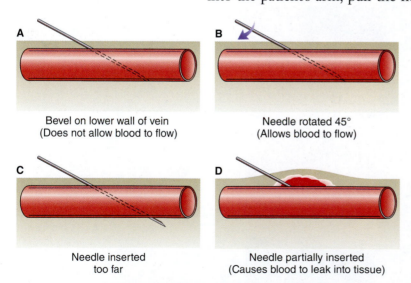

A　Bevel on lower wall of vein (Does not allow blood to flow)

B　Needle rotated 45° (Allows blood to flow)

C　Needle inserted too far

D　Needle partially inserted (Causes blood to leak into tissue)

Figure 8-11 Problematic needle positions within the vein: (A) blood may not flow into the needle if the bevel is lying against the vessel wall; (B) rotating the needle 45 degrees (a quarter of a turn) will move the bevel off the vessel wall so it is open to the lumen of the vein, allowing blood to flow into the needle; (C) the needle is inserted too far; and (D) the needle is partially inserted, causing a hematoma.

Collecting the Specimen

It is important to hold the venipuncture assembly steady during the entire tube-filling procedure (see Figure 8-13). Grasp the flange (short wings) of the tube holder with your index and middle fingers. Use your thumb to push the tube to the end of the adapter. If the needle is properly positioned in the vein, blood will flow freely into the evacuated tube. During the filling process, keep the needle as motionless as possible. Some phlebotomists release the tourniquet once collection has started; others wait until the entire draw is finished to ensure that there is no **venous reflux** (backflow). Either way is acceptable. However, many practicing phlebotomists would suggest releasing the tourniquet when the last tube is about one-half full. A tourniquet should not be left on the patient during specimen collection for longer than 1 minute. If blood flow stops once you release the tourniquet, you may reapply the tourniquet and leave it on for three or four tubes (approximately 1 minute). The reapplying of a tourniquet is difficult without help. If you are using an elastic strip, you would need both hands to reapply it.

Collection tubes are filled according to the order of draw outlined in the *Blood Collection Equipment* chapter. Continue filling the evacuated tube until the blood flow stops inside the tube. Blood flow will stop once the vacuum is gone from inside the evacuated tube. The amount of vacuum inside each tube has been designed so that a consistent amount of blood is drawn into each evacuated tube. Overfilling an evacuated tube is not possible unless the stopper is removed and blood is added. Never remove a tube cap to fill a tube or force blood through the cap with a syringe assembly. Always use a syringe transfer device. Underfilling an evacuated tube is possible if it is removed from the assembly before it is completely filled. When an evacuated tube is full, the proper dilution or mixture of additive to blood has been achieved. Overfilling and underfilling change the ratio of blood to anticoagulant required not only to keep the blood anticoagulated but also to maintain the ratio required for laboratory tests.

To change tubes during collection, brace your thumb against the flange of the holder and use a pulling motion while removing the tube (see Figure 8-14).

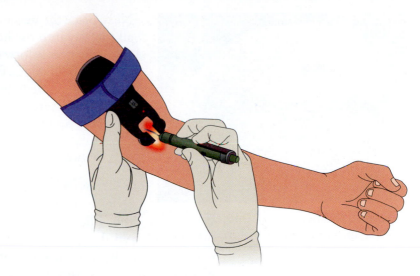

Figure 8-12 A venoscope uses a high intensity light to make the veins of the arm easier to locate.

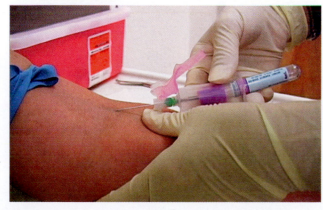

Figure 8-13 Hold the assembly steady while collecting the blood. Do not leave the tourniquet on for more than 1 minute.

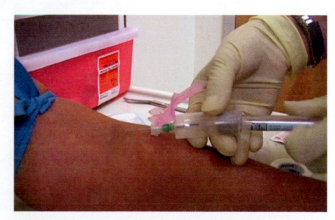

Figure 8-14 Hold the needle steady while removing and replacing tubes during the blood collection.

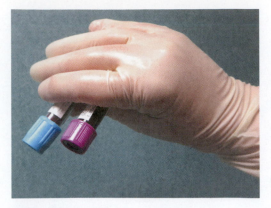

Figure 8-15 When necessary, mix the specimen by inversion.

Next, place the new tube into the holder and gently push the tube all the way into the holder and onto the needle. Take care not to move the needle forward or pull the needle out of the patient's arm during tube changes. Fill all necessary tubes for the tests requested. Mix them immediately the number of times recommended by the manufacturer, usually as determined by the additives inside each tube and the type of container (vacuum or microcollection). Most tubes with additives need to be gently inverted 3 to 10 times (see Figure 8-15).

Removing the Needle

Release the tourniquet at this point, if you did not do so during tube filling. Remove the last tube from the holder and, with your other hand, fold the gauze in half or in quarters; then gently place it directly over the area where the needle enters the skin. Do not apply pressure on the gauze or skin because this will cause pain to the patient before and during needle removal. Using one smooth motion and maintaining a 15- to 30-degree angle, withdraw the needle from the patient's arm. Engage the safety mechanism as the needle is withdrawn. Exact timing for engaging the safety mechanism depends on the manufacturer's recommendations (see Figure 8-16).

Immediately apply gentle pressure to the site for 3 to 5 minutes, or until bleeding stops. The arm should remain straight (not bent at the elbow) to prevent ecchymosis and hematoma formation. **Ecchymosis** is bruising or discoloration caused by blood seeping beneath the skin, and it can spread over a large area. A **hematoma** is a bloody mass that forms when blood seeping beneath the skin remains localized to the immediate area.

Be sure to instruct the patient not to disturb the platelet plug that is forming at the venipuncture site. It is common for a patient to want to bend the arm after needle removal, but tell the patient not to bend the arm upward. Bending the arm may cause bruising. The patient should not touch, blot, or wipe the venipuncture site. Have the patient gently press on the gauze while you are labeling the specimens. Ensure that bleeding has stopped before leaving the patient.

If pressure is not applied to the venipuncture site after removing the needle, a hematoma may form. If the tourniquet is left on and the needle is removed, blood will be forced out of the hole the needle left into the

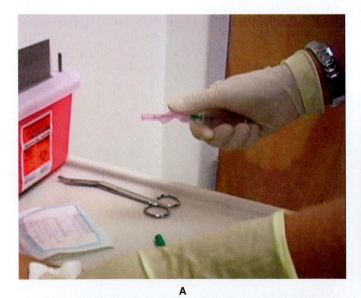

A

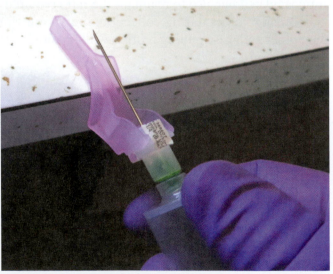

B

Figure 8-16 While holding pressure to the puncture site, engage the needle safety mechanism immediately using the manufacturer's instructions. For example, use (A) your thumb or (B) the edge of a table.

surrounding tissue and into the layer of skin, resulting in a hematoma. Some patients may be on **anticoagulants** (substances that slow the process of clotting, erroneously referred to as blood thinners) and will bleed for a longer time than other patients. Do not leave the patient if bleeding has not stopped; and do not let outpatients leave if the puncture site is still bleeding.

After the Venipuncture

A few more steps are needed to complete the phlebotomy procedure. A phlebotomist's first responsibility is to the patient. You may ask the patient to hold pressure on the gauze while you are completing the final tasks. Make sure the patient is comfortable with holding pressure on the venipuncture site (see Figure 8-17). If the patient is unable to hold pressure, you should do so until the bleeding stops. Then proceed to disposing of the needle and labeling the specimen. Apply a bandage to the venipuncture site after all tubes are labeled and bleeding has stopped. Documenting specimen collection and delivering the specimen to the appropriate laboratory section are the final steps in the phlebotomy process.

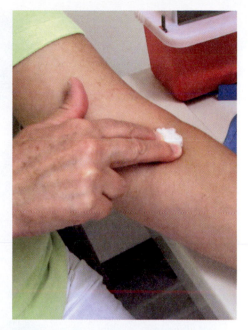

Figure 8-17 Have the patient apply firm pressure to the venipuncture site.

Disposing of the Equipment

The current Needlestick Prevention Act requires that the needle and adapter be disposed of as one unit. Do not unscrew the needle from the adapter to discard it. Keep your opposite hand and arm back and away from the contaminated needle and drop the needle and adapter assembly into the sharps container (Figure 8-18). Never place your hand inside the sharps container.

Sharps containers should be made of a puncture-resistant material and display the biohazard symbol. Pay close attention when disposing of sharp materials. Never overfill the sharps container. Once the sharps container is two-thirds to three-fourths full, put the lid on tightly and place the container in an appropriate biohazard box for disposal, or follow the specific policy at your facility. Remember to check the sharps container before the blood collection procedure so that you are not left with a contaminated needle and no place to discard it. The sooner a contaminated needle enters the sharps container, the less chance of an accidental needlestick.

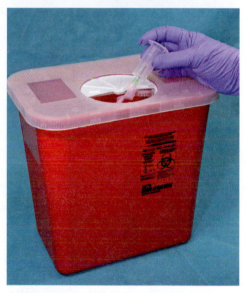

Figure 8-18 Carefully dispose of the needle and adapter in the sharps container.

Labeling the Specimen

As discussed in the chapter *Patient and Specimen Requirements*, all specimens must be labeled properly before leaving the patient's room or blood collection area or before allowing an outpatient to leave. Properly labeled collection tubes include the patient's full name, medical record number, date, time of collection, and your initials or employee ID code (see Figure 8-19).

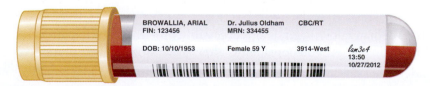

BROWALLIA, ARIAL   Dr. Julius Oldham   CBC/RT
FIN: 123456   MRN: 334455

DOB: 10/10/1953   Female 59 Y   3914-West   lam3e4
                                                           13:50
                                                            10/27/2012

Figure 8-19 Properly labeled collection tubes include the patient's full name, medical record number, date, the time of collection, and your initials or employee ID code.

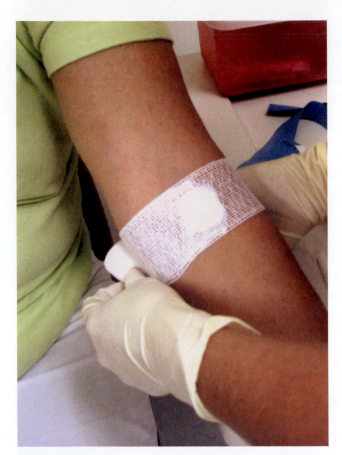

Applying the Bandage

First check the patient's arm to verify that bleeding has stopped. At a minimum, bleeding usually stops after 3 minutes. This is approximately the time it takes to properly label the specimen tubes and dispose of the used needle. Discard the gauze pad and apply a new gauze pad by folding it in half or quarters, placing it on the site, and applying an adhesive bandage or paper tape over the folded gauze. The patient can remove the bandage after 15 minutes. If the patient is allergic to bandages or tape, the patient may apply pressure for a while longer, and paper tape may be placed over the gauze. Other options include wrapping roller gauze completely around the arm or applying a Coban® (elastic) dressing (see Figure 8-20); however, some facilities do not use Coban® on acute (inpatient) collections. If the patient is elderly and the skin tends to tear when tape or bandages are applied, hold pressure a little longer to ensure that bleeding has stopped. To prevent injury, do not use tape on anyone with thin or fragile skin. Notify the patient's healthcare provider, so that he or she can recheck the venipuncture site. Pressure to the venipuncture site should never be removed until bleeding has stopped—not just on the surface but at the vein level. Bleeding may no longer be present on the skin, but this does not mean that a clot has completely formed in the vein. Once a clot has formed, no bandage is needed. Although a bandage is recommended in most cases, it is the patient's decision as to whether one is applied. Keep in mind that small bandages are not recommended for small children, who may choke on or swallow them.

Figure 8-20 Apply a bandage to the site to avoid disturbing the platelet plug and causing further bleeding.

Next, properly put away and dispose of all other supplies and equipment used in the venipuncture procedure. Place the unused evacuated tubes back in their proper places. Dispose of used alcohol pads, dirty gauze, trash from the needle assembly, and adhesive bandages in the trash receptacle. Remove and dispose of gloves in the biohazard trash receptacle or regular trash, depending on your facility's policy, and wash your hands. Thank the patient and leave the phlebotomy area as it was before the procedure.

If an inpatient specimen was collected, replace the bedrail in the same position as it was before the procedure. Move any other items you may have moved for the venipuncture procedure back into their original place. Dispose of non-sharp, noncontaminated items in the patient's trash can, but any tubes or glass slides must be disposed of properly in the laboratory. Thank the patient and, if the door was closed when you entered, close the door when you exit. Use the competency checklist *Routine Venipuncture (Evacuated Tube System)* at the end of this chapter to review and practice the procedure.

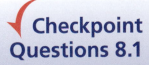

Checkpoint Questions 8.1

1. If the median cubital vein is not accessible on either of the patient's arms, which veins might you consider as alternative sites for venipuncture?
2. Under what circumstances should you avoid using adhesive bandages or tape to bandage a patient's arm?
3. What is the difference between repositioning a needle and probing?

8.2 Difficult Blood Draws

Although routine venipuncture using evacuated tubes and tube holder is the most commonly used procedure for obtaining blood specimens, situations will arise that require the use of alternate blood collection methods. Patients may have very small or difficult-to-access veins or have a condition that causes uncontrollable tremors or shaking. Or the patients may be children who have a difficult time keeping still. Blood collection in these situations often requires the use of a butterfly needle and either an evacuated tube adapter or a syringe.

Butterfly Needle Set

The butterfly needle set, or winged infusion set, has been reported to be less painful to patients. However, the use of the butterfly needle set results in more accidental needlesticks. Thus, the butterfly needle set should only be chosen when a standard venipuncture cannot be performed. Figure 8-21 shows one type of butterfly assembly. Butterfly needle sizes range from 21- to 25-gauge in diameter and ½ to ¾ inch in length. Butterfly needles may be used with either evacuated tubes or syringes. Figure 8-22 shows a blood collection using the butterfly assembly with an evacuated tube.

While evacuated tubes are most commonly used with butterfly needles, a syringe is more appropriate in certain situations. Infants, children, and some adults have small veins that require using a butterfly needle set with a syringe. If a small amount (less than 10 mL) of specimen is needed, a safety needle attached directly to a syringe may be used. When a butterfly is used with evacuated tubes, a small or delicate vein can collapse, stopping the specimen collection process (this is referred to as a **collapsed vein**). A syringe does not have a vacuum, so the phlebotomist can control the amount of pressure applied to small or delicate veins. A luer adapter attaches the butterfly needle set to the syringe. See Figure 8-23.

Performing the Venipuncture

When performing a venipuncture using a syringe attached to a needle or butterfly needle set, follow the general steps for routine venipuncture. However, you should be aware of some differences. Equipment setup includes selecting the evacuated tubes needed for specimen transfer from a syringe. Place the evacuated tubes in the correct order of transfer into the collection rack. Collection

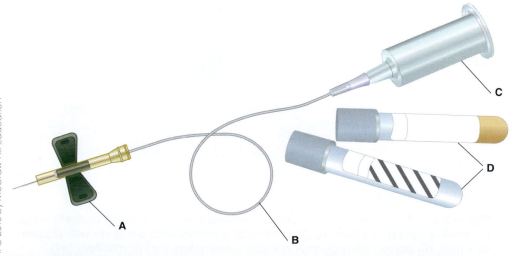

Figure 8-21 This butterfly assembly includes (A) a safety needle with butterfly wings, (B) connecting tubing, (C) an evacuated tube holder, and (D) evacuated tubes.

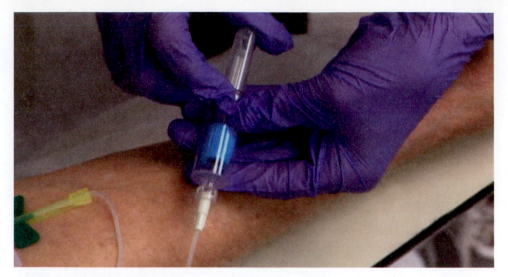

Figure 8-22 Venipuncture using butterfly assembly.

tubes are filled from the syringe using a transfer device. Put all other necessary venipuncture equipment within arm's reach before starting the procedure.

Next, remove the syringe from the sterile packaging and push the plunger in and out to ensure free and smooth movement during the venipuncture procedure. Before beginning, make sure the plunger is pushed completely in. While maintaining aseptic conditions, attach the syringe to a safety needle or butterfly setup. Make sure the plunger is pushed all the way in and perform the venipuncture procedure as described earlier in this chapter. Hold the syringe in the same manner as you would hold the tube holder. The first sign of a successful venipuncture is blood in the hub, or clear area, of the needle. Carefully pull the plunger back, so that you do not accidentally withdraw the needle from the arm. The barrel of the syringe will fill with blood as you pull the plunger out. Complete the syringe collection in the same manner as routine venipuncture.

When using a syringe, take care that the specimen is not hemolyzed, which means that the red blood cells are destroyed or broken apart. If the plunger is pulled back too hard or fast, the cells racing through the needle will be hemolyzed. These cells will rupture (break apart) and release their contents,

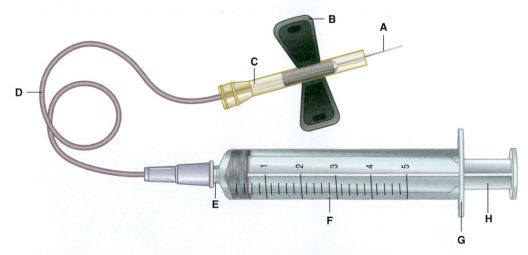

Figure 8-23 This butterfly assembly includes (A) a needle with (B) butterfly wings, (C) a slide-type safety device, (D) connecting tubing, and a syringe with (E) luer-lock hub, (F) barrel with markings in cubic centimeters (cc) or milliliters (ml), (G) a flange for ease of gripping, and (H) a plunger to create suction. After successful entry into the vein, the plunger is pulled back until the desired amount of blood is obtained; it is never pulled completely out while drawing blood.

TABLE 8-1 Laboratory Tests Affected by Hemolysis

Severely Affected	Considerably Affected	Barely Affected
APTT—activated partial thromboplastin time	ALT—alanine aminotransferase	Acid phosphatase
AST—aspartate aminotransferase	ANA—antinuclear antibodies	Albumin
CBC—complete blood count	Fe—iron	Ca—calcium
K—potassium	Folate	Mg—magnesium
LD—lactate dehydrogenase	TSH—thyroid stimulating hormone	P—phosphorus
PT—prothrombin time	Vitamin B_{12}	TP—total protein

resulting in a hemolyzed specimen that is unsuitable for most laboratory tests (see Table 8-1). Also, if the plunger is pulled back too hard, the vein may collapse due to the vacuum created by the syringe and the plunger.

Transferring the Specimen to Tubes

Immediately after removing the needle from the patient's arm, transfer the blood collected in the syringe to evacuated tubes using a blood transfer safety device (see Figure 8-24). Evacuated tubes are filled from the syringe in the same order of draw as outlined in the chapter *Blood Collection Equipment*. When using a blood transfer device, first you must remove the needle from the syringe. Before doing so, make sure the safety mechanism is engaged, so that the needle is not exposed. Attach the device to the syringe and then insert the evacuated blood collection tube into the transfer device. Allow the blood to transfer using the vacuum in the tube. Do not depress the plunger, as this may result in hemolysis. When the tubes are filled, mix them according to the manufacturer's recommendation and dispose of the transfer device and syringe in the appropriate sharps container. Use the competency checklist *Transferring Specimens to Tubes* at the end of the chapter to review and practice the procedure.

Using a Butterfly Needle Set with Evacuated Tubes

A butterfly needle set can be used with an evacuated tube adapter. Evacuated tube adapters come in two sizes, one for regular-size tubes and one for

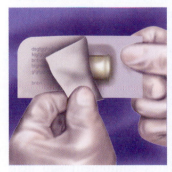
1. Peel off backing from transfer device.

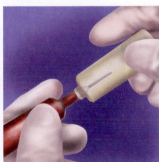
2. Insert syringe tip into hub and rotate syringe clockwise to secure.

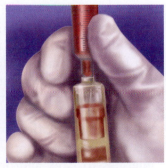
3. Hold the syringe facing down and push the evacuated tube into the holder. Do not depress the plunger of the syringe.

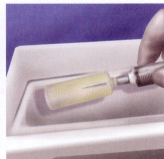
4. After removing the evacuated tube, discard the tube holder and syringe in an approved sharps container.

Figure 8-24 Using a syringe transfer device.

pediatric-size tubes. A butterfly needle set has tubing that attaches the needle to the evacuated tube adapter area. Tubes are pushed into the adapter in the same manner as in routine venipuncture.

Disposing of a Syringe and Butterfly Needle Set

Extra care should be taken when disposing of the entire butterfly needle set in the sharps container. When the needle is removed from the arm, the needle tends to hang from the butterfly assembly tubing, exposing both the phlebotomist and the patient to a potential needlestick injury. Be certain to use the safety device, which should be employed immediately on withdrawal from the vein, and, in some cases, before the needle is withdrawn from the patient. Some safety devices have a hard plastic cover that snaps into place after withdrawing the needle. Other safety devices retract the needle into a special holder. A safety device should always be present and engaged as soon as possible after blood collection. Use the competency checklists *Routine Venipuncture (Syringe)*, *Venipuncture Using a Butterfly and Syringe*, and *Venipuncture Using a Butterfly and Evacuated Tube Adaptor* at the end of this chapter to review and practice these procedures.

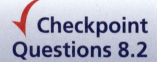

Checkpoint Questions 8.2

1. Under what conditions would you consider drawing a patient's blood using a butterfly needle set?
2. When transferring blood from a syringe to evacuated tubes, in what order should you fill the tubes?

8.3 Venipuncture Complications

Most venipuncture procedures proceed without complication. However, some do not. Complications include events involving the patient and situations that affect the quality of the specimen collected.

Patient Complications

Phlebotomists must be aware of various patient reactions to and complications of the venipuncture procedure. Being prepared to handle complications will help you provide the best customer service, if and when complications occur. Patient complications include choking, fainting, nausea, vomiting, seizures, post-procedure bleeding, formation of petechiae or hematomas, accidental arterial puncture, infection or injury, and additive reflux. Documentation of patient complications is essential for patient follow-up and assurance of quality healthcare delivery. Documentation may need to be recorded at the nurse's station or in the patient's EHR, the laboratory computer, the phlebotomy department log books, the variance forms, and the risk management forms. Always follow the requirements of your facility for documentation of patient complications. Quality assurance is discussed in more detail in the chapter *Quality Essentials*.

Allergic Reactions
Recall from the chapter *Infection Control and Safety* that some patients have allergies to latex and/or alcohol. Using only nonlatex equipment will help patients avoid such reactions. If the phlebotomist knows that the patient has an allergy to alcohol, he/she should use an alternate antiseptic. Rarely is a patient allergic to many types of antiseptics. In that case, use warm water on a gauze pad to cleanse the puncture site.

Choking

A patient should not be drinking, eating, or chewing gum during the phlebotomy procedure. Any foreign object in the mouth during phlebotomy can cause choking.

Syncope

During phlebotomy, **syncope** (fainting) can occur. The symptoms to look for in the patient are heavy perspiration, pale skin, and shallow or fast breathing. Following this, the patient experiences drooping eyelids, rapid and weak pulse, and finally unconsciousness. If the patient does have a syncopal episode, immediately remove the tourniquet and needle; then call for help. Apply pressure to the venipuncture site. Do not attempt to handle this situation alone and do not leave the patient. Position yourself in front of the phlebotomy chair or next to the bedside to block the patient from falling or sliding out of the chair or bed. If the patient is sitting, lower the patient's head and arms by placing both the head and arms between the patient's knees. If a sink is near the patient, wipe the patient's forehead and back of the neck with a cold compress. Some patients who faint also experience nausea and vomiting. Be prepared to provide the patient with a trash can or other container. In rare cases, seizures or convulsions occur during a fainting episode. Protect the patient from injury and notify the appropriate personnel to assist and administer first aid.

Petechiae

Petechiae, or small, nonraised red spots on the skin due to a minute hemorrhage, can result if a tourniquet is left on too long. Petechiae may be seen in normal patients and in patients with coagulation disorders. The presence of these small purple or red spots leaves the patient with a negative, lasting impression of the phlebotomy procedure. Any form of temporary or permanent disfigurement must be avoided, so be sure to remove the tourniquet in a timely manner and keep pressure on the site as long as necessary to stop the bleeding.

Bleeding

A patient may say that the bleeding has stopped, leave the phlebotomy area, and remove the arm gauze but return a few moments later with blood dripping down the arm. In this case, the following has occurred: the venipuncture wound appeared to be closed and the bleeding stopped, but movement of the arm caused it to open back up. This will not happen if proper procedures are followed. You must check the puncture site to determine if bleeding has stopped and apply a bandage before leaving the patient or allowing outpatients to leave. Advise the patient to apply additional pressure for several minutes before taking off the bandage or gauze. In addition, caution the patient not to use the venipuncture arm to push off with, open doors, or lift heavy objects, such as a purse.

Hematoma

A hematoma, or mass of blood caused by leakage of blood into the tissues, will occur if the tourniquet is left on the arm too long after the needle has

Syncope

After the initial steps of introducing yourself, identifying the patient, and obtaining consent to the procedure, it is a good idea to ask the patient about past experiences with having blood drawn. The patient may convey the tendency to faint during blood-drawing procedures. If fainting is a concern for an outpatient, have him or her lie down on a hospital bed or an exam table during blood collection.

Patient Education & Communication

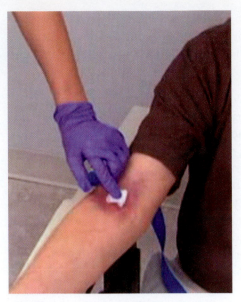

Figure 8-25 Hematomas form underneath the skin if the needle is not inserted completely into the vein or if the needle slips out.

been taken out (see Figure 8-25). A hematoma will occur if the needle has gone through the vein or if the bevel of the needle is not inserted fully into the vein. If you notice the formation of a hematoma, release the tourniquet, pull the needle out, and apply firm pressure at the site. If the patient complains of discomfort, apply ice to the hematoma.

Iatrogenic Anemia and Exsanguination

Patients who have repeated blood collections may develop an anemic condition in response to the removal of a large amount of blood over time. This phlebotomy-induced condition is known as **iatrogenic anemia.** If the amount of blood removed for testing—at one time or over a short period of time—exceeds 10% of the patient's total blood volume, it could become life-threatening. This later condition is called **exsanguination** and can easily occur in patients of smaller size, children, and infants.

Infection

Puncture site infections are rare, but they do occur. Be careful to ensure the sterility of all the equipment you use. Do not remove the cap from the needle until you are ready to insert the needle into the vein. Never remove a needle cap or lancet cover and then set the needle or device on the bed or other surface. Do not touch the puncture site once it has been cleansed. Ask the patient to keep the bandage on the puncture site until bleeding has completely stopped. Never perform a venipuncture or dermal puncture through a previously used site. It may be difficult because of possible scar formation, and microorganisms may be present in scar tissue and can be introduced deeper into the puncture site.

Injury

Injury to the patient can occur if a venipuncture site is poorly selected. A vein that feels very tight and stringy may not be a vein but, rather, a tendon. Nerves lie close to blood vessels. If you insert the needle too deeply, you may intersect a nerve. Probing after an unsuccessful venipuncture may also cause nerve or tendon damage.

Additive Reflux

Additive reflux is the flowing of blood mixed with tube additive back into the patient's vein. Additives can cause adverse reactions in the patient. To avoid additive reflux, you should always have the patient's arm and evacuated tubes in a downward position while performing venipuncture.

Situations That Affect the Quality of the Specimen

Accidental Arterial Puncture

It is important for phlebotomists to be able to differentiate between veins and arteries. Recall that a vein feels bouncy and an artery feels firmer and pulsates. If an artery is punctured by mistake, the blood will appear bright red and will flow with greater force and may even pulsate into the tube. If this occurs, release the tourniquet immediately, withdraw the needle, and apply firm pressure for at least 5 minutes (longer if there is still active bleeding). Then, apply a taut gauze dressing. Instruct the patient to keep the arm relatively still for a short period to minimize the flow of blood and immediately notify a nurse or other licensed professional, who can assist you in preventing hematoma formation. When arterial blood is given to the laboratory for testing, it must be labeled as "arterial" because the normal values for many blood test results are different for arterial and venous blood. In most cases arterial blood is not used for testing and venous blood will need to be collected.

Hemoconcentration

Hemoconcentration is a rapid increase in the ratio of blood components to plasma. Imagine berries in a jar of liquid that contains five berries per ounce of liquid. Removing some of the liquid, but none of the berries, will increase the amount of berries per ounce of fluid. Hemoconcentration is similar; water can slowly leave the vein, causing the concentration of cells and chemicals to increase. Hemoconcentration can be caused if the patient vigorously pumps (rapidly opens and closes) the fist, if the phlebotomist leaves the tourniquet on for longer than 1 minute, or if the tourniquet is too tight. Hemoconcentration happens long before the patient notices it, usually in 3 to 5 minutes. Pain, pressure, or a "falling asleep" sensation of the arm can occur. Hemoconcentration should be avoided because it can cause erroneous results for some laboratory tests, such as protein levels, cell counts, and coagulation studies.

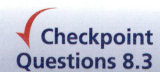

Checkpoint Questions 8.3

1. List seven complications that may affect the patient during phlebotomy.
2. How will you know if an artery is accidently punctured instead of a vein?
3. How can you prevent hemoconcentration while drawing a patient's blood?

Chapter Summary

Learning Outcome	Key Concepts/Examples	Related NAACLS Competency
8.1 Summarize the steps necessary to perform a competent/effective venipuncture. Pages 204–218.	Venipuncture sites are selected based on their location and appearance and with consideration of the patient's age, the accessibility of appropriate veins, and varying patient situations. Venipuncture is typically performed in the antecubital area of the arm. Each step of the venipuncture procedure is crucial in providing the patient with a successful venipuncture experience. 1. Obtain and verify the correct tubes and supplies. 2. Introduce yourself and identify the patient. 3. Explain procedure to the patient. 4. Wash hands and put on gloves. 5. Apply the tourniquet. 6. Select the venipuncture site. 7. Release the tourniquet the first time. 8. Cleanse the venipuncture site. 9. Reapply the tourniquet. 10. Anchor the vein. 11. Insert the needle into the patient's vein. 12. Engage the first tube. 13. Remove tube, and insert the next tube if multiple tubes are needed (mix each tube as the next is filling). Remove and mix the last tube. 14. Release the tourniquet the second time. 15. Remove needle apparatus. 16. Cover venipuncture site loosely with gauze. 17. Apply pressure to puncture site. 18. Label tubes. 19. Thank the patient.	5.00, 5.5, 5.6, 6.00, 6.1, 6.2, 6.3, 6.4, 6.5, 6.10, 6.11
8.2 Describe special procedures needed for venipuncture on difficult-to-draw veins. Pages 219–222.	Difficult blood draws may require selection of alternate puncture sites, equipment, and techniques. A butterfly needle set is normally a last resort when attempting blood collection; however, it may become necessary in certain circumstances.	5.00, 5.5, 5.6, 6.00, 6.5, 6.7, 6.10
8.3 Describe signs and symptoms of venipuncture complications. Pages 222–225.	Phlebotomists must be aware of and prepared to handle possible complications of venipuncture. Some patient complications include allergic reactions, bleeding and hematoma formation, choking, syncope, pain, injury, and infection. Complications that can affect the quality of the specimen collected include accidental puncture of an artery and hemoconcentration due to prolonged tourniquet application.	6.8, 6.9

Chapter Review

A: Labeling

Label the venipuncture equipment pictured in the image below.

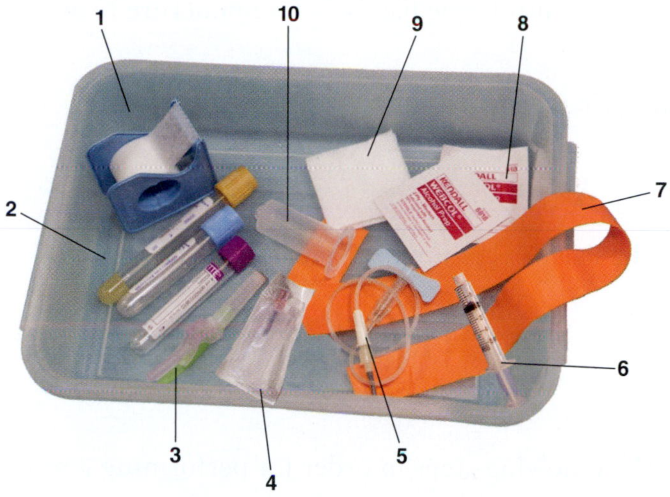

1. [LO 8.1] ______________________________
2. [LO 8.1] ______________________________
3. [LO 8.1] ______________________________
4. [LO 8.1] ______________________________
5. [LO 8.1] ______________________________
6. [LO 8.1] ______________________________
7. [LO 8.1] ______________________________
8. [LO 8.1] ______________________________
9. [LO 8.1] ______________________________
10. [LO 8.1] ______________________________

B: Matching

Match each definition with the correct term.

___**11.** [LO 8.3] additive reflux

___**12.** [LO 8.3] collapsed vein

___**13.** [LO 8.3] ecchymosis

___**14.** [LO 8.3] hemoconcentration

___**15.** [LO 8.3] hematoma

___**16.** [LO 8.3] petechiae

___**17.** [LO 8.3] arterial puncture

___**18.** [LO 8.3] syncope

a. abnormal caving in of the vessel walls, stopping blood flow

b. fainting

c. increase in ratio of blood components to plasma

d. large bruise caused by blood under the skin

e. mass formed by leakage of blood under the skin

f. results in bright red blood flowing with greater force

g. tiny red spots caused by minor hemorrhaging in underlying tissue

h. flow of blood mixed with tube additive back into a patient's vein

C: Fill in the Blank

19. [LO 8.1] A(n) _____ can be used to visualize the veins during phlebotomy.

20. [LO 8.1] When performing venipuncture, the _____ of the needle should face upward.

21. [LO 8.1] The cap of the needle should not be removed until immediately before puncture to avoid _____.

22. [LO 8.2] If the vacuum in the tube is too great for the vein to handle, it may _____.

23. [LO 8.1] A tube will not fill completely if it has lost its _____.

24. [LO 8.3] If the tourniquet is not released before the needle is removed from the vein, a(n) _____ may form.

D: Sequencing

Based on what you have learned in this chapter, put the following steps in order for performing a routine venipuncture by numbering them from 1 to 18 in the spaces provided.

25. [LO 8.1] _____ Anchor vein.

26. [LO 8.1] _____ Apply pressure to puncture site.

27. [LO 8.1] _____ Apply tourniquet.

28. [LO 8.1] _____ Cleanse venipuncture site.

29. [LO 8.1] _____ Cover venipuncture site loosely with gauze.

30. [LO 8.1] _____ Engage the first tube.

31. [LO 8.1] _____ Explain the procedure to the patient.

32. [LO 8.1] _____ Identify the patient.

33. [LO 8.1] _____ Insert needle into the patient's arm.

34. [LO 8.1] _____ Introduce yourself.

35. [LO 8.1] _____ Label tubes.

36. [LO 8.1] _____ Reapply tourniquet.

37. [LO 8.1] _____ Release tourniquet first time.

38. [LO 8.1] _____ Release tourniquet second time.

39. [LO 8.1] _____ Remove needle apparatus.

40. [LO 8.1] _____ Remove tube and mix.

41. [LO 8.1] _____ Select venipuncture site.

42. [LO 8.1] _____ Thank the patient.

43. [LO 8.1] _____ Wash hands and put on gloves.

E: Case Study/Critical Thinking

44. [LO 8.3] You encounter a patient with very small veins. You make one attempt and miss; you make another attempt and miss. What should be your next step after the second failed attempt to obtain a specimen?

45. [LO 8.3] An outpatient informs you that he has had several bad experiences with fainting during blood collection procedures. What should you do?

46. [LO 8.3] A patient tells you that it is very difficult to obtain blood from her veins. You are not able to palpate any appropriate vein in the antecubital area. What is your next step?

47. [LO 8.3] During a venipuncture procedure, the blood stops flowing into the tube. What may have happened and how can you save the draw?

F: Exam Prep

Choose the best answer for each question.

48. [LO 8.2] When is a phlebotomist allowed to perform a venipuncture on an ankle vein?

   a. Never

   b. When the patient has IVs in both arms

   c. During an emergency

   d. When all other options have been exhausted and the physician has given approval

49. [LO 8.1] The most important step in performing a venipuncture is

   a. removing the tourniquet before taking the needle out.

   b. drawing the correct amount of blood.

   c. inserting the needle in the vein properly.

   d. identifying the patient.

50. [LO 8.1] The vein most frequently used for venipuncture is the

   a. cephalic vein.

   b. dorsal arch vein.

   c. median cubital vein.

   d. saphenous vein.

51. [LO 8.2] A blood specimen in which the red blood cells are destroyed or broken apart is said to be

   a. arterial.

   b. hemolyzed.

   c. clotted.

   d. hemoconcentrated.

52. [LO 8.3] When a patient develops syncope during venipuncture, the phlebotomist should first

   a. lower the patient's head.

   b. remove the tourniquet and needle and call for help.

   c. complete the venipuncture as quickly as possible.

   d. none of these.

53. [LO 8.1] Which action is appropriate when cleaning the puncture site?

   a. Blow on the applied alcohol to hasten drying.

   b. Do not allow the alcohol to dry prior to puncture.

   c. Rub the alcohol pad in concentric circles from inside out.

   d. Use 70% isopropanol on the site before and after puncture.

54. [LO 8.2] What part of a butterfly needle set should be disposed of in a sharps container?

   a. The needle

   b. The needle and tubing

   c. The entire butterfly needle set

   d. The needle and safety device

55. [LO 8.1] The angle at which you enter the vein should be

   a. bevel up at a 15- to 30-degree angle.

   b. bevel up at a 45- to 60-degree angle.

   c. bevel down at a 15- to 30-degree angle.

   d. bevel down at a 45- to 60-degree angle.

56. [LO 8.2] Why is a butterfly needle set used only when a standard venipuncture cannot be performed?

a. Butterfly needle sets have a tendency to cause veins to collapse.

b. Using a butterfly needle set results in more accidental needlesticks.

c. Butterfly needle sets cannot be used with patients who are shaking or have tremors.

d. Safety devices cannot be used with butterfly needle sets.

57. [LO 8.1] Advancing the stopper of a collection tube past the mark or ridge on the adapter during equipment setup will

a. cause hemolysis in the specimen collected.

b. help ensure that the evacuated tube is working properly.

c. make the venipuncture less painful for the patient.

d. cause a loss of the vacuum in the tube.

58. [LO 8.3] Which of the following laboratory tests is *severely* affected by hemolyzed blood?

a. Magnesium (Mg)

b. Calcium (Ca)

c. Potassium (K)

d. Phosphorus (P)

59. [LO8.2] When using a blood transfer device to transfer blood from a syringe into evacuated tubes, what is the *first* thing you should do?

a. Make sure the safety mechanism is engaged.

b. Remove the needle from the syringe.

c. Attach the blood transfer device to the syringe.

d. Insert the evacuated blood collection tube into the transfer device.

60. [LO 8.3] Another phlebotomist tells you that the patient you are about to draw tends to develop hematomas very easily. This means that

a. the area around the tourniquet will show small, red spots.

b. the venipuncture site may swell and fill with blood.

c. the patient will faint and should be lying down.

d. you should not apply a bandage because the patient has allergies.

61. [LO 8.1] Which veins are appropriate for routine venipuncture? *(Choose all that apply.)*

a. Cephalic vein

b. Dorsal arch vein

c. Median cubital vein

d. Metacarpal plexus veins

62. [LO 8.1] Which action is appropriate when cleaning the puncture site? *(Choose all that apply.)*

a. Clean the site with antiseptic, moving back and forth over the site.

b. Start at the top of the puncture site and wipe downward.

c. Start at the bottom of the puncture site and wipe upward.

d. Rub the alcohol pad in concentric circles from inside out.

63. [LO 8.2] Which veins may a phlebotomist access during difficult venipuncture procedures? *(Choose all that apply.)*

a. Ankle veins

b. Dorsal arch vein

c. Femoral vein

d. Metacarpal plexus veins

64. [LO 8.3] You are informed that a specimen you delivered to the laboratory has to be re-collected due to hemolysis. What might have caused this specimen to hemolyze? *(Choose all that apply.)*

a. Not waiting for the alcohol to dry

b. Leaving the tourniquet on too long

c. Vigorously mixing the specimen

d. Removing the tourniquet while the tubes were filling

65. [LO 8.2] Which of the following is another name for a butterfly needle set?

a. Evacuated tube set

b. Pediatric set

c. Blood transfer device

d. Winged infusion set

66. [LO 8.3] Reflux during a venipuncture procedure is a condition in which

a. the patient is experiencing heartburn.

b. the patient is jerking his or her arm.

c. the tube additive is being pulled into the patient's vein.

d. the needle is slipping out of the vein.

67. [LO 8.1] During a venipuncture, the blood stops flowing into the tube. You change tubes, and blood flows into the second tube, but then it stops again before the tube is filled. What may be causing this to happen? *(Choose all that apply.)*

a. The tubes are expired and have partially lost vacuum.

b. The vein collapses and expands when the tube is removed.

c. The tube selected is a pediatric draw tube and fills only part of the way.

d. The needle is too far into the vein.

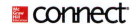

Enhance your learning by completing these exercises and more at connect.mheducation.com.

References

Clinical and Laboratory Standards Institute. (2007). *Procedures for the collection of diagnostic blood specimens by venipuncture; approved standard.* (6th ed.). H3-A6. 27(26). Wayne, PA. CLSI.

Dale, J. C., & Novis, D. A. (2002). Outpatient phlebotomy success and reasons for specimen rejection. *Archives of Pathology & Laboratory Medicine, 126,* 416–419.

Masoorli, S., Angeles, T., & Barbone, M. (1998). Danger points: How to prevent nerve injuries from venipuncture. *Nursing, 28,* 34–39.

National Accrediting Agency for Clinical Laboratory Sciences. (2010). *NAACLS entry-level phlebotomist competencies.* Rosemont, IL. NAACLS.

Niwinski, N. (2009). Capillary blood collection: Best practices. *BD LabNotes. 20*(1). Becton, Dickinson and Company.

Product FAQs. (2011). *Venous blood collection.* Becton, Dickinson and Company. Retrieved April 12, 2011, from www.bd.com/vacutainer/faqs/

Wilson, D. D. (2008). *McGraw-Hill manual of laboratory and diagnostic tests.* New York: McGraw-Hill.

COMPETENCY CHECKLIST: ROUTINE VENIPUNCTURE (EVACUATED TUBE SYSTEM)

Procedure Steps	Practice			Performed		
	1	2	3	Yes	No	Master
Preprocedure						
1. Examines the requisition.						
2. Greets the patient; introduces self.						
3. Identifies the patient verbally using two identifiers, including comparing the identification band with the requisition.						
4. Explains the procedure to the patient.						
5. Verifies dietary restrictions or instructions.						
6. Washes hands and puts on gloves.						
7. Selects the correct equipment and supplies.						
8. Assembles the equipment and supplies properly.						
9. Conveniently places the equipment.						
10. Reassures the patient.						
11. Positions the patient's arm comfortably.						
12. Applies the tourniquet.						
13. Identifies a vein by palpation.						
14. Selects a venipuncture site.						
15. Releases the tourniquet.						
16. Cleanses the venipuncture site.						
17. Allows the site to air dry.						
Procedure						
18. Reapplies the tourniquet.						
19. Confirms the venipuncture site visually.						
20. Anchors the vein below the puncture site.						
21. Smoothly inserts the needle at the correct angle.						
22. Inserts the needle with the bevel up.						
23. Inserts the tubes without causing pain.						
24. Allows the tubes to fill completely.						
25. Removes the tubes.						
26. Mixes the tubes by inversion (as recommended by the manufacturer).						
27. Collects the tubes in correct order.						
28. Does not move the needle between tubes.						
29. Removes the last tube from the holder.						
30. Releases the tourniquet.						

Procedure Steps	Practice			Performed		
	1	2	3	Yes	No	Master
Procedure						
31. Places gauze over the puncture site.						
32. Withdraws the needle smoothly.						
33. Activates the safety engineering control device.						
Postprocedure						
34. Applies pressure to the venipuncture site.						
35. Disposes of the needle and tube adaptor in the correct container.						
36. Labels the tubes correctly (including date, time, and phlebotomist identification).						
37. Observes special handling instruction.						
38. Checks the venipuncture site.						
39. Applies a bandage.						
40. Thanks the patient.						
41. Disposes of used supplies appropriately.						
42. Removes gloves and washes the hands.						
43. Transports specimens to the laboratory.						
44. Documents specimen collection.						

COMMENTS: _____
_____
_____
_____

SIGNED

EVALUATOR: _____

STUDENT: _____

COMPETENCY CHECKLIST: ROUTINE VENIPUNCTURE (SYRINGE)

Procedure Steps	Practice			Performed		Master
	1	2	3	Yes	No	
Preprocedure						
1. Examines the requisition.						
2. Greets the patient; introduces self.						
3. Identifies the patient verbally using two identifiers, including comparing the identification band with the requisition.						
4. Explains the procedure to the patient.						
5. Verifies dietary restrictions or instructions.						
6. Washes hands and puts on gloves.						
7. Selects the correct equipment and supplies.						
8. Assembles the equipment and supplies properly.						
9. Checks the plunger movement of the syringe.						
10. Conveniently places the equipment.						
11. Reassures the patient.						
12. Positions the patient's arm comfortably.						
13. Applies the tourniquet.						
14. Identifies a vein by palpation.						
15. Selects the venipuncture site.						
16. Releases the tourniquet.						
17. Cleanses the venipuncture site.						
18. Allows the site to air dry.						
Procedure						
19. Reapplies the tourniquet.						
20. Confirms the venipuncture site visually.						
21. Anchors the vein below the puncture site.						
22. Smoothly inserts the needle at the correct angle.						
23. Inserts the needle with the bevel up.						
24. Collects the appropriate amount of the sample.						
25. Releases the tourniquet.						
26. Places gauze over the puncture site.						
27. Withdraws the needle smoothly.						
28. Activates the safety engineering control device.						

Procedure Steps	Practice			Performed		Master
	1	2	3	Yes	No	
Postprocedure						
29. Applies pressure to the venipuncture site.						
30. Uses a safe technique to fill the tubes.						
31. Fills the tubes in correct order.						
32. Mixes anticoagulated tubes by inversion.						
33. Disposes of the needle and syringe in the correct container.						
34. Labels the tubes correctly (including date, time, and phlebotomist identification).						
35. Observes special handling instruction.						
36. Checks the venipuncture site.						
37. Applies a bandage.						
38. Thanks the patient.						
39. Disposes of used supplies appropriately.						
40. Removes gloves and washes the hands.						
41. Transports the specimens to the laboratory.						
42. Documents specimen collection.						

COMMENTS: _____

_____

_____

_____

SIGNED

EVALUATOR: _____

STUDENT: _____

COMPETENCY CHECKLIST: VENIPUNCTURE USING A BUTTERFLY AND SYRINGE

Procedure Steps	Practice			Performed		
	1	2	3	Yes	No	Master
Preprocedure						
1. Examines the requisition.						
2. Greets the patient; introduces self.						
3. Identifies the patient verbally using two identifiers, including comparing the identification band with the requisition.						
4. Explains the procedure to the patient.						
5. Verifies dietary restrictions or instructions.						
6. Washes hands and puts on gloves.						
7. Selects the correct equipment and supplies.						
8. Assembles the equipment and supplies properly.						
9. Checks the plunger movement of the syringe.						
10. Conveniently places the equipment.						
11. Reassures the patient.						
12. Positions the patient's arm comfortably.						
13. Applies the tourniquet.						
14. Identifies a vein by palpation.						
15. Selects the venipuncture site.						
16. Releases the tourniquet.						
17. Cleanses the venipuncture site.						
18. Allows the site to air dry.						
Procedure						
19. Reapplies the tourniquet.						
20. Confirms the venipuncture site visually.						
21. Anchors the vein below the puncture site.						
22. Holds the butterfly needle with the wings upward and bevel up.						
23. Inserts the needle smoothly at the correct angle.						
24. Collects the appropriate amount of the sample.						
25. Releases the tourniquet.						
26. Places gauze over the puncture site.						
27. Withdraws the needle smoothly.						
28. Activates the safety engineering control device.						

Procedure Steps	Practice			Performed		Master
	1	2	3	Yes	No	
Postprocedure						
29. Applies pressure to the venipuncture site.						
30. Uses safe technique to fill tubes.						
31. Fills the tubes in correct order.						
32. Mixes anticoagulated tubes by inversion.						
33. Disposes of the needle and syringe in the correct container.						
34. Labels the tubes correctly (including date, time, and phlebotomist identification).						
35. Observes special handling instruction.						
36. Checks the venipuncture site.						
37. Applies a bandage.						
38. Thanks the patient.						
39. Disposes of used supplies appropriately.						
40. Removes the gloves and washes hands.						
41. Transports the specimens to the laboratory.						
42. Documents the specimen collection.						

COMMENTS: _____

_____

_____

_____

SIGNED

EVALUATOR: _____

STUDENT: _____

COMPETENCY CHECKLIST: VENIPUNCTURE USING A BUTTERFLY AND EVACUATED TUBE ADAPTOR

Procedure Steps	Practice			Performed		
	1	2	3	Yes	No	Master
Preprocedure						
1. Examines the requisition.						
2. Greets the patient; introduces self.						
3. Identifies the patient verbally using two identifiers, including comparing the identification band with the requisition.						
4. Explains the procedure to the patient.						
5. Verifies diet restrictions or instructions.						
6. Washes hands and puts on gloves.						
7. Selects the correct equipment and supplies.						
8. Assembles the equipment and supplies properly.						
9. Conveniently places the equipment.						
10. Reassures the patient.						
11. Positions the patient's arm comfortably.						
12. Applies a tourniquet.						
13. Identifies a vein by palpation.						
14. Selects a venipuncture site.						
15. Releases the tourniquet.						
16. Cleanses the venipuncture site.						
17. Allows the site to air dry.						
Procedure						
18. Reapplies the tourniquet.						
19. Confirms the venipuncture site visually.						
20. Anchors the vein below the puncture site.						
21. Holds the butterfly needle with wings upward and bevel up.						
22. Inserts the needle smoothly at the correct angle.						
23. Collects tubes in the correct order of draw.						
24. Mixes the tubes by inversion (as recommended by the manufacturer).						
25. Releases the tourniquet.						
26. Places gauze over the puncture site.						
27. Withdraws the needle smoothly.						
28. Activates the safety engineering control device.						

Procedure Steps	Practice			Performed		
	1	2	3	Yes	No	Master
Postprocedure						
29. Applies pressure to the venipuncture site.						
30. Disposes of the needle and holder in the correct container.						
31. Labels the tubes correctly (including date, time, and phlebotomist identification).						
32. Observes special handling instruction.						
33. Checks the venipuncture site.						
34. Applies a bandage.						
35. Thanks the patient.						
36. Disposes of used supplies appropriately.						
37. Removes gloves and washes hands.						
38. Transports specimens to the laboratory.						
39. Documents the specimen collection.						

COMMENTS: _____

_____

_____

_____

SIGNED

    EVALUATOR: _____

    STUDENT: _____

NAME: _____ DATE: _____

COMPETENCY CHECKLIST: TRANSFERRING SPECIMEN TO TUBES

Procedure Steps	Practice			Performed		
	1	2	3	Yes	No	Master
Preprocedure						
1. Prepares for specimen transfer after the venipuncture preprocedure but prior to the venipuncture procedure.						
2. Selects the correct equipment and supplies (blood transfer device).						
3. Conveniently places the equipment.						
4. Performs the specimen transfer procedure immediately after removing the needle from the vein.						
Procedure						
5. Inserts the syringe into the transfer device hub.						
6. Transfers the specimen into tubes.						
7. Uses safe technique to fill the tubes.						
8. Fills the tubes in correct order.						
9. Allows the tubes to fill naturally.						
10. Mixes anticoagulated tubes by inversion.						
Postprocedure						
11. Disposes of the transfer device and syringe in the correct container.						
12. Continues with the venipuncture postprocedure.						

COMMENTS: _____

_____

_____

_____

SIGNED

EVALUATOR: _____

STUDENT: _____

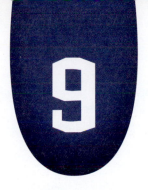

9

essential terms

calcaneus
interstitial fluid
osteomyelitis
palmar
plantar

Dermal/Capillary Puncture

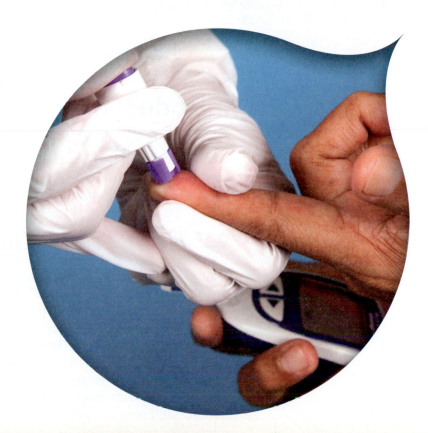

Learning Outcomes

9.1 Explain why dermal/capillary puncture is used instead of routine venipuncture for some patients.

9.2 Select an appropriate site for dermal puncture and identify the equipment needed.

9.3 Carry out the procedure for performing a dermal puncture.

9.4 Apply the procedure for collecting a capillary specimen.

Related NAACLS Competencies

5.00 Demonstrate knowledge of collection equipment, various types of additives used, special precautions necessary, and substances that can interfere in clinical analysis of blood constituents.

5.5 List and select the types of equipment needed to collect blood by venipuncture and capillary (dermal) puncture.

5.6 Identify special precautions necessary during blood collections by venipuncture and capillary (dermal) puncture.

6.00 Follow standard operating procedures to collect specimens.

6.1 Identify potential sites for venipuncture and capillary (dermal) puncture.

6.2 Differentiate between sterile and antiseptic techniques.

6.3 Describe and demonstrate the steps in the preparation of a puncture site.

6.4 List the effects of tourniquet, hand squeezing, and heating pads on specimens collected by venipuncture and capillary (dermal) puncture.

6.6 Describe and perform correct procedure for capillary (dermal) collection methods.

6.7 Describe the limitations and precautions of alternate collection sites for venipuncture and capillary (dermal) puncture.

6.10 List the steps necessary to perform a venipuncture and a capillary (dermal) puncture in order.

6.12 Demonstrate a successful capillary (dermal) puncture following standard operating procedures.

Introduction

Dermal/capillary puncture is frequently used when collecting blood from infants and children as well as when an alternative to venipuncture is necessary for difficult draws on adults. This chapter outlines reasons why dermal/capillary puncture is used, the equipment needed, and the techniques for performing it.

9.1 The Dermal/Capillary Puncture

Venipuncture is more difficult in infants and children than in adults. Because of a child's smaller size, it is difficult to locate a vein that is large enough to withstand the vacuum present in evacuated collection tubes without collapsing. Furthermore, children do not enjoy venipuncture and usually do not remain still for the length of time this procedure requires. Dermal/capillary puncture is therefore the preferred blood collection technique for infants (heel) and very small children (finger).

Dermal puncture may also be used as an alternate method of blood collection for adult patients with whom venipuncture procedures are too difficult. In some cases, patients who are obese, elderly, or severely burned have veins that are difficult to locate. These patients are often candidates for dermal puncture. Be certain to check the policy at your facility as well as the laboratory tests ordered. Blood for some laboratory tests, such as coagulation tests, cannot be collected using dermal puncture. See Table 9-1 for a comparison of blood collection methods.

The blood specimen obtained during dermal puncture is a mixture of capillary blood, venous blood, arterial blood, and **interstitial fluid** (fluid between cells and tissues). However, new and developing technology in laboratory instrumentation allows tests to be performed on capillary blood. The most notable exceptions are blood cultures and erythrocyte sedimentation rate (ESR) because both of these tests require a relatively large amount of blood. An ESR is the measurement of the erythrocyte settling rate. One drawback of a dermal puncture for the laboratory is the small amount of blood collected. This small quantity usually leaves an insufficient sample if the test requires a large amount of blood or needs to be repeated.

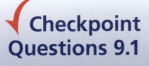

✓ Checkpoint Questions 9.1

1. For what types of patients is dermal puncture often the preferred method?
2. What components make up blood specimens obtained by dermal puncture?

TABLE 9-1 Comparison of Collection Methods

Method	When to Use	Pros	Cons

Evacuated tube	Routine collection
	Whenever possible
		Fast
		Relatively safe
		Best specimen quality
		Large collection amount possible
			May not work with
			  small veins
			  fragile veins
			  difficult draws
			  small children
			  hand veins

Butterfly assembly	Small veins Fragile veins Difficult draw Small children	Least likely to collapse vein Less painful for patient Least likely to pass through small veins	Syringe not as safe: tube transfer Specimen may be hemolyzed Expense Increased risk of needlestick
Dermal puncture	Children Infants Elderly patients Oncology patients Severely burned patients Obese patients Inaccessible veins Extremely fragile veins Home testing by patient Procedure requiring capillary specimen only	Easy to perform Requires small amount of specimen	Not good for dehydrated patient Not good for patient with poor circulation Cannot collect for certain tests, such as blood cultures, ESRs, and coagulation tests

9.2 Preparing for Dermal Puncture

Preparation steps must be performed before you begin the dermal puncture procedure. These steps are the same as those used in venipuncture. The main differences between venipuncture and dermal puncture are the site selection and the equipment assembled (see Figure 9-1).

Competency Check 9-1

Dermal Puncture Preparation

1. Acquire and examine the requisition slip.
2. Greet and identify the patient.
3. Explain the procedure.
4. Verify any dietary restrictions.
5. Wash your hands.
6. Put on gloves.

Selecting the Site for Dermal Puncture

The skin should be warm, pink, and free from scars, cuts, rashes, or bruises. The sites to consider for dermal puncture are the distal regions of the middle finger (third finger) and ring finger (fourth finger) in children and adults and the medial or lateral regions of the plantar surface of the heel in infants. The

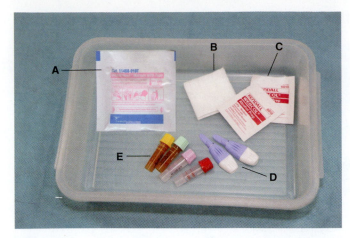

FIGURE 9-1 Equipment for dermal puncture includes (A) tissue warmer, (B) gauze, (C) alcohol prep pads, (D) lancets, and (E) microcollection containers.

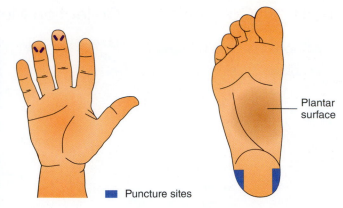

■ Puncture sites

FIGURE 9-2 The dark areas (in blue) indicate correct sites for finger and heel dermal puncture.

blue-shaded areas in Figure 9-2 show the proper and most common sites for dermal puncture blood collection. In rare cases, it may be necessary to perform a dermal puncture on a toe of a patient. For example, this may occur for an adult with burns.

For a finger puncture, do not use the thumb (first finger), pinkie (fifth finger), or pointer finger (second finger); they are poor choices because the area is often too thick and callused. Always puncture across the grain (across the lines) of the fingerprint lines. Do not use the end or tip of the finger.

In infants of less than 1 year who are not walking, the heel is the recommended puncture site. Never perform a dermal puncture on an infant who has begun to walk because of the potential for pain at the site. Examine the infant's heel and choose the lateral surface for dermal puncture. Do not use the arch of the foot, the back of the heel, or the **plantar** area (bottom surface, or sole) of the foot. If an infant has several old puncture sites, attempt to find an unused area. The site chosen for puncture should be well away from the area of the **calcaneus,** or heel bone. If the calcaneus is punctured, it can cause **osteomyelitis,** an infection of the bone. In premature infants, the calcaneus is less than 2.0 mm below the surface of the skin and a lancet length of less than 2.0 mm should be used.

For children and adults, the preferred site for dermal puncture is the **palmar** (palm side) surface of the finger. Usually, the ring or middle finger of the non-dominant hand is chosen. The dermal puncture site of choice is the side of the fingertip. Slightly warming the finger with a warm cloth (or the heel with a heel warmer) enhances blood flow.

Life Span Considerations

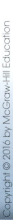

Selecting Age-Appropriate Dermal Puncture Sites

For blood collection on neonates (newborns), always use the heel. Their tiny fingers are much too small for maintaining a safe distance from the bone during puncture. Heelsticks may continue to be used until the young child begins to walk. Remember never to puncture through a previous puncture site. When performing fingerstick blood collections on children and adults, remember that the third and fourth fingers are the most appropriate to use because they are the least likely to cause pain and discomfort afterward.

TABLE 9-2 Dermal Puncture Site Selection Summary

Recommended Areas	Areas *Not* Recommended
Heel; medial and lateral plantar surfaces	Back of heel, bottom of foot, arch of foot
Central fleshy area of third and fourth fingers	Callused finger (usually index finger), thumb, or pinkie
Across fingerprint lines	Along fingerprint lines
	Areas with visible damage or edema
	Sites previously used for dermal puncture

The finger to be punctured or cut for a dermal puncture should not be edematous. Edema is caused by a buildup of fluids, with the result that the specimen will contain an abnormal amount of interstitial fluid, which will cause abnormal laboratory results. Look at the other hand to see if it is also edematous. If both hands are edematous, a venipuncture should be attempted. Table 9-2 summarizes the recommended sites (and those to avoid) for dermal puncture.

Equipment for Dermal Puncture

The equipment needed for dermal puncture is the same as that used for venipuncture, with the exception of the puncture device and the collection containers. You will need a requisition slip, an alcohol prep pad, gauze, gloves, an adhesive bandage or tape, a sharps container, a computer label, and a permanent marker or pen. You will also need a safety dermal puncture device or lancet and microspecimen containers.

Microspecimen containers vary in size and shape. Some collection devices have a strawlike apparatus attached to the end. Capillary action—the force that causes fluids to rise into tubes with small diameters—helps these devices fill with a pulling action. These strawlike tubes are typically held horizontally during collection. Some microcollection devices appear to fill by themselves once the end is brought near the drop of blood. If the opening is narrow, this phenomenon could also be due to capillary action. Microspecimen containers with wide openings fill by the action of gravity; blood flows downward into the container.

Safety dermal puncture devices have a blade or puncture point that retracts after the device is used. These devices are frequently spring-loaded to control the depth and to ensure that the blade retracts to prevent accidental needlesticks. However, safety devices operate differently, depending on the manufacturer and the location of the puncture. If you are unsure how to use a dermal puncture device, always check the manufacturer's directions before you attempt the actual dermal puncture.

Devices are chosen according to the age and size of the patient. Special devices have been developed for newborns and premature newborns. Other devices are used mostly on children or adults.

1. What are the preferred dermal puncture sites for infants, children, and adults?
2. What equipment is needed for a dermal puncture?

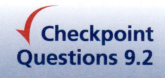

Checkpoint Questions 9.2

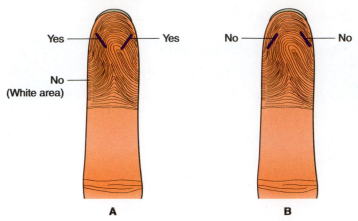

Yes — Yes
No (White area)
No — No

FIGURE 9-3   For a correct dermal puncture, **(A)** cut across the fingerprint; **(B)** do not cut in the same direction as the fingerprint.

9.3 Performing a Dermal Puncture

When a dermal puncture is performed, a cut is made into the layers of the dermal (skin) surface. The finger should be held in such a way that the skin is stretched tightly. For a finger dermal puncture, the cut is made across the fingerprint lines. Cutting across the fingerprint delivers the best possible blood flow and droplet formation for a dermal puncture (see Figure 9-3). If the cut is made between the fingerprint lines (parallel to the fingerprints), the blood flow is less, and the blood tends to flow down the fingerprint instead of forming drops.

Safety & Infection Control

Dermal Puncture Depth

Improper technique during dermal puncture can cause bone infection. This is especially true in infants. It can be considered malpractice if the calcaneus is punctured by mistake, creating a site for bacterial infection. This infection can lead to further infection of the surrounding bone, cartilage, and bone marrow. Thus, puncture depth should never be greater than 2 mm and should never be performed at the center of the heel, where the calcaneus is most likely to be punctured.

Clean the finger with an alcohol pad and allow the finger to dry thoroughly. It is very important to allow the site to dry prior to collecting the dermal puncture specimen. This will prevent hemolysis of the blood due to contact with the alcohol. Apply slight pressure; then puncture the site with the proper safety device (see Figure 9-4).

Do not use spring-loaded devices designed for glucose monitoring when performing a routine dermal puncture. These lancets produce a smaller puncture and only two or three drops of blood. Most microcollection containers need more than two or three drops to fill.

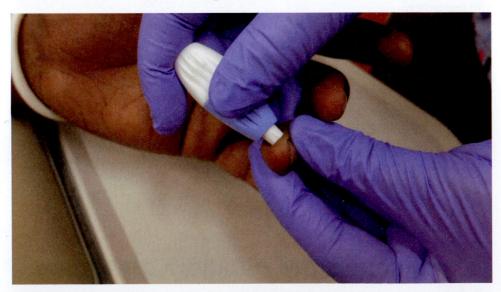

FIGURE 9-4   Hold the finger downward and apply pressure to puncture the site. Be sure the puncture is made across the fingerprint lines.

Use the device correctly. Check the directions. No matter which device or site (finger or heel) you use, dermal puncture will cause pain. It is better to make the first puncture deep enough, using the proper technique, than to have to puncture a second time to obtain sufficient blood. Use the competency checklists *Dermal Puncture on Finger* and *Dermal Puncture on Heel* at the end of the chapter to review and practice the procedure.

✓ **Checkpoint Questions 9.3**

1. Why should you position the lancet or dermal puncture device so that the blade cuts across the fingerprint lines?
2. What is the maximum allowable depth for a dermal puncture?

9.4 Collecting the Capillary Specimen

At the puncture site, a drop of capillary blood forms. Before collecting the blood in the microcollection container, wipe away the first drop of blood. This drop contains interstitial fluid and damaged tissue cells, which will contaminate the blood specimen. After the next drop has formed, touch the open end (collection tube or scoop) of the microcollection container to the drop of blood. The microcollection container will fill by gravity or capillary action, depending on the size of the collection area (see Figure 9-5). Capillary tubes are typically collected horizontally using capillary action and require very little blood. However, more than 0.5 mL of capillary blood can be collected by dermal puncture if the puncture is performed properly.

Correct dermal puncture collection involves allowing free-flowing drops to enter the collection device. The blood flows onto the tip and then down the walls of the microcollection container. Do not "milk" the finger. This will not enhance blood flow but will contaminate the specimen with interstitial fluid, causing hemolysis or clotting. Also, do not scrape the collection container against the skin because this may cause the blood to either hemolyze or clot before it can be mixed with the anticoagulant in the microcollection container. The resulting clotted specimen is unsuitable for testing. Instead, gently squeeze and release the site periodically, allowing for capillary refill, until an adequate amount of blood is obtained. Keep the site below the level of the heart to increase blood flow.

Recall that some microcollection containers have an anticoagulant additive. After each drop enters the container, gently tap the container on a hard surface to mix the blood with the anticoagulant. Tapping should cause the blood to flow down the side or wall. Most microcollection containers have a fill line. It is critical to collect to the fill line, especially if the container has an anticoagulant. Do not underfill or overfill the container. After the container is

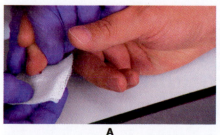
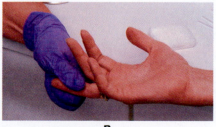
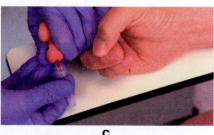

A   B   C

FIGURE 9-5 For a dermal puncture, (A) the first drop of blood is wiped away to avoid contaminating the specimen with tissue fluid, (B) the finger is positioned so that drops of blood form freely and fall away from the puncture site, and (C) each drop is collected in a microcollection container and the container is gently tapped after each drop to ensure mixing with the anticoagulant (if present).

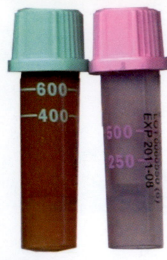

FIGURE 9-6 Blood microcollection containers with markings for acceptable minimum and maximum fill levels.

correctly filled, apply the cap to the container and mix by inverting the container according to the manufacturer's instructions. Follow the order of the draw as outlined in the chapter *Blood Collection Equipment* when more than one microcollection container is used.

Complications of Dermal Puncture

Care must be taken when performing dermal punctures because several complications may occur as a result of improper technique. It is important NOT to puncture through a previous site. Using the same site on the heel of an infant or the finger on a child or adult may cause the site to become infected if microorganisms are present in the scar tissue from the previous puncture. Care must also be taken to ensure the puncture is not so deep as to puncture the bone. Doing so may cause osteochondritis (inflammation of bone and cartilage) or osteomyelitis (inflammation of bone marrow and adjacent bone).

Minimum and Maximum Blood Volumes

Phlebotomists must be aware of the minimum amount of blood required for each laboratory test, which may require asking the testing laboratory for specific volumes. This is very important when collecting blood from infants and small children because phlebotomists must not only be certain that enough blood is collected but also ensure that the blood collection for these patients does not exceed the maximum allowed for the day or over time. Most blood microcollection containers display markings for acceptable minimum and maximum fill levels (see Figure 9-6). The amounts vary by manufacturer and type of additive present. In the example in Figure 9-6, the PST tube (light green) shows that the acceptable amounts of blood for this tube are from 400 to 600 microliters, while the EDTA tube (lavender) shows an acceptable fill range of 250 to 500 microliters. Filling between these two marks and mixing adequately will ensure a quality specimen is collected.

Some facilities require anyone collecting blood specimens from infants to record the amount withdrawn in the patient's health record or on a special document maintained at the nursing unit. Hospital neonatal units may have guidelines established for the maximum amount of blood that can be collected from infants and who is responsible for monitoring these volumes. See Table 9-3 for

TABLE 9-3 Example Guidelines for Maximum Blood Collection Volumes*

Body Weight (kg)	Body Weight (lbs)	Maximum allowable volume (mL) in one blood draw (2.5% of total blood volume)	Total maximum allowable volume (mL) drawn over 30 days
1	2.2	2.5	5
2	4.4	5	10
3	6.3	6	12
4	8.8	8	16
5	11	10	20
6	13.2	12	24
7	15.4	14	28
8	17.6	16	32
9	19.8	18	36
10	22	20	40

* Based on blood volumes of 100mL/kg for preterm infants and 80ML/kg for term infants. Always follow the guidelines for your facility.

an example of maximum blood volume guidelines. Always abide by the protocols of your facility. Paying careful attention to the amount collected from infants and children will reduce the occurrence of iatrogenic anemia and exsanguination in these patients. Recall that iatrogenic anemia is a result of drawing too much blood for hospital tests or other medical procedures. If the amount of blood removed for testing exceeds 10% of the patient's total blood volume, it could become life-threatening and is known as exsanguination. These conditions can easily occur in patients of smaller size, children, and infants.

Just the Right Amount

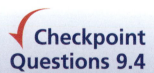

Critical Thinking

Pay very close attention to blood volumes in microcollection containers to ensure the collection of a quality specimen by dermal puncture. An underfilled container may contain too much anticoagulant for the amount of blood collected, which alters the anticoagulant to blood ratio and affects test results. An overfilled container will not have enough anticoagulant for the volume of blood collected and will result in microclot formation or the entire specimen may clot. Both situations will result in the need for recollection of the specimen. If daily maximum blood collection levels have been reached, testing and treatment will be delayed. To avoid over- and underfilling microcollection containers, fill the containers to between the minimum and maximum volume markings found on the container. See Figure 9-6.

After the Dermal Puncture

After you complete the dermal puncture, mix the specimens (if necessary). Dispose of the contaminated safety lancet in the sharps container. Label the microcontainers and observe any specimen handling instructions. Check the site of puncture and apply a bandage, when appropriate. Small children should not have bandages applied to their fingers because they have a tendency to put their fingers in their mouth and run the risk of swallowing or choking on the bandage. In addition, infants have delicate skin that can tear when adhesive bandages are removed. Collect and dispose of your supplies appropriately. Clean the area. Provide for safety, then thank and dismiss the patient, if appropriate. Remove your gloves and transport the specimen to the laboratory.

1. Why is it important to wipe away the first drop of blood from a dermal puncture?
2. An adult patient objects to having a dermal puncture because her job involves typing on a keyboard all day. What might you say to reassure this patient?
3. What physical principles are involved in the proper collection of microcollection containers?

Checkpoint Questions 9.4

Chapter Summary

Learning Outcome	Key Concepts/Examples	Related NAACLS Competency
9.1 Explain why dermal/capillary puncture is used instead of routine venipuncture for some patients. Pages 242–243.	Although routine venipuncture is usually the preferred method for obtaining blood specimens, dermal puncture may be performed on the following patients: • infants and young children • adults whose veins are difficult to find or are unsuitable; these patients may include those who are obese, elderly, or severely burned	5.00, 6.7
9.2 Select an appropriate site for dermal puncture and identify the equipment needed. Pages 243–245.	Skin at the site of a dermal puncture should be warm, pink, and free from scars, cuts, rashes, or bruises. For children and adults, dermal puncture sites include the distal regions of the middle finger (third finger) and ring finger (fourth finger). For infants, the medial or lateral regions of the plantar surface of the heel are used. The equipment for dermal puncture is the same as that for venipuncture, except dermal puncture requires a safety dermal puncture device and microspecimen containers as well.	5.00, 5.5, 6.1, 6.3
9.3 Carry out the procedure for performing a dermal puncture. Pages 246–247.	Clean the finger with an alcohol pad and allow the finger to dry thoroughly before performing the dermal puncture. Apply slight pressure and then use the dermal puncture device to puncture the skin so that the cut crosses the fingerprint lines. Be aware of the minimum volume required for testing as well as the maximum allowed blood collection volume.	5.6, 6.12
9.4 Apply the procedure for collecting a capillary specimen. Pages 247–249.	The general steps for performing a capillary/dermal puncture and collecting a specimen include the following: 1. Introduce yourself. 2. Identify the patient. 3. Explain procedure to the patient. 4. Wash hands and put on gloves. 5. Select an appropriate site. 6. Cleanse the capillary puncture site. 7. Firmly hold the finger or foot. 8. Properly position and engage the safety lancet device. 9. Wipe away the first drop of blood. 10. Collect blood specimens into microcollection containers using proper order of draw as required. 11. Cover the puncture wound with gauze. 12. Apply pressure to the puncture site. 13. Appropriately dispose of sharps and trash. 14. Label the tubes. 15. Clean the area. 16. Thank the patient and provide for safety if necessary.	5.6, 6.00, 6.4, 6.6, 6.10, 6.12

Chapter Review

A: Labeling

Label the blood collection equipment pictured in the image below.

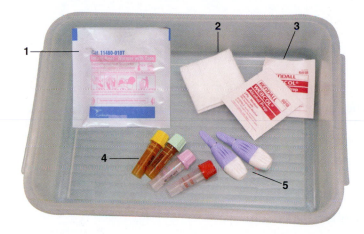

1. [LO 9.2] _____

2. [LO 9.2] _____

3. [LO 9.2] _____

4. [LO 9.2] _____

5. [LO 9.2] _____

B: Matching

Match each definition with the correct term.

_____**6.** [LO 9.2] calcaneus

_____**7.** [LO 9.2] edema

_____**8.** [LO 9.1] interstitial fluid

_____**9.** [LO 9.2] osteomyelitis

____**10.** [LO 9.2] palmar

____**11.** [LO 9.2] plantar

a. infection of the bone

b. heel bone

c. bottom surface

d. caused by a buildup of fluids

e. fluid between cells and tissues

f. palm side or surface

C: Fill in the Blank

12. [LO 9.1] New and developing technology in laboratory instrumentation allows some tests to be performed on blood obtained from _____, instead of the traditional venous blood.

13. [LO 9.2] The preferred sites for dermal puncture in an infant are the medial or lateral regions of the _____ surface of the infant's heel.

14. [LO 9.2] Finger punctures are not usually performed on the first finger, fifth finger, or _____ because the skin is often too thick or calloused.

15. [LO 9.2] To increase blood flow to a dermal puncture site, a _____ may be applied.

16. [LO 9.1] For infants and small children, _____ is the preferred method of blood collection.

17. [LO 9.3] Controlling the depth of puncture when using a lancet is important in preventing an infection of the bone called _____.

D: Sequencing

Based on what you have learned in this chapter, put the following steps for performing a routine capillary/dermal puncture in order by numbering them from 1 to 14 in the spaces provided.

18. [LO 9.3] _____ Apply pressure to the puncture site.

19. [LO 9.3] _____ Cleanse the capillary puncture site.

20. [LO 9.4] _____ Collect blood samples into microcollection containers.

21. [LO 9.3] _____ Cover puncture wound with gauze.

22. [LO 9.3] _____ Engage the safety lancet device.

23. [LO 9.3] _____ Explain the procedure to the patient.

24. [LO 9.3] _____ Firmly hold the finger or foot.

25. [LO 9.3] _____ Identify the patient.

26. [LO 9.3] _____ Introduce yourself.

27. [LO 9.4] _____ Label the tubes.

28. [LO 9.3] _____ Select an appropriate site.

29. [LO 9.3] _____ Thank the patient.

30. [LO 9.3] _____ Wash hands and put on gloves.

31. [LO 9.3] _____ Wipe away the first drop.

E: Case Study/Critical Thinking

32. [LO 9.2] When asked to collect blood from an infant in the special care nursery, you notice that there are several lancet scars on both heels. What site will you choose and why?

33. [LO 9.3] While performing a dermal puncture on a finger, you are having difficulty forming a good drop of blood. Instead, the blood seems to be running along the fingerprint and going everywhere except into the collection tube. What caused this to happen and what should you have done?

34. [LO 9.3] Several EDTA microcollection containers from different infants were found to have microclots in them. The CBC on these specimens is not reliable and the specimens must be recollected. What may have caused these specimens to clot? How can this situation be avoided? What harm could it cause the patients?

35. [LO 9.4] You have been asked to collect more blood on an infant that has had blood collected multiple times every day for several days. What precautions should be taken in this situation?

F: Exam Prep

Choose the best answer for each question.

36. [LO 9.3] To produce a rounded drop of blood, finger punctures should be made

    a. before the alcohol is dry.

    b. across the fingerprint.

    c. along or on the fingerprint.

    d. on the index finger.

37. [LO 9.2] What is the effect of warming the site prior to dermal puncture?

    a. It may cause hemolysis in the specimen.

    b. It increases blood flow to the area.

    c. It makes the puncture less painful.

    d. It causes hemoconcentration.

38. [LO 9.4] During a fingerstick collection, excessive milking can cause

    a. irritation at the site.

    b. excessive bleeding.

    c. contamination of the specimen with tissue fluid.

    d. introduction of an infection.

39. [LO 9.3] According to guidelines, the depth of a heelstick lancet should be no more than

    a. 1 mm.

    b. 1.8 mm.

    c. 2 mm.

    d. 2.4 mm.

40. [LO 9.4] Why should the first drop of blood be wiped during a dermal puncture?

    a. To remove any interstitial fluid contamination

    b. To limit the amount of blood released

    c. To increase the amount of blood released

    d. To decrease the possibility of bloodborne pathogen transmission

41. [LO 9.4] A fingerstick specimen was found to be clotted. What might have caused this specimen to be clotted? *(Choose all that apply.)*

    a. Not waiting for the alcohol to dry

    b. Scraping the blood off the finger

    c. Mixing the specimen after each drop

    d. Aggressively squeezing the finger

42. [LO 9.1] Which of the following patients is the most likely candidate for a dermal puncture to obtain blood for laboratory testing?

    a. 30-year-old pregnant woman

    b. 2-week-old infant with pneumonia

    c. 17-year-old boy with influenza

    d. 46-year-old man with asthma

43. [LO 9.1] For which blood tests is dermal puncture *not* recommended? *(Choose all that apply.)*

    a. Erythrocyte sedimentation rate

    b. Potassium level

    c. Blood culture

    d. Complete blood count

44. [LO 9.1] Which of the following is an advantage of dermal puncture, relative to other blood specimen collection methods?

    a. It allows a large amount of blood to be drawn.

    b. It provides the best specimen quality.

    c. It requires transferring the blood to micro-specimen containers.

    d. It is easy to perform.

45. [LO 9.2] Why should a dermal puncture *not* be performed on the heel of a 2-year-old toddler?

    a. If the site becomes infected, osteomyelitis may result.

    b. Walking on the puncture site may cause pain.

    c. The skin around the plantar surface of the foot may be calloused.

    d. Osteomyelitis may occur if the puncture site becomes dirty.

46. [LO 9.2] Why do phlebotomists avoid using the fingers of a newborn for dermal puncture?

    a. The potential for pain is greater in the fingers than in the heel.

    b. A greater volume of blood can be obtained from the infant's heel.

    c. The fingers are too small for maintaining a safe distance from bone.

    d. The fingerprint is not yet well enough developed to cut across.

47. [LO 9.2] Which of the following areas of the heel are recommended for dermal puncture? *(Choose all that apply.)*

a. Back of heel

b. Medial plantar surface

c. Lateral plantar surface

d. Arch of foot

48. [LO 9.3] Which of the following describes the proper way to hold a finger for a dermal puncture?

a. Stretch the skin tightly across the surface to be punctured.

b. Pinch the area to be punctured to elevate it above the rest of the finger.

c. Allow the skin to rest naturally, without touching it.

d. Hold the finger firmly above the level of the heart.

49. [LO 9.3] Why is a dermal puncture performed so that the cut runs across the fingerprint lines?

a. To prevent hemolysis

b. To prevent the puncture from piercing too deep

c. To direct the blood along the lines of the fingerprint

d. To deliver the best possible blood flow

50. [LO 9.4] After the skin has been punctured, the next step in collecting a capillary blood specimen is to

a. clean the puncture using an alcohol prep pad.

b. wipe away the first drop of blood.

c. touch the open end of the container to the blood drop.

d. "milk" the finger to obtain the specimen.

51. [LO 9.4] If you are having trouble obtaining enough blood from a puncture site, which of the following is the *best* alternative for obtaining the proper specimen?

a. Gently squeeze and release the finger, allowing for capillary refill.

b. Perform a second dermal puncture to obtain the rest of the blood.

c. "Milk" the finger to enhance the blood flow.

d. Scrape the container against the puncture site.

52. [LO 9.4] If the microspecimen container has an anticoagulant, how should you mix the blood with the anticoagulant?

a. Shake the microspecimen container vigorously.

b. Invert the microspecimen container according to the manufacturer's instructions.

c. Use a micropipette to stir the blood in the container.

d. Process the microspecimen container in a centrifuge at a low speed.

53. [LO 9.4] How should you dispose of the safety lancet after performing a dermal puncture?

a. Wrap it in a tissue and place it in the garbage.

b. Place it in a biohazardous waste container.

c. Place it in a sharps container.

d. Send it to a medical reprocessing unit for cleaning.

54. [LO 9.2] Which of the following may cause osteomyelitis?

a. Puncturing the middle of the pad of the finger

b. Failing to clean the site of the puncture with alcohol

c. Puncturing the calcaneus

d. Choosing a calloused site for the dermal puncture

55. [LO 9.2] A swollen finger should not be used for dermal puncture because

a. this would increase the amount of interstitial fluid in the specimen.

b. the site cannot be properly prepared due to the edema.

c. the fingerprint is not sufficiently visible on a swollen finger.

d. pain is greatly increased in an edematous area.

References

Clinical and Laboratory Standards Institute. (2007). *Procedures for the collection of diagnostic blood specimens by venipuncture; approved standard.* (6th ed.). H3-A6. 27(26). Wayne, PA. CLSI.

Dale, J. C., & Novis, D. A. (2002). Outpatient phlebotomy success and reasons for specimen rejection. *Archives of Pathology & Laboratory Medicine, 126,* 416–419.

Masoorli, S., Angeles, T., & Barbone, M. (1998). Danger points: How to prevent nerve injuries from venipuncture. *Nursing, 28,* 34–39.

National Accrediting Agency for Clinical Laboratory Sciences. (2010). *NAACLS entry-level phlebotomist competencies.* Rosemont, IL. NAACLS.

Niwinski, N. (2009). Capillary blood collection: Best practices. *BD LabNotes. 20*(1). Becton, Dickinson and Company.

Product FAQs. (2011). *Capillary blood collection.* Becton, Dickinson and Company. Retrieved April 12, 2011, from www.bd.com/vacutainer/faqs/

Wilson, D. D. (2008). *McGraw-Hill manual of laboratory and diagnostic tests.* New York: McGraw-Hill.

COMPETENCY CHECKLIST: DERMAL PUNCTURE ON FINGER

Procedure Steps	Practice			Performed		Master
	1	2	3	Yes	No	
Preprocedure						
1. Examines the requisition.						
2. Greets the patient (and parents, if the patient is a child); introduces self.						
3. Identifies the patient verbally using two identifiers, including comparing the identification band with the requisition.						
4. Explains the procedure to the patient.						
5. Verifies diet restrictions or instructions.						
6. Washes hands and puts on gloves.						
7. Selects the correct equipment and supplies.						
8. Assembles the equipment and supplies properly.						
9. Conveniently places the equipment.						
10. Reassures the patient.						
11. Selects the appropriate finger.						
12. Warms the finger, if necessary.						
13. Selects the dermal puncture site.						
14. Cleanses the puncture site.						
15. Allows the site to air dry.						
Procedure						
16. Applies the lancet across the fingerprints.						
17. Uses adequate pressure when activating the lancet.						
18. Wipes away the first drop of blood.						
19. Collects the sample without scraping.						
20. Collects the sample without milking the site.						
21. Collects an appropriate amount of sample.						
22. Mixes Microtainer® or seals capillary tubes.						
23. Cleanses the site of excess blood.						
24. Places gauze over the puncture site.						
25. Applies pressure to the puncture site.						
26. Removes all items from the collection area.						
27. Disposes of the puncture device correctly.						
28. Labels the tubes correctly.						

Procedure Steps	Practice			Performed		
	1	2	3	Yes	No	Master
Postprocedure						
29. Observes special handling instructions.						
30. Checks the patient's finger.						
31. Applies a bandage (unless the patient is a small child).						
32. Thanks the patient (and parents, if present, for small children).						
33. Disposes of used supplies appropriately.						
34. Removes gloves and washes hands.						
35. Transports specimens to the laboratory.						
36. Documents the specimen collection.						

COMMENTS: _____

_____

_____

_____

SIGNED

EVALUATOR: _____

STUDENT: _____

COMPETENCY CHECKLIST: DERMAL PUNCTURE ON HEEL

Procedure Steps	Practice			Performed		Master
	1	2	3	Yes	No	
Preprocedure						
1. Examines the requisition.						
2. Greets the parents; introduces self.						
3. Identifies the patient verbally using two identifiers, including comparing the identification with the requisition. (If nursery collection, confirms identity with nursing staff and the identification band.)						
4. Explains the procedure to the parents (if present).						
5. Verifies diet restrictions or instructions.						
6. Washes hands and puts on gloves.						
7. Selects the correct equipment and supplies.						
8. Assembles the equipment and supplies properly.						
9. Conveniently places the equipment.						
10. Reassures the patient (and parents).						
11. Warms the heel, if necessary.						
12. Selects an appropriate site on the heel.						
13. Cleanses the puncture site.						
14. Allows the site to air dry.						
Procedure						
15. Avoids previously punctured sites.						
16. Applies the lancet at the appropriate place and angle on the heel.						
17. Uses adequate pressure when activating the lancet.						
18. Wipes away the first drop of blood.						
19. Collects without scraping the site.						
20. Collects an appropriate amount of sample.						
21. Mixes Microtainer® or seals capillary tubes.						
22. Cleanses the site of excess blood.						
23. Places gauze over the puncture site.						
24. Applies pressure to the puncture site.						
25. Removes all items from the collection area.						
26. Disposes of the puncture device correctly.						
27. Labels the tubes correctly.						

Procedure Steps	Practice			Performed		Master
	1	2	3	Yes	No	
Postprocedure						
28. Observes special handling instructions.						
29. Checks the patient's heel.						
30. Applies a bandage (optional).						
31. Thanks the parents, if present.						
32. Disposes of used supplies appropriately.						
33. Removes gloves and washes hands.						
34. Transports specimens to the laboratory.						
35. Documents the specimen collection.						

COMMENTS: _____
_____
_____
_____

SIGNED

EVALUATOR: _____

STUDENT: _____

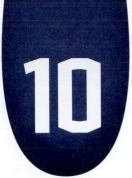

10

Blood Specimen Handling

essential terms

additive-to-blood ratio
aerosol
aliquoting
autoantibodies
centrifuging
chain of custody
cold agglutinins
delta check
glycolysis

icteric
light-sensitive
lipemia
pneumatic tube system
pre-examination error
real-time tracking
reference
  laboratory
STAT

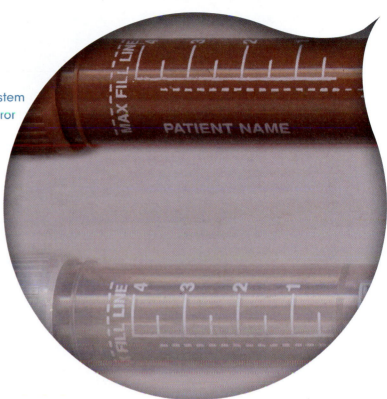

Learning Outcomes

10.1 Explain methods for transporting and processing blood specimens for routine and special testing and reference laboratories.

10.2 Recognize criteria for special specimen handling.

10.3 List the circumstances that would lead to re-collection or rejection of a patient sample.

Related NAACLS Competencies

7.00 Demonstrate understanding of requisitioning, specimen transport, and specimen processing.

7.3 Explain methods for transporting and processing blood specimens for routine and special testing.

7.4 Explain methods for processing and transporting blood specimens for testing at reference laboratories.

7.5 Identify and report potential pre-analytical errors that may occur during specimen collection, labeling, transporting, and processing.

7.6 Describe and follow the criteria for specimens and test results that will be used as legal evidence, i.e., paternity testing, chain of custody, blood alcohol levels, etc.

Introduction

Once a specimen is collected, special care must be taken to maintain its quality. This chapter includes the ways in which specimens reach the testing laboratory, the handling of specimens requiring special conditions during transport, the processing of specimens using centrifugation, and the causes for specimen rejection.

10.1 Specimen Transport

The process of venipuncture and dermal puncture involves more than just the collection of a blood sample. The way in which blood specimens destined for testing are handled within the healthcare setting is of crucial importance to the phlebotomist, the laboratory personnel, and, of course, the patient. One minor mistake may result in a large error that could end up causing harm to the patient. Equally important is how the sample is obtained and handled after the collection. All specimens must be transported to the laboratory in a timely manner.

Transporting Specimens Within the Facility

In some laboratories, the outpatient phlebotomy area is part of the laboratory, so transporting may simply require a walk to the next room. However, sometimes the phlebotomy area is in a different part of the building, so transportation becomes more important. Some medical facilities use **pneumatic tube systems** or other devices to expedite the process of transporting specimens to the laboratory. A pneumatic tube system moves tubes with a vacuum, just like the tube system at the bank drive-through window (see Figure 10-1). Other devices for transporting specimens include a dumbwaiter (small elevator), automated tracks, robotics, or a series of conveyor belts. The effects that transporting specimens by these systems may have on laboratory test results should be studied by each laboratory considering adopting one of these methods. For example, some pneumatic tube systems may agitate or disturb the specimen, resulting in hemolysis or other adverse effects. Automated systems may require facilities to provide a clearance for the installation of tracks or robotic sensors. Laboratories should validate all methods of specimen transport prior to establishing a policy that allows for alternate ways of delivering specimens to the laboratory.

There are many reasons for rapid delivery of specimens. Some tests are ordered as **STAT** (immediately) and must be performed immediately on arrival at the laboratory. Results for tests ordered STAT are expected within 1 hour after they are ordered. Some specimens require centrifugation and separation of plasma or serum from cells within a specified amount of time. Ideally, the specimen should be taken to the laboratory within 45 minutes and centrifuged within 1 hour. CSLI standards recommend a limit of 2 hours between collection and separation of serum or plasma by centrifugation. Operation of the centrifuge is discussed later in this chapter. If you are unsure of specimen requirements, look them up in the procedure manual. If the blood is not taken to the laboratory in the necessary length of time, the test results will be inaccurate.

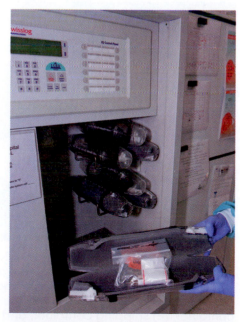

Figure 10-1 Pneumatic tube system.

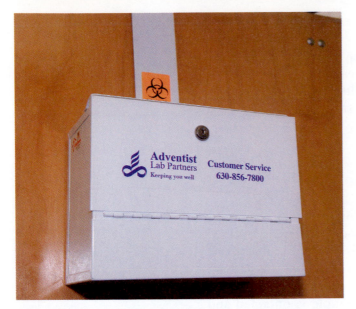

Figure 10-2 Courier specimen pickup lockbox.

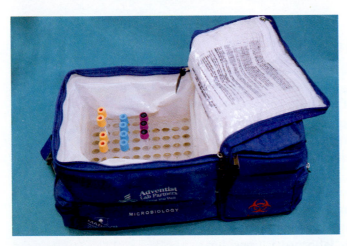

Figure 10-3 Courier transport container.

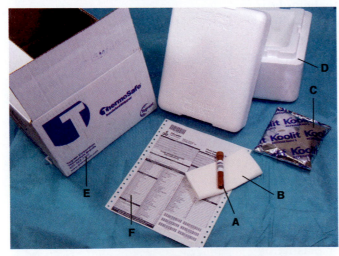

Figure 10-4 The requirements for specimen packaging include (A) the specimen or its aliquot in a properly labeled primary leak-proof container, (B) absorbent material, (C) a coolant, (D) secondary container, (E) shipping container, and (F) paperwork including patient, specimen, and test information.

Transporting Specimens from Outside the Facility

Outpatient facilities present a different challenge with regard to transportation of laboratory specimens. Usually, a courier service transports the specimens from the collection facility to the reference laboratory. Specimens may need to be processed at the outpatient facility before being transported to the reference laboratory. You may be required to follow special handling procedures for the specimens drawn. Specimens for pickup from outpatient facilities are often placed in courier pickup lockboxes just inside or outside the facility (see Figure 10-2). Policies should be in place concerning the length of time these specimens stay in these boxes, as well as how to protect them from extreme temperatures. Couriers should follow a predetermined pickup schedule and ensure specimen integrity by maintaining specific specimen requirements, which include the use of proper transport containers (see Figure 10-3).

Transporting Specimens to Other Facilities

Some tests that physicians order must be sent to a **reference laboratory** or another facility because the hospital's laboratory does not offer the tests. Reference laboratories usually offer a larger variety of laboratory tests than the average community hospital laboratory. Depending on the location of the reference laboratory, it may provide its own courier service, or specimens may have to be shipped to the laboratory. Specimens sent in the mail or through express delivery services, such as FedEx, must comply with local, state, and federal laws governing special packaging and biohazard identification. In general, packages containing clinical specimens must include the following:

- A watertight primary container
- An original specimen tube or a plastic screw-cap transfer tube
- Absorbent material
- A watertight secondary container, such as a ziplocked bag, plastic canister, or Styrofoam box
- Sturdy outer packaging, such as a fiberboard box or mailing tube, wooden box, or rigid plastic container (see Figure 10-4)

The primary container holding the specimen should be labeled the same as the original specimen. This container is then wrapped with the absorbent material and placed in a secondary container. Any accompanying paperwork is affixed to or enclosed in

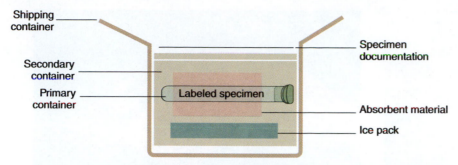

Figure 10-5 Cross-sectional diagram of specimen shipping packaging.

the secondary container and must include specimen identification along with appropriate biohazard labels attached. A coolant (ice packs or dry ice) may be required in the secondary container for refrigerated or frozen specimens. The secondary container is then placed in the outer package for shipping, which must display appropriate biohazard warning labels in addition to the sender and recipient addresses. Carrier documentation is affixed to the shipping container and must include the weight of dry ice, if present. Figure 10-5 shows a cross-sectional view of a specimen properly packaged for shipping. Facilities must package and ship specimens according to regulations set by the agency governing the type of specimen that is being shipped. Table 10-1 lists agencies that regulate the transportation of medical specimens.

Protecting Personnel

Protecting personnel is important when transporting specimens. Tubes containing specimens are usually placed in biohazard bags for safe transport. If a specimen is dropped and the tube breaks, the blood or body fluid will stay contained inside the bag. If specimens are sent by pneumatic tube or automated systems, they, too, should first be placed inside biohazard bags. When opening the pneumatic tube to receive a specimen in the laboratory, phlebotomists should wear personal protective equipment (PPE), including gloves, a lab coat, and face protection. The specimen container may have broken in transit and the specimen may have spilled into the carrier tube. If this is the case, you must follow your facility's policies and procedures for proper decontamination of the pneumatic carrier tube.

Safety & Infection Control

TABLE 10-1 Agencies That Regulate the Transport of Medical Specimens

Agency	Acronym	Website
Centers for Disease Control and Prevention	CDC	www.cdc.gov
Department of Transportation	DOT	www.dot.gov
Federal Aviation Administration	FAA	www.faa.gov
Food and Drug Administration	FDA	www.fda.gov
International Air Transport Association	IATA	www.iata.org
International Civil Aviation Organization	ICAO	www.icao.int
Occupational Safety and Health Administration	OSHA	www.osha.gov
Transportation Safety Administration	TSA	www.tsa.gov

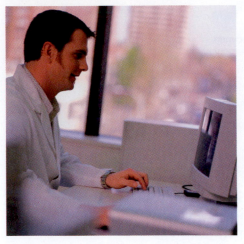

Figure 10-6 Phlebotomist entering collection data into the LIS.

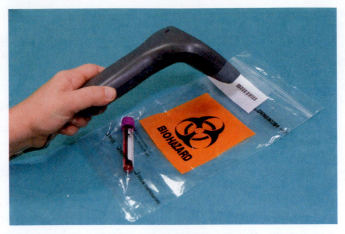

Figure 10-7 Courier bar-coding specimen delivery confirmation data.

Tracking Specimen Transit

Documentation of specimen collection and transport is essential for proper record keeping. If test results are questionable, the collection and transport information can provide valuable clues as to the cause of invalid results. For example, if a specimen is hemolyzed, knowing how long it sat in a courier pickup box or courier vehicle may help explain the cause of the hemolysis. In addition to recording collection information on the specimen label, phlebotomists must enter specific data into the patient's electronic health record (EHR) using the laboratory information system (LIS), including the date and time of collection, the phlebotomist's identification code, and any comments that might aid in specimen analysis, such as "collected from right arm with I.V." (see Figure 10-6). This information is readily accessible and provides a specimen tracking system. Couriers also enter information into the LIS regarding the pickup and drop-off of specimens. Some facilities require phlebotomists and couriers to scan bar codes on specimens with a device that communicates with the LIS to provide **real-time tracking** (see Figure 10-7). Real-time tracking of laboratory specimens is similar to how the U.S. Postal Service and United Parcel Service track packages. Real-time tracking allows laboratory personnel to estimate when they will have the specimen, so that they can inform physicians or nurses, who may call for results, of the approximate time the test results will be ready.

> ✓ **Checkpoint Questions 10.1**
>
> 1. According to CSLI standards, what is the maximum allowable time between obtaining a blood specimen and centrifugation?
> 2. List two reasons for tracking specimens.
> 3. Explain why leaving a specimen in an outdoor courier box may not be the best practice for maintaining a quality laboratory specimen.

10.2 Special Specimen Handling

The way a specimen is collected and how it is handled are essential to an acceptable specimen and accurate results. Special handling applies to specimens that are to be kept warm, cool, or protected from light. Special handling

TABLE 10-2 Common Laboratory Tests That Require Special Handling

Laboratory Test	Special Handling
Acid phosphatase	Deliver to lab within 1 hour. Separate, and freeze serum after clotting.
Adrenocorticotropic hormone (ACTH)	Place in ice-water mixture.*
Alcohol, blood	Use antiseptic other than alcohol prep pad to cleanse venipuncture site.
Ammonia	Place in ice-water mixture.*
Beta-carotene	Protect from light.**
Bilirubin, total or direct	Protect from light.**
Catecholamines	Place in ice-water mixture.*
Clot retraction	Incubate at 37° C until clotted.
Cold agglutinins	Warm tube, incubate at 37° C until clotted. Separate immediately after clotting.
Complement, C4	Separate, freeze serum after clotting.
Complement, total (CH50)	Let clot in refrigerator. Separate immediately, and freeze serum.
Complement, total (CH100)	Let clot in refrigerator. Separate immediately, and freeze serum.
Gastrin	Place in ice-water mixture.*
Gentamicin	Label peak or trough.
Glucose tolerance	Label tubes with time interval.
Human leukocyte antigen (HLA-B27)	Maintain at room temperature. Do *not* refrigerate or freeze. Record date and time collected.
Lactic acid	Place in ice-water mixture.*
Parathyroid hormone (PTH)	Place in ice-water mixture.*
pH/blood gas	Place in ice-water mixture.*
Porphyrins	Protect from light.**
Prostate-specific antigen (PSA)	Deliver to lab within 1 hour. Separate, and freeze serum after clotting.
Prostatic acid phosphatase	Deliver to lab within 1 hour. Separate, and freeze serum after clotting.
Pyruvate	Place in ice-water mixture.*
Thioridazine (Mellaril®)	Protect from light.**
Tobramycin	Label peak or trough.
Vancomycin	Label peak or trough.
Vitamin A	Protect from light.**
Vitamin B_6	Protect from light.**
Vitamin B_{12}	Protect from light.**

*Place in ice-water mixture = place tube in a cup with a mixture of ice and water.
**Protect from light = protect by wrapping the tubes in aluminum foil or using plastic amber tubes.

also includes processes such as special identification for legal specimens as well as centrifugation and separation prior to specimen delivery. Table 10-2 presents a list of common laboratory tests that require special handling.

Temperature-Sensitive Specimens

Some specimens for laboratory testing must be maintained at a specific temperature range, either warm or cool. They are placed in the appropriate environment immediately upon collection and are kept there until delivery to the laboratory.

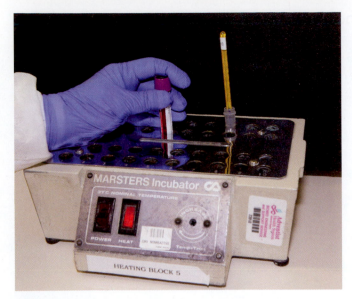

Figure 10-8 Specimens that need to be kept warm can be placed into a heating block set at the correct temperature.

Specimens Requiring Warmth During Transit

Testing for **cold agglutinins,** or antibodies that react at cooler temperatures, is done for patients suspected of having conditions such as atypical pneumonia. People with atypical pneumonia are infected with *Mycoplasma pneumoniae* and can produce **autoantibodies** (antibodies against oneself). These antibodies, also known as immunoglobulins, attack the patient's own body as if the body were foreign.

Cold agglutinins react with red blood cells at temperatures lower than body temperature, which has a normal range of 97.6°F to 99.6°F (36.5°C to 37.6°C). The cold temperature reaction is the principle of the laboratory test for atypical pneumonia. After a blood sample is drawn, it begins to cool, or drop below body temperature. At temperatures lower than body temperature, cold agglutinins in the plasma attach to red blood cells, causing clumping. Collection tubes for cold agglutinins may be red-topped tubes that contain no additives or lavender-topped EDTA tubes, depending on specific laboratory requirements. In addition, the following requirements must be followed when working with collection tubes for cold agglutinins:

- The tubes must be pre-warmed by placing them in a container of 37°C water or other warming device, such as a heel warmer, before collection and kept warm throughout the process.

- The tubes must be delivered directly to the laboratory section responsible for performing this test and placed in an incubator or water bath in the laboratory, set at 37°C (98.6°F) (see Figure 10-8). Care should be taken to keep the sample at 37°C (98.6°F). Failure to keep the sample warm will result in erroneous laboratory results.

- Cold agglutinin test samples must be kept at body temperature until the serum or plasma can be separated from the cells, which must be done within 1 hour.

Routine venipuncture procedures are followed, with the noted addition of the warmed collection tube.

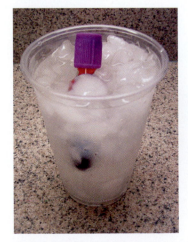

Figure 10-9 Special handling procedures may involve placing the tube in a cup of ice-water mixture.

Specimens Requiring Chilling During Transit

Unlike testing for cold agglutinins, some specimens must be chilled immediately after collection. Chilling specimens slows down the metabolic process, keeping analyte levels as close as possible to those found in the blood stream. Tests such as arterial blood gases, ammonia, and lactic acid require chilling. Blood collected for these tests is placed in a container with a slurry of crushed ice and water, as shown in Figure 10-9; however, the specimen must not be allowed to freeze, as this will cause hemolysis. Specimens may even require collection in a pre-chilled evacuated tube. Refer to the policy at your place of employment to determine what special handling must be given each blood test you will be collecting. Use the competency checklist *Specimen Handling: Temperature-Sensitive Specimens* at the end of this chapter to review and practice the procedure.

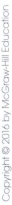

Light-Sensitive Specimens

Some substances are **light-sensitive,** meaning that they break down when exposed to light. Specimens collected to test for these substances must be covered in foil or placed in a special container to protect them from light (see Figure 10-10). Microcollection containers, as shown in Figure 10-11, are available in amber plastic, which protects specimens from light. The amber plastic container protects the specimen similarly to how tinted glasses protect eyes from sunlight. Substances such as bilirubin and carotene require protection from light because light (especially sunlight) can alter their chemical composition. Use the competency checklist *Specimen Handling: Light-Sensitive Specimens* at the end of this chapter to review and practice the procedure.

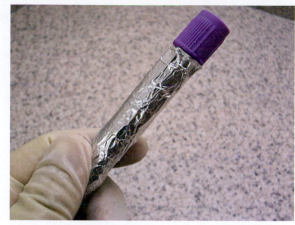

Figure 10-10 Specimens for measurement of substances that are affected by light are usually wrapped in foil.

Neonatal Bilirubin

Life Span Considerations

Bilirubin levels are commonly performed on newborn infants. Infants normally have an increased level of red blood cells at birth. As the extra red blood cells break down, bilirubin forms and may be deposited in tissues. If too much is in the infant's body tissue, it must be removed by placing the infant under ultraviolet light. It is very important to turn off the ultraviolet light when collecting blood from an infant under this light because leaving the light on will destroy some of the bilirubin in the sample as you are collecting it. This may falsely lower the bilirubin result when the blood is tested. Be sure to turn the light back on after you finish collecting the specimen and safely remove it from under the lamp.

Blood Alcohol, Forensic Testing, and Toxicology Specimens

Certain phlebotomy procedures, such as blood alcohol testing, forensic testing, and toxicology, require extra considerations regarding the patient, collection, and specimen handling. Test results obtained for these procedures may be used in a court of law.

Specimens of a legal matter require special handling. Blood and other specimens are often collected from a victim, a suspect, or another person—dead or alive—involved in a legal matter. These specimens must be correctly identified and under the uninterrupted control of authorized personnel to ensure their validity. Accurately identifying a specimen and making sure it has not been altered or replaced is called establishing a **chain of custody.** This procedure is required for medicolegal specimens for which test results are needed in court cases, such as evidence of rape or drug tests for illicit drug use. If the chain of custody between the victim and/or suspect and the specimen cannot be proved to have remained unbroken, the specimen and any tests performed on this specimen will be considered invalid.

The first link in the chain of custody is collecting the specimen. During this process, make sure to collect the specimen from the correct patient and guard against tampering. The chain-of-custody form (see Figure 10-12) must be completed correctly and the patient may be required to sign or initial the form. The chain-of-custody procedure dictates that each person who handles the specimen must sign

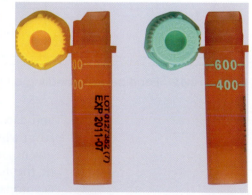

Figure 10-11 Amber-colored microcollection containers.

LABORATORY CHAIN-OF-CUSTODY FORM (EXAMPLE FORM)

Submitter:

(Complete Sections 1 and 2 before collection and document transfer of samples/evidence in Section 3.)

Section 1

Investigator name:	Date submitted:
Agency:	Agency case no.:

Address:		

City/County:	State:	ZIP code:

Phone no.:	Fax no.:	E-mail:

Emergency contact:	Phone no.:

Submitter: (Print name):	Agency: Telephone: ( ) -	Date:

Section 2

Sampling site:	Site address:

Collected by:	Date collected:	Agency:

Submitter description: Include the number of containers, identification number(s), and a physical description of each sample submitted for testing. {Relinquish sample(s) on page 2.}

Submitter comments:

Lockbox evidence seal number:

Section 3

Chain of custody: Persons relinquishing and receiving evidence: Provide signature, organization, and date/time to document evidence transfers. (Start with Box Number 1 below.)

Relinquished by (submitter)	Organization	Date/time	Received by	Organization	Date/time
1.			2.		

Relinquished by	Organization	Date/time	Received by	Organization	Date/time
3.			4.		

Relinquished by	Organization	Date/time	Received by	Organization	Date/time
5.			6.		

Figure 10-12 Each person handling a legal specimen must complete and sign the chain-of-custody form.

and date the legal document. The document indicates the name of the person from whom the specimen was received, the person to whom the specimen was given, and the length of time each person had the specimen. Multiple copies of the form are used as a safeguard system. One copy, usually the original, accompanies the specimen in a sealed envelope. Another copy is attached to the outside of the envelope, so that each person who handles the specimen can initial the form. A third copy is usually retained in the patient's file.

In addition, the specimen must be kept in a locked container and/or the tube must be sealed with a tamper-proof label or wax at all times to prevent unauthorized personnel from tampering with the sample. The chain of custody accounts for the specimen from the time of collection to the final disposition of the specimen and guarantees the integrity of the specimen in a court of law. These general procedures help maintain an intact chain of custody. Always refer to the procedure at your facility to make sure you are meeting all relevant requirements.

Legal Blood Alcohol Specimens

It is critical for the phlebotomist to understand that the patient has the right to refuse to give a blood alcohol specimen unless that right has been legally removed by an appropriate legal action. If it is being required due to an accident or possible litigation, there must be a legal document, signed by the proper authorities, authorizing the draw. It is up to the phlebotomist to determine if these legalities have been completed before the draw. If not, the phlebotomist can be sued for assault and battery. If the specimen is being ordered for possible litigation, a chain-of-custody form must also be filled out and the top of the tube must be sealed with a tamper-proof label or wax.

Blood Alcohol Testing

The police may request a blood alcohol level because of a charge of driving under the influence (DUI). Before the test can be performed, the patient must consent to having the test done, and the patient can refuse the test. If the phlebotomist attempts to collect a specimen for the test without written consent from the patient or a court order, the phlebotomist can be found guilty of assault and battery and the test is not admissible in court.

An employer may request a blood alcohol level because an employee appears to be intoxicated. Care must be taken when collecting a blood alcohol specimen because these specimens are often needed for legal reasons. The chain-of-custody procedure must be followed. The collection procedure is the same as routine venipuncture, with the noted exception of the cleaning agent. Although the alcohol used in an alcohol prep pad is different from the alcohol used for human consumption, an alcohol prep pad must *not* be used because its use will cause the legal system to question the blood alcohol result. Thus, the venipuncture site must be cleaned with a *disinfectant* (a solution containing an agent intended to kill microorganisms) other than alcohol, such as green surgical soap or hydrogen peroxide. Do not use iodine swabs because they also contain alcohol.

Following Protocols

The phlebotomist's job also includes ensuring that all collection protocols are followed during a procedure. If you collect a blood alcohol level, you must take extra care that the site is cleaned with a nonalcohol cleanser. A contaminated or false-positive result could cause the police officer to lose the court case or a person to lose his or her job or even go to jail. A phlebotomist involved in collecting a blood alcohol specimen for legal reasons can be summoned to appear in court, so the phlebotomist needs to be especially diligent in following all established collection protocols.

Forensic Testing

Forensic specimens usually involve testing specimens for legal cases. Forensic and legal specimens must follow the chain-of-custody procedure. The types of specimens listed in Table 10-3 are commonly obtained and used for forensic purposes. The primary aim of forensic testing is to provide evidence that may help prove or disprove a link between an individual and objects, places, or other individuals.

Competency Check 10-1

Forensic Testing Guidelines

1. Avoid contamination by wearing gloves at all times.

2. Collect the specimen as soon as possible.

3. Ensure that the specimen is packed, stored, and transported correctly. In general, fluids are refrigerated and other specimens are kept dry and at room temperature.

4. Label each specimen with the patient's name and date of birth, the name of the person collecting the specimen, the type of specimen, and the date and time of the collection.

5. Make sure the specimen is packed securely and is tamper-proof. Only authorized people should touch the specimen.

6. Record all handling of the specimen, most commonly on a chain-of-custody form.

Check for guidelines specific to your place of employment. In some cases, you will use a special evidence kit (see Figure 10-13). Know the specific procedure and only perform it if you have had the proper training to collect forensic specimens.

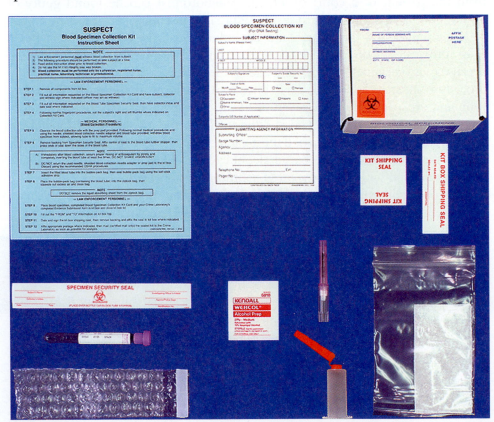

Figure 10-13 A forensic specimen kit such as this one may be used at your facility.

Toxicology Specimens

Toxicology is the scientific study of poisons, drugs, and medications. Toxicologists study the detection of poisons, the action of poisons on the human body, and the treatment of the medical conditions that poisons can cause. Toxicology may also include testing for trace elements, such as aluminum, lead, mercury, and zinc. Some toxicology specimens are performed in the chemistry section of the laboratory, whereas others require testing at a reference laboratory. For toxicology specimens, it is critical to follow your laboratory's protocol for collection, type of specimen, and equipment usage. Oil or bacteria from hands, glass, or plastic materials will contaminate or even react with some of the analytes.

Special Handling During Venipuncture

For some laboratory specimens, special handling is part of the venipuncture procedure. Examples of special handling during blood collection include

- not using alcohol (explained previously)
- not using a tourniquet
- collecting blood for special coagulation tests

No Tourniquet/Lactic Acid Blood Collection Procedure

To assess levels of lactic acid in the blood, some facilities require that venipuncture be performed without a tourniquet. Lactic acid forms in the muscles during carbohydrate metabolism and its blood level can be affected by

- exercise
- vigorous hand pumping prior to blood collection
- the application of a tourniquet during blood collection

A tourniquet may be applied for no longer than 1 minute in order to locate a vein, but it must be removed prior to collection. The arm from which the blood is to be collected must be at rest for at least 2 minutes after the tourniquet is removed. The patient should not make a fist or pump the hand. A sodium fluoride tube (gray stopper) is collected, placed in a mixture of ice and water for transport, and delivered to the laboratory STAT. As explained in the chapter *Blood Collection Equipment*, sodium fluoride minimizes the effects of **glycolysis,** which changes glucose into lactic acid. Placing the specimen in a mixture of ice and water also helps slow this process. Be aware that the protocols for some laboratories may require specimens for lactic acid be collected using another additive. As always, follow the protocol at your facility.

Specimens for Special Coagulation Studies

As we have already learned, the order of draw is critical when collecting blood for coagulation tests, especially when using a butterfly needle assembly. Recall from the chapter *Blood Collection Equipment* that when a butterfly needle is used, a nonadditive discard tube—one that is never used for testing—must be collected first, followed by a light-blue-topped tube used for coagulation tests. The light-blue tube should never be collected after any tube containing additives. When special coagulation studies are needed, a detailed procedure must be followed to collect the specimen. Phlebotomists must follow the procedure used by the facility where they work. The following are general guidelines for special coagulation collection:

- In addition to following a strict order of draw, special coagulation venipunctures must be performed using a large-bore needle (nothing smaller than a 21 gauge).

Copyright © 2016 by McGraw-Hill Education

TABLE 10-3

Samples Collected for Forensic Purposes

- Blood
- Bones
- Hair
- Nails
- Saliva
- Skin
- Sperm
- Sweat
- Teeth
- Mud
- Vegetation

TABLE 10-4 Coagulation Studies Often Requiring Special Handling

Coagulation Study	Specific Tests	Special Handling
Coagulation factor assays	Factors I, II, V, VII, VIII, IX, X, XI, XII, XIII, von Willebrand Factor	• May require discard tube • Centrifugation, separation, shipped frozen to reference lab
Coagulation inhibitor assays	Anti-thrombin III Antiphospholipids Lupus inhibitor Proteins S and C	• May require discard tube • Centrifugation, separation, shipped frozen to reference lab
Platelet function studies	Platelet antibodies Platelet inhibition	• May require discard tube • Centrifugation, separation, shipped frozen to reference lab
	Platelet function assay (PFA), platelet response (aspirin and/or Plavix®)	• Requires discard tube • Immediate delivery to laboratory

- The procedure must be performed quickly to minimize the amount of time the tourniquet is applied.
- Each tube collected must be gently inverted the required number of times while the next tube is filling.

Sometimes phlebotomists assist nurses in collecting blood for coagulation studies through a venous access device. A phlebotomist may be asked to provide the needed equipment at the appropriate time in the procedure, transfer the specimen to evacuated tubes, and ensure adequate mixing. Blood collection from the line attached to the venous access device requires that the line first be flushed with saline and then that at least 10–20 milliliters (mL) of fluid and blood be drawn by syringe and discarded. A new syringe is used to collect the required amount of blood, which is immediately transferred into blue-stoppered tubes using a syringe transfer device. The tubes are then gently inverted the required number of times.

Specimens for special coagulation studies must be delivered to the laboratory immediately, so that proper processing and testing can occur in a timely manner. Table 10-4 lists special coagulation studies that may require special collection procedures.

Separated Specimens

Some laboratory tests require that specimens be separated as soon as possible after collection. In some facilities, phlebotomists are expected to process these specimens. Specimen processing can be a separate section of a large laboratory, and for the phlebotomist, this presents an opportunity to aid in the testing procedure. Processing patient samples involves **centrifuging** (spinning down or separating the cells from the liquid portion of the blood) and **aliquoting** (dividing or separating specimens into separate containers). For most laboratory tests that require serum or plasma, it is recommended that specimens be separated within 2 hours of collection. If samples are not centrifuged or aliquoted within 2 hours, the laboratory test results may be altered. Potassium and glucose blood tests are most affected. If blood cells are left in contact with the serum or plasma, glucose can be decreased and potassium can significantly increase. Blood cells use glucose to keep alive and nourished, whereas potassium can slowly leak out of red blood cells.

Using the Centrifuge

Centrifuges come in many different styles: refrigerated, floor models, and table-top models. The speed of rotation (revolutions per minute, or rpm) and the radius of the rotor head determine the relative centrifugal force (RCF) of a centrifuge. The relative centrifugal force is expressed as gravity (g). Centrifugal force used in a centrifuge is similar to that used by the spin cycle of a clothes washing machine. Centrifuges typically have dials for speed of rotation and time.

Laboratory centrifuges are designed to spin blood specimens, separating the cells from the liquid portion. Cells are pushed to the bottom while the liquids remain on top. If a gel separator is used, the gel will migrate to the middle and form a barrier between the cell and liquid layers. Nonadditive tubes and serum separator tubes (SSTs) must be completely clotted prior to centrifugation. Figure 10-14 shows specimens before and after centrifugation.

Most laboratory specimens are centrifuged at 1,000 to 3,000 revolutions per minute for 15 minutes. Times and speeds depend on the specimen requirement and the manufacturer's recommendation. Tubes of various sizes can be spun in the same centrifuge at the same time. Be sure to place tubes of equal size and volume directly across from each other (see Figure 10-15). Also, make sure that the levels of sample are the same, so that the centrifuge will be balanced. If you do not have an even number of blood tubes to spin, you can balance the centrifuge with a similar tube filled with water or saline. An unbalanced centrifuge is similar to a washing machine that is heavier on one side than the other. It will jump around, will make unusual noises, and may damage the specimens or injure the phlebotomist. Figure 10-16 compares balanced and unbalanced tube placement within a centrifuge. Centrifuges are available that can handle several specimens at one time. Specimens in these centrifuges must also be distributed evenly according to volume and weight (see Figure 10-17).

After the lid has been securely closed, turn the centrifuge on and set the timer for the time designated in your procedure manual (usually 10–15 minutes). Wait until the centrifuge has reached its running speed before leaving the area. If the centrifuge is loaded with samples that are not balanced, the centrifuge will vibrate and make noise. If you are nearby, you can turn off the

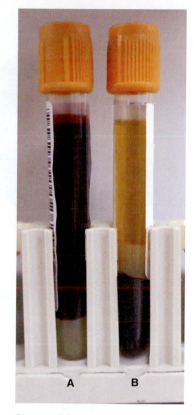

Figure 10-14 Serum separator tubes (A) uncentrifuged and (B) after centrifugation. Upon centrifugation, the separator gel forms a barrier between the blood cells (on the bottom) and the serum (on the top).

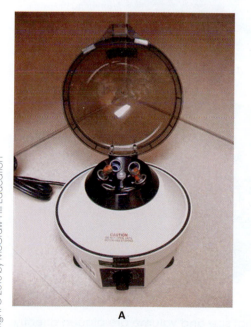

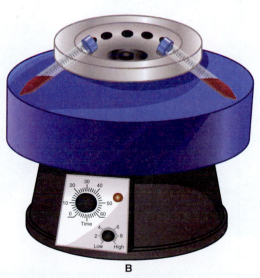

Figure 10-15 (A) Common style counter-top centrifuge. (B) Centrifuge showing tube placement.

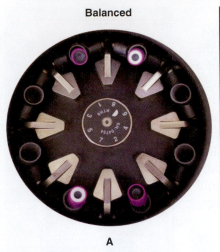

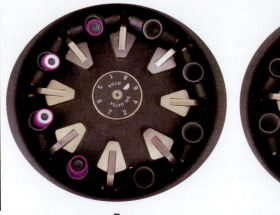

Balanced   **Not Balanced**

A   B   C

Figure 10-16 Small centrifuges with a few specimens. (A) Tubes of equal size and volume are placed directly across from each other. (B) Tubes placed all to one side and (C) tubes of unequal size and volume placed across from each other will cause damage to the centrifuge and may result in harm to the operator. Although image (C) appears balanced, remember that Bio-One tubes with dark rings are standard volume tubes while those with white rings draw less volume.

centrifuge before the unbalanced samples are broken. The centrifuge must be calibrated regularly to ensure proper centrifugation (discussed further in the chapter *Waived Testing and Collection of Non-Blood Specimens*).

Improper use of a centrifuge can be dangerous to the user and can ruin laboratory specimens. If a tube is broken, the cup containing the broken tube must be completely emptied into a sharps container and disinfected.

Never open a centrifuge lid until the rotor has come to a complete stop. There might be a glass tube that shattered during the centrifuge process. If you open the lid before it stops, you run the risk of being injured by flying glass or debris. Use the competency checklist *Centrifuge Operation* at the end of this chapter to review and practice the procedure.

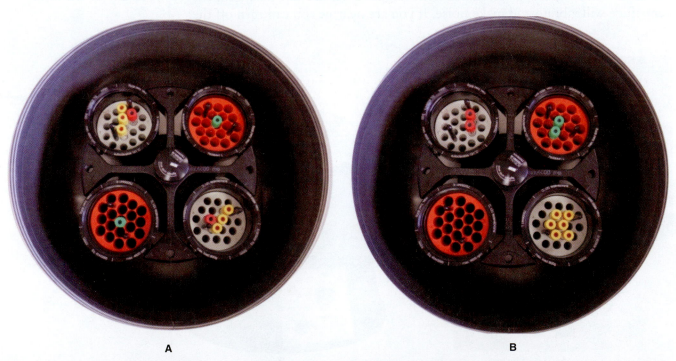

A   B

Figure 10-17 Large centrifuges for multiple specimens. (A) Tubes of equal size and volume are placed directly across from each other. (B) Tubes grouped by type result in unequal placement and will cause damage to the centrifuge. They also may result in harm to the operator.

Avoiding Aerosol Exposure

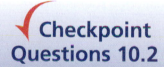

The prevention of **aerosols** (mists that travel in the air) escaping when stoppers are removed or in uncovered centrifuged tubes is a major concern of laboratory personnel. Aerosols are similar to the droplets of moisture produced by a sneeze, but they are smaller and may not be easily detected. Aerosols can contain viruses and can endanger a person if inhaled. Shields (see Figure 10-18) are available for use when opening centrifuges or tubes; they act as a barrier between the person and the aerosol. Always follow the manufacturer's recommendations and your facility's policies when opening containers that may produce aerosols.

Safety & Infection Control

Aliquoting Specimens

Aliquoting is the process of transferring a portion of a specimen into one or more containers. Careful attention to detail is imperative when aliquoting patient specimens. Mixing up patient samples is one of the greatest concerns of all laboratory workers. Before you begin to aliquot a sample, make sure the transfer tube is properly labeled by comparing it to the label on the specimen tube that was used for collection. A pipet (a graduated tube with a suction bulb) is used to transfer the serum or plasma to the transfer tube (see Figure 10-19). Be sure to check the specimen requirements before selecting an appropriate transfer tube. Some transfer tubes are clear plastic, whereas others are amber-colored for light-sensitive specimens. The person processing the specimen must also ensure that aliquoted specimens are stored properly prior to and during delivery to the laboratory section or reference laboratory.

1. You need to centrifuge three tubes of blood. Two of the tubes are adult-size and the other is pediatric-size. Explain how you will balance the centrifuge.
2. Describe two methods of protecting a light-sensitive specimen from light.

✓ **Checkpoint Questions 10.2**

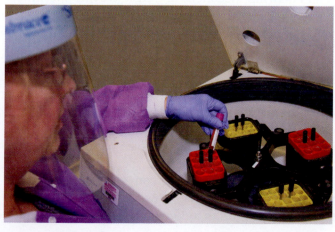

Figure 10-18 Phlebotomist using a face shield while opening a centrifuge.

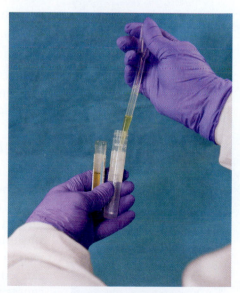

Figure 10-19 Phlebotomist transferring a specimen from a collection tube to a transfer tube.

10.3 Specimen Rejection

Laboratory test results are only as good as the specimens from which they are obtained. Specimen collection and handling are pre-examination variables that only those collecting and transporting the specimen can control. Any error made before the specimen is analyzed is known as a **pre-examination error.** There is nothing medical laboratory technicians and scientists can do to the specimen to obtain quality results from inappropriately collected or handled specimens.

Furthermore, unless obvious characteristics are present (hemolysis, clots, underfilled tubes), errors in collection or handling may go unnoticed by those performing testing procedures. As a result, questionable results may be reported. Questionable or inaccurate results can affect patient care negatively. For this reason, phlebotomists should know the causes for specimen rejection and how to minimize the occurrence of poor-quality specimens. The following paragraphs contain more detailed information about the specific reasons for specimen rejection and re-collection.

Hemolysis

Hemolysis is the destruction of red blood cells (RBCs). The hemoglobin inside the RBCs is released into the plasma or serum and gives it a reddish color (see Figure 10-20). This color may interfere with some laboratory tests. Other substances found in RBCs, such as potassium and calcium, cause erroneous results for various laboratory tests when hemolysis is present. Although some patient conditions (such as hemolytic anemia and transfusion reactions) can lead to hemolysis, more commonly a hemolyzed specimen is the result of improper collection or handling. The following are common causes of hemolysis:

- Not allowing the alcohol to dry prior to puncture
- Continuing to draw blood during hematoma formation
- Forcefully squeezing during dermal puncture
- Vigorously mixing the collection tube
- Forcing blood when using a syringe transfer procedure by pushing on the plunger
- Roughly handling the specimen during transport (such as turbulence in a pneumatic tube system)
- Freezing and thawing specimens in transit (leaving specimens in outdoor courier pickup boxes or an unheated courier vehicle for long periods of time)

Clotted Anticoagulated Specimens

If laboratory tests require whole blood, plasma, or cells, the specimen is collected in a tube containing an anticoagulant, which is designed to prevent clotting. However, if the specimen in an anticoagulated tube does clot (see Figure 10-21), the specimen must be re-collected. If clots are not discovered by testing personnel, the results will be erroneous and, if reported, can jeopardize patient safety. The following is a list of common causes for specimen clotting in anticoagulant tubes:

- Incorrect order of draw (clot activator tube drawn before light-blue-topped tube)

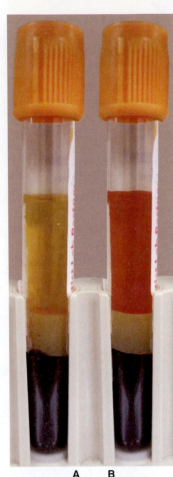

Figure 10-20
Centrifuged specimens with (A) normal serum and (B) hemolyzed serum.

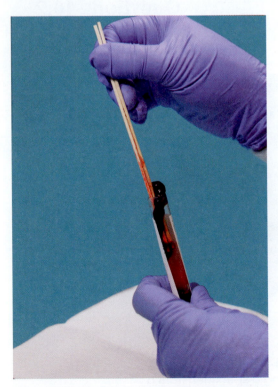

Figure 10-21 Clotted specimen.

- Failure to mix each tube as it is removed from the holder or to tap a microcollection container between each drop
- Delay in transferring specimens from a syringe to an evacuated tube
- Difficult blood draws in which the blood flows very slowly into the tube
- Use of an expired tube

Incomplete Collection

An incomplete collection is often rejected as "quantity not sufficient" (QNS), meaning there is not enough specimen to perform the test (see Figure 10-22). Sometimes a QNS specimen does contain the minimum amount of blood required to run a test but is rejected because of an improper **additive-to-blood ratio** (the balance between the amount of additive or anticoagulant and the amount of blood). This imbalance will produce erroneous results, such as abnormal chemistry values, coagulation test results, and blood counts. Always check with the laboratory prior to collecting specimens from difficult-to-draw patients so that you know what the minimum amounts are you must collect. For example, 1

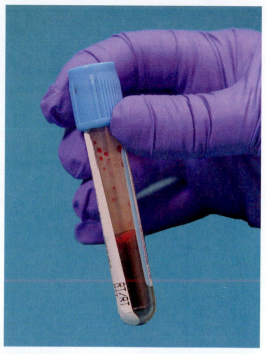

Figure 10-22 Underfilled specimen tube.

mL may be adequate for performing a CBC, but not for an erythrocyte sedimentation rate (ESR), and definitely not if both are ordered. A citrate tube must always be filled to the fill level indicated on the label. The following can cause incomplete collection:

- Loss of vacuum during venipuncture
- Loss of vacuum during shipping
- Failure to purge air out of butterfly needle tubing using a discard tube
- Use of expired tubes
- Removal of the tube before its fill level is reached
- Veins collapsing during venipuncture
- Dermal puncture site that becomes clotted before enough specimen is obtained

Incorrect Tube Collected

Specimens collected must be appropriate for the laboratory tests to be performed. If a specimen is collected using the incorrect type of tube, the specimen will be rejected and will need to be re-collected. The following are causes for incorrect collections:

- The procedure manual was not consulted or information was misinterpreted.
- The tube was delivered to the wrong laboratory section (a switch occurred).
- The wrong tube was collected by mistake.
- The requisition was misinterpreted.

Incorrect Order of Draw

As you know, the order of draw is designed to prevent specimens from being contaminated with additives that may cause erroneous results. Correct tube placement is of the utmost importance for coagulation testing. Although current CLSI standards allow for coagulation tests to be drawn without a discard tube, this applies when the phlebotomist can ensure that the venipuncture is uncomplicated and no contamination of the light-blue-topped tube will occur. Recall from the chapter *Blood Collection Equipment* that coagulation tests are usually collected in a light-blue-topped tube that is not the first tube collected and does not follow other anticoagulant tubes. A discard tube (red, nonadditive or another light blue tube) may be drawn before the light blue tube that will be used for coagulation testing. Alternately, if a sterile specimen is to be collected during the same draw, it should be collected first, followed by the light blue tube (the discard tube is skipped). Phlebotomists should follow the protocol established at their facility. The following are causes of an incorrect order of draw:

- The procedure manual was not consulted or information was misinterpreted.
- The tubes were collected in the wrong order by mistake.

Hemoconcentration or Contamination

The effects of hemoconcentration (prolonged tourniquet application, discussed in the chapter *Venipuncture*) and contamination by intravenous (IV) fluids (collecting blood from a site above an IV) are not easily detected. Laboratory personnel may question phlebotomists about collection procedures when they obtain results that do not make sense or do not pass **delta check.** The delta check is when results of the same test are compared with previous results on the same patient. If laboratory personnel suspect hemoconcentration or contamination, the specimen will need to be re-collected. If no apparent cause can be determined for questionable results, the specimen may still need to be re-collected.

Icterus and Lipemia

Two interfering substances over which the phlebotomist has no control are icterus and lipemia. **Icteric** plasma and serum appear dark-yellow to greenish-yellow in color due to the presence of an increased amount of bilirubin, the substance made during the breakdown of red blood cells. This abnormal color may interfere with some chemistry tests, such as creatinine. **Lipemia** is the presence of abnormal amounts of fats in the blood and can make plasma or serum appear cloudy. This cloudiness can interfere with laboratory tests, such as hemoglobin levels. Figure 10-23 compares normal serum with lipemic and icteric sera.

Special Requirements Not Followed

As discussed earlier, some laboratory tests require special specimen handling. If these requirements are not followed, the specimen will be rejected and then it must be re-collected. The following are special handling requirements:

- The specimen must be protected from light.
- The specimen must be kept at the appropriate temperature.
- Alcohol must not be used during site preparation.
- A tourniquet must not be used during specimen collection.
- The specimen must be centrifuged and separated within the required timeframe.

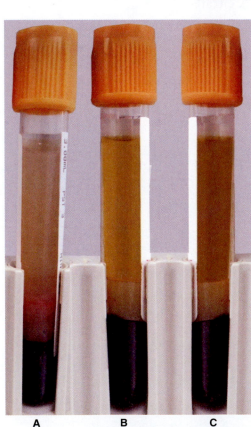

Figure 10-23 Comparison of serum color and transparency: (A) lipemic serum appears milky, (B) normal serum is clear and yellow in color, and (C) icteric serum may be clear but has an olive-green color due to the presence of excessive amounts of bilirubin.

Documentation Errors

As you may recall from the chapter *Blood Collection Equipment*, specimens must be labeled with certain required information. The laboratory may reject specimens with inadequate or missing documentation, depending on the severity of the omission. In addition, misidentified specimens will be rejected. If a specimen is obtained from the wrong patient, not only will the specimen be labeled incorrectly, but the error may also go undetected. This can result in delay of treatment for one patient and inappropriate treatment being given to the other. Sometimes a labeling error is detected at the time of test performance, if the test result produces a delta check error (described earlier in this chapter). Unexplained delta checks will initiate a rejection and re-collection of the specimen. Reasons for specimen rejection due to documentation include the following:

- An unlabeled specimen
- A mislabeled specimen (labeled with another patient's identification information)
- A specimen with two labels containing different patient information
- Missing documentation for a chain-of-custody specimen
- Labels placed on the wrong tubes for the same patient (for example, a CBC label on a chemistry tube and vice versa, which can usually be resolved without re-collecting the specimen)
- A special labeling procedure that was not followed (such as blood bank labeling, which is discussed in the chapter *Special Phlebotomy Procedures*)

Specimen Rejection and Customer Satisfaction

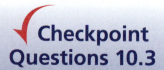

Critical Thinking

Many factors contribute to the need for rejecting specimens. Taking the time to collect, handle, and process specimens correctly will ensure accurate and timely reporting of test results. Consider the patient's feelings when you must repeat a blood collection. The patient may be angry at the need for a repeat collection or may express doubt about your ability to perform the procedure properly. Customer satisfaction with your laboratory and facility may suffer if patients perceive that they are not receiving quality care. Thus, your role as the phlebotomist includes making sure your customer (your patient) is comfortable in your presence and confident in your ability to provide adequate care.

1. How can a phlebotomist help ensure that a blood specimen does not become hemolyzed?
2. How does a delta check help laboratory personnel determine whether hemoconcentration has occurred in a blood specimen?

✓ **Checkpoint Questions 10.3**

Documentation Errors

As you may recall from the chapter *Blood Collection Equipment*, specimens must be labeled with certain required information. The laboratory may reject specimens with inadequate or missing documentation, depending on the severity of the omission. In addition, misidentified specimens will be rejected. If a specimen is obtained from the wrong patient, not only will the specimen be labeled incorrectly, but the error may also go undetected. This can result in delay of treatment for one patient and inappropriate treatment being given to the other. Sometimes a labeling error is detected at the time of test performance, if the test result produces a delta check error (described earlier in this chapter). Unexplained delta checks will initiate a rejection and re-collection of the specimen. Reasons for specimen rejection due to documentation include the following:

- An unlabeled specimen
- A mislabeled specimen (labeled with another patient's identification information)
- A specimen with two labels containing different patient information
- Missing documentation for a chain-of-custody specimen
- Labels placed on the wrong tubes for the same patient (for example, a CBC label on a chemistry tube and vice versa, which can usually be resolved without re-collecting the specimen)
- A special labeling procedure that was not followed (such as blood bank labeling, which is discussed in the chapter *Special Phlebotomy Procedures*)

Specimen Rejection and Customer Satisfaction

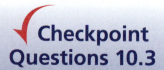

Critical Thinking

Many factors contribute to the need for rejecting specimens. Taking the time to collect, handle, and process specimens correctly will ensure accurate and timely reporting of test results. Consider the patient's feelings when you must repeat a blood collection. The patient may be angry at the need for a repeat collection or may express doubt about your ability to perform the procedure properly. Customer satisfaction with your laboratory and facility may suffer if patients perceive that they are not receiving quality care. Thus, your role as the phlebotomist includes making sure your customer (your patient) is comfortable in your presence and confident in your ability to provide adequate care.

1. How can a phlebotomist help ensure that a blood specimen does not become hemolyzed?
2. How does a delta check help laboratory personnel determine whether hemoconcentration has occurred in a blood specimen?

✓ **Checkpoint Questions 10.3**

Chapter Summary

Learning Outcomes	Key Concepts/Examples	Related NAACLS Competency
10.1 Explain methods for transporting and processing blood specimens for routine and special testing and reference laboratories. Pages 261–264.	• Blood and other specimens must be transported to the laboratory in a timely manner by hand-delivery, a pneumatic tube system, or automated transport systems. • Packaging specimens for transport to the laboratory from client sites or to reference laboratories must meet safety standards for specimen handling and transport. • Proper documentation of specimen collection and transport allows laboratory and other healthcare personnel to track the specimen and approximate a test completion time.	7.3, 7.4

10.2 Recognize criteria for special specimen handling. Pages 264–275.	• Correct specimen handling and processing requirements include temperature control, exposure to light, and use of special draw techniques (no alcohol, no tourniquet, coagulation).
	• Specimen handling for legal specimens must follow established practices for maintaining the chain of custody.
	  • For blood alcohol testing to be performed, the patient must consent or a legal document must be obtained. The venipuncture site should be cleaned with something other than alcohol.
	  • A forensic specimen is collected as evidence to help prove or disprove a link between an individual and objects, places, or other individuals. Toxicology specimens are collected to detect poisons, drugs, and medications.
	• Proper separation of specimens may require centrifugation and aliquoting of specimens, which involves the safe use of a centrifuge and careful attention to labeling and documentation.
		7.3, 7.4, 7.6

10.3 List the circumstances that would lead to re-collection or rejection of a patient sample. Pages 276–279.	Specimen rejection may occur due to improper collection technique or handling and processing errors. Reasons for specimen rejection include clots, contamination, hemoconcentration, hemolysis, incomplete collection, incorrect tube or order of draw, inadequate or missing documentation, failure to follow special requirements, and delta checks due to unexplainable changes in test results and specimen collection from the wrong patient.	7.5

Chapter Review

A: Labeling

Label the essential parts of a properly packaged specimen for shipping to an out-of-state reference laboratory.

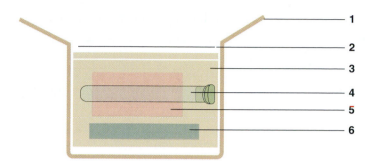

1. [LO 10.1] _____

2. [LO 10.1] _____

3. [LO 10.1] _____

4. [LO 10.1] _____

5. [LO 10.1] _____

6. [LO 10.1] _____

B: Matching

Match each definition with the correct term.

_____**7.** [LO 10.2] aerosol

_____**8.** [LO 10.2] aliquot

_____**9.** [LO 10.2] centrifuging

____**10.** [LO 10.3] clotted

____**11.** [LO 10.3] delta check

____**12.** [LO 10.3] hemolyzed

____**13.** [LO 10.2] glycolysis

____**14.** [LO 10.2] light-sensitive

____**15.** [LO 10.3] pre-examination

____**16.** [LO 10.1] STAT

a. amount of change in a test from one time to the next on the same patient

b. errors that occur prior to specimen testing

c. fine mist

d. obtain or process immediately

e. portion of a specimen

f. process to separate cells from the liquid portion of blood

g. specimens in which plasma has changed to serum and now contains a solid mass of cells

h. specimens in which red blood cells have been destroyed

i. specimens in which presence of light causes chemical changes

j. conversion of glucose to lactic acid

C: Fill in the Blank

Complete each statement.

17. [LO 10.1] Specimens within a hospital facility can be hand-delivered to the hospital laboratory or sent in the _____ system.

18. [LO 10.1] Information for specimen tracking is entered, by phlebotomists and couriers, into the _____.

19. [LO 10.2] Testing for cold agglutinins is done for patients suspected of having conditions such as atypical pneumonia; these patients may be infected with the organism _____.

20. [LO 10.2] Specimens that need to be transported chilled should be _____.

21. [LO 10.2] The lid on the _____ machine should remain properly closed during the specimen separation process.

22. [LO 10.2] The specimen separation process includes _____ and then _____ into transfer tubes.

23. [LO 10.1] Specimens on critically ill patients may need to be collected first and immediately delivered to the laboratory. These specimens are usually labeled as _____.

D: Sequencing

Place the following events in chronological order from 1 to 10 for the processing of specimens for shipping to a reference laboratory.

24. [LO 10.1] _____ Attach specimen information to container.

25. [LO 10.1] _____ Centrifuge the specimen, if required.

26. [LO 10.1] _____ Label the transfer tube.

27. [LO 10.1] _____ Obtain original specimen.

28. [LO 10.1] _____ Pipet specimen aliquot into transfer tube.

29. [LO 10.1] _____ Place ice pack into Styrofoam container.

30. [LO 10.1] _____ Place package into shipping container.

31. [LO 10.1] _____ Place wrapped transfer tube into Styrofoam container.

32. [LO 10.1] _____ Seal transfer tube.

33. [LO 10.1] _____ Wrap tube in absorbent material.

E: Case Study/Critical Thinking

34. [LO 10.3] You are working in the laboratory's processing area and notice that a specimen you were just given was drawn over 2 days ago. This is the same blood sample for which a doctor just called for the results. He was upset and wanted the results immediately. What would you do?

35. [LO 10.2] You have finished labeling all of Mrs. Diaz's blood tubes when you notice that one sample was supposed to be put on ice immediately. You have been talking to Mrs. Diaz for the last 10 minutes. What would you do?

36. [LO 10.3] You need to collect a lactic acid on a patient who has had blood drawn before. He is pumping his fist in preparation for the blood collection. What should you do and why?

37. [LO 10.2] You need to collect a specimen for cold agglutinins on a patient. How will you maintain the specimen at the correct temperature while transporting it to the laboratory? What will you do once you arrive at the laboratory section that is responsible for this test?

38. [LO 10.2] You must collect blood for an alcohol level that may be used in a court of law. What procedures do you need to follow for this blood collection and why?

F: Exam Prep

Choose the best answer for each question.

39. [LO 10.1] Pneumatic tube systems are used to transport specimens from a
    a. hospital unit to the laboratory.
    b. physician office to a hospital laboratory.
    c. hospital laboratory to a reference lab.
    d. courier's vehicle to the laboratory.

40. [LO 10.1] Specimens for tests that are ordered STAT must be
    a. verified with the laboratory manager prior to collection.
    b. collected by the physician.
    c. delivered to the laboratory immediately.
    d. collected last when drawing several patients.

41. [LO 10.1] Specimen lockboxes are used
    a. when dropping off specimens at the main laboratory.
    b. by clients to store specimens for courier pickup and delivery to the laboratory.
    c. to transport specimens in courier vehicles.
    d. to hand-deliver specimens from within the facility.

42. [LO 10.1] Which of the following does NOT represent proper data documentation for specimen tracking?
    a. Bar-coding specimen information upon delivery to the laboratory
    b. Centrifuging specimens within 5 minutes of collection
    c. Entering collection information into the computer
    d. Recording the time of collection and initials on the specimen container

43. [LO 10.1] Containers for specimen transport must be
    a. airtight.
    b. light-tight.
    c. microbe-free.
    d. watertight.

44. [LO 10.1] Which of the following specimen transport methods will have the LEAST effect on specimen quality?
    a. Leaving a specimen in a pickup box located outside during winter months
    b. Leaving a specimen in the courier's vehicle for several hours during summer months
    c. Shipping specimens on dry ice to a reference laboratory
    d. Using the facility's nonvalidated pneumatic tube system

45. [LO 10.2] When aliquoting specimens, a shield or splashguard is used to protect the phlebotomist from
    a. aerosols.
    b. bacteremia.
    c. normal flora.
    d. septicemia.

46. [LO 10.2] Which statement describes proper centrifuge operation?
    a. Centrifuge specimens within 5 minutes of collection.
    b. Balance specimens by placing tubes of equal size and volume opposite each other.
    c. Never centrifuge plasma specimens with serum specimens.
    d. Remove tops from tubes before centrifuging.

47. [LO 10.2] Which of the following specimens must be placed on ice during transport to the laboratory?
    a. Cold agglutinins
    b. Lactic acid
    c. Specimens sent via pneumatic tube
    d. Tubes that will be centrifuged

48. [LO 10.2] Protecting a specimen from the effects of heat can be accomplished by *(Choose all that apply)*

    a. collecting the specimen in an amber microcollection container.

    b. wrapping the specimen tube with foil.

    c. wrapping the specimen tube with absorbent material.

    d. placing the specimen on ice.

49. [LO 10.2] Transporting a specimen for cold agglutinin testing includes *(Choose all that apply)*

    a. placing the specimen in a portable heating block.

    b. wrapping the specimen tube with foil.

    c. wrapping the specimen tube with a heel warmer.

    d. placing the specimen on ice.

50. [LO 10.2] Substances that need protection from the effects of light include *(Choose all that apply)*

    a. alcohol.

    b. bilirubin.

    c. calcium.

    d. carotene.

51. [LO 10.2] Alcohol pads are not used during blood collection for alcohol mainly because

    a. alcohol from alcohol pads will interfere with the test.

    b. patients may be allergic to alcohol.

    c. evidence presented in a court of law will be invalidated.

    d. alcohol pads will absorb the alcohol from the patient.

52. [LO 10.2] Contamination of the specimen by additional lactic acid during blood collection for lactic acid may occur when

    a. a tourniquet is not used during collection.

    b. an alcohol prep pad is used during collection.

    c. the patient makes a tight fist during collection.

    d. the specimen is placed on ice after collection.

53. [LO 10.3] Tubes that are not completely filled may be rejected because

    a. all the vacuum is not used up in the tube.

    b. the extra airspace makes sampling difficult.

    c. the ratio of blood to anticoagulant is out of balance.

    d. all tests require absolutely filled tubes.

54. [LO 10.3] Hemolysis occurs due to

    a. allowing alcohol to air-dry prior to puncture.

    b. forcing syringe-drawn specimens into evacuated tubes.

    c. gently massaging a dermal puncture site.

    d. mixing the collection tube too slowly.

55. [LO 10.3] Clotting of specimens occurs due to

    a. not allowing alcohol to air-dry prior to puncture.

    b. quickly transferring syringe blood into evacuated tubes.

    c. placing collection tubes into a test tube rack without mixing.

    d. tapping microcollection containers on a hard surface during collection.

56. [LO 10.3] Inadequately filled tubes may result from *(Choose all that apply)*

    a. loss of vacuum during venipuncture.

    b. veins collapsing during venipuncture.

    c. premature clotting of a dermal puncture site.

    d. use of expired evacuated blood collection tubes.

57. [LO 10.3] Test results that do not compare with previous results *(Choose all that apply)*

    a. may be due to contamination with IV fluids.

    b. may result from prolonged tourniquet application.

    c. fail the delta check test.

    d. usually have no apparent cause.

58. [LO 10.3] Specimens that are rejected for documentation errors include *(Choose all that apply)*

    a. unlabeled specimens.

    b. specimens whose label is missing the phlebotomist's identification.

    c. specimens labeled with another patient's information.

    d. specimens whose label is upside-down.

connect

Enhance your learning by completing these exercises and more at connect.mheducation.com

References

Adventist Lab Partners. (2013). *Adventist Lab Partners test directory.* Retrieved July 29, 2013, from www.keepingyouwell.com/care-services/lab-services/adventist-lab-partners-test-directory

ARUP Laboratories. (2011). *Specimen preparation and transport.* Retrieved April 10, 2011, from www.aruplab.com/Specimen-Handling/index.jsp

Burtis, C. A., Ashwood, E. R., & Bruns, D. E. (Eds.). (2005). *Tietz textbook of clinical chemistry and molecular diagnostics* (4th ed.). Philadelphia: W.B. Saunders.

Federal Express. (2013) *HealthCare Solutions.* Retrieved July 29, 2013, from http://healthcare.van.fedex.com/

National Accrediting Agency for Clinical Laboratory Sciences. (2010). *NAACLS entry-level phlebotomist competencies.* Rosemont, IL. NAACLS.

Sodi, R., Darn, S., & Stott, A. (2004). Pneumatic tube system induced haemolysis: Assessing sample type susceptibility to haemolysis. *Annals of Clinical Biochemistry, 41,* 237–240.

COMPETENCY CHECKLIST: SPECIMEN HANDLING: TEMPERATURE-SENSITIVE SPECIMENS

Procedure Steps	Practice			Performed		
	1	2	3	Yes	No	Master
Preprocedure						
1. Examines the requisition.						
2. Performs the patient identification procedure.						
3. Performs site selection and the preparation procedure.						
4. Prepares an ice bath or specimen warming equipment.						
5. Performs the specimen collection procedure.						
6. Performs the postcollection patient care procedure.						
Procedure						
7. Places the labeled specimen immediately into the correct temperature control equipment.						
8. Labels the outside of the ice bath or warming device.						
Postprocedure						
9. Immediately transports the specimen to the laboratory.						
10. Ensures that cooling or warming is maintained while transporting the specimen.						
11. Places the specimen in the appropriate laboratory device (incubator, water bath, refrigerator, etc.).						
12. Alerts laboratory staff of the temperature-sensitive specimen.						
13. Documents the specimen collection.						

COMMENTS: _____

_____

_____

_____

SIGNED

EVALUATOR: _____

STUDENT: _____

NAME: _____ DATE: _____

COMPETENCY CHECKLIST: SPECIMEN HANDLING: LIGHT-SENSITIVE SPECIMENS

Procedure Steps	Practice			Performed		
	1	2	3	Yes	No	Master
Preprocedure						
1. Examines the requisition.						
2. Performs the patient identification procedure.						
3. Performs the site selection and preparation procedure.						
4. Prepares foil for the evacuated tubes or uses an amber microcollection container.						
5. Performs the specimen collection procedure.						
6. Performs the postcollection patient care procedure.						
Procedure						
7. Wraps the labeled specimen with foil.						
8. Labels the outside of the oil.						
Postprocedure						
9. Immediately transports the specimen to the laboratory.						
10. Ensures that the specimen remains protected from light.						
11. Alerts laboratory staff of the light-sensitive specimen.						
12. Documents the specimen collection.						

COMMENTS: _____
_____
_____
_____

SIGNED

EVALUATOR: _____

STUDENT: _____

COMPETENCY CHECKLIST: CENTRIFUGE OPERATION

Procedure Steps	Practice			Performed			
	1	2	3	Yes	No	Master	
Preprocedure							
1. Puts on gloves.							
2. Transports the specimen to the centrifuge area.							
3. Safely and conveniently places the specimens.							
4. Opens the lid of the centrifuge.							
Procedure							
5. Inserts the tubes so that they are balanced.							
6. Does not remove the caps from the tubes.							
7. If a cap is missing, covers the end of the tube.							
8. Closes the centrifuge lid.							
9. Locks the lid in place.							
10. Sets the centrifuge time and speed correctly.							
Postprocedure							
11. Allows the centrifuge to stop completely.							
12. Opens the lid after the centrifuge has stopped.							
13. Observes special handling instructions.							
14. If tubes are broken, cleans appropriately.							
15. Disposes of used supplies appropriately.							
16. Removes gloves and washes hands.							

COMMENTS: _____

_____

_____

_____

SIGNED

EVALUATOR: _____

STUDENT: _____

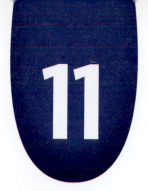

11

Special Phlebotomy Procedures

essential terms

aerobic
anaerobic
antibiotic removal
 device (ARD)
arterial puncture
autologous
bacteremia
biotinidase
cannula
congenital
culture media
cystic fibrosis
diabetes mellitus
differential
false-negative
false-positive

fistula
galactosemia
gestational diabetes
glycolysis
hemochromatosis
heparin lock
hypothyroidism
normal flora
phenylketonuria
 (PKU)
polycythemia vera
septicemia
sickle cell disease
therapeutic
 phlebotomy

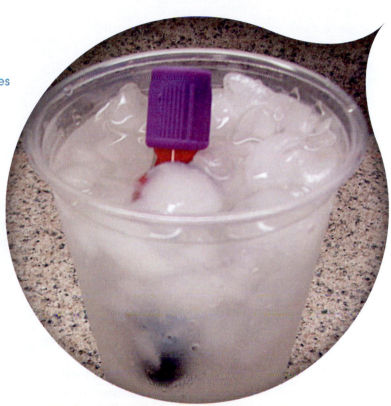

Learning Outcomes

11.1 Recognize the requirements of special collection procedures.

11.2 Identify steps to competent and effective arterial puncture.

11.3 Classify venous access sites and their uses.

Related NAACLS Competencies

2.00 Demonstrate knowledge of infection control and safety.

4.00 Demonstrate understanding of the importance of specimen collection and specimen integrity in the delivery of patient care.

4.2 Describe the types of patient specimens that are analyzed in the clinical laboratory.

4.3 Define the phlebotomist's role in collecting and/or transporting these specimens to the laboratory.

4.4 List the general criteria for suitability of a specimen for analysis, and reasons for specimen rejection or re-collection.

4.5 Explain the importance of timed, fasting, and stat specimens, as related to specimen integrity and patient care.

5.00 Demonstrate knowledge of collection equipment, various types of additives used, special precautions necessary, and instances that can interfere in clinical analysis of blood constituents.

289

5.3 Describe the proper order of draw for specimen collections.

5.4 Describe substances that can interfere in clinical analysis of blood constituents and ways in which the phlebotomist can help avoid these occurrences.

6.00 Follow standard operating procedures to collect specimens.

6.2 Differentiate between sterile and antiseptic techniques.

6.3 Describe and demonstrate the steps in the preparation of a puncture site.

6.7 Describe the limitations and precautions of alternate collection sites for venipuncture and capillary (dermal) puncture.

7.00 Demonstrate understanding of requisitioning, specimen transport, and specimen processing.

7.3 Explain methods for transporting and processing blood specimens for routine and special testing.

9.7 Follow written and verbal instructions.

Introduction

Some laboratory tests require specimens collected in a manner that is different than routine venipuncture or dermal/capillary puncture. This chapter includes tests that need specialized techniques, equipment, processes, or patient preparation for the collection of the required blood specimen. Making peripheral blood smears, which is sometimes part of the phlebotomist's duties, is included.

11.1 Special Procedures

Although routine blood collection is the most common procedure performed by phlebotomists, on occasion, special protocols must be followed depending on the reason for the collection or analyte (substance) to be tested. Special procedures that phlebotomists may perform include

- collection of blood cultures
- glucose tolerance specimens
- collection for neonatal blood screening
- preparation of blood smears
- special identification procedures for type and cross-match specimens
- collection of donor blood

Blood Cultures

A blood culture is the testing of blood for the presence of infection. Blood culture samples are frequently requested for patients who have a fever of unknown origin (FUO). The purpose of a blood culture test is to isolate any microorganisms present in the patient's blood sample to determine which organism is causing the fever. Strict sterile technique and attention to detail are required for preparation of the blood culture site. In addition, blood cultures must be obtained in tubes or bottles that contain **culture media,** which enhance microorganism growth. The evacuated tubes designed for blood cultures are the yellow-stoppered SPS (sodium polyanethol sulfonate) tubes. Blood culture bottles are usually larger and more cumbersome to handle than normal venipuncture tubes. However, blood culture bottles may be preferred, depending on the method used for blood cultures in the microbiology section.

Some blood culture containers include an **antibiotic removal device (ARD).** An ARD is a resin that absorbs any antibiotic found in the specimen. ARD bottles are used for patients who are on antibiotics at the time of collection and provide for more accurate results.

Blood is normally sterile, so the presence of microorganisms in the blood (**bacteremia**) can be very serious and result in death. **Septicemia** (the presence of pathogenic microorganisms in the blood) will usually cause a person to have a fever. The largest number of organisms will be present in the blood right before a patient has a sudden increase in temperature or spikes a fever. Because the number of microorganisms causing the fever is still very small, it is difficult to isolate them with only one sample. Therefore, a licensed practitioner may order the blood cultures to be drawn in sets of two or three. Samples will be placed in an

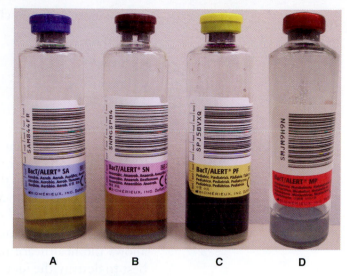

Figure 11-1 Blood culture bottles from left to right: (A) aerobic, (B) anaerobic, (C) pediatric, and (D) *Mycobacterium*.

incubator (an environmentally controlled device, usually set at 37° C) to allow time for microorganisms to grow, if present. Blood culture samples are often collected in pairs of bottles (see Figure 11-1A and B). One bottle is an **anaerobic** (without oxygen or air) specimen and the other bottle is an **aerobic** (with oxygen or air) specimen. Each subsequent set should be obtained from different sites and/or at different time intervals. Special blood culture bottles are sometimes used to test for *Mycobacterium* (the causative agent of tuberculosis or TB) (see Figure 11-1D). Blood cultures are usually requested STAT when a patient has a serious fever because antibiotics need to be administered. The most effective antibiotic cannot be determined until the samples are collected and processed to identify the pathogen. Pathogens are microorganisms capable of producing diseases.

Accurate Blood Cultures

A pathogenic (disease-producing) organism in the blood is a serious condition that must be treated. However, sometimes the blood culture result indicates the presence of a pathogen in the blood when the specimen was actually contaminated during the collection procedure. When a blood specimen is contaminated with organisms that did not originate in the blood, this result is called a **false-positive.** These organisms can get into the blood culture specimen by the following actions:

Safety & Infection Control

- Inadequately cleaning the puncture site
- Not allowing the cleaning agent to dry thoroughly
- Using contaminated equipment or specimen containers
- Touching the puncture site after it has been cleaned

The phlebotomist drawing the blood cultures is responsible for ensuring that the cultures are not contaminated during the process by strictly adhering to the blood culture procedure. Blood culture contamination is serious and may need to be reported to the state health department.

The most common classifications of pathogens are

- bacteria
- viruses
- fungi
- protozoa

Many groups of microorganisms exist under each of these classifications. If the isolated causative agent is identified as a bacterium, it can be from one of several groups of bacteria. The blood culture helps identify the specific microorganism that is causing the infection. For example, a culture helps differentiate between the bacterium *Streptococcus pyogenes*, which causes strep throat, and the bacterium *Streptococcus pneumoniae*, which is one agent responsible for pneumonia. Isolating the causative agent (microorganism) from the blood culture allows the healthcare provider to prescribe the antimicrobial that will work best to destroy the identified microorganisms.

Blood Culture Site Cleaning Procedure

The collection of a blood culture sample is similar to routine venipuncture, with added steps to ensure that the skin is as clean as possible. Cleaning the venipuncture site is the most important part of this collection procedure. Once the site is selected, release the tourniquet. Cleanse the site using sterile technique and the appropriate antiseptic. Routine venipuncture cleansing involves swabbing the area with a 70% alcohol prep pad. Sterile technique used for blood cultures typically requires a two-step process. If sterile technique is not followed, **normal flora** (skin surface microorganisms, such as normal bacteria and fungi) could be introduced into the blood culture sample and interfere with the patient's results.

Competency Check 11-1

Cleaning the Blood Culture Site
1. Cleanse the site with 70% or 90% alcohol prep, or other cleansing agents, such as 0.5% chlorhexidine gluconate, 2% iodine, Betadine, or benzalkonium chloride (Zephiran Chloride) (see Figure 11-2). Be aware that some products are not used on infants and children. Always check the manufacturer's directions.
2. Start in the center of the puncture site and continue outward, in concentric circles, using firm pressure. Do not allow the strokes to go back toward the center area as this would bring contaminants toward the selected puncture site.
3. Clean the site with friction for at least 60 seconds to ensure that the normal flora and contaminants are removed from the area.
4. Allow the site to air-dry, so that the antiseptic has time to kill the germs.
5. When using alcohol, once the initial cleansing area has air-dried, a second cleansing step may be required. A circular cleansing pattern is used, this time with a swab or applicator containing 0.5% chlorhexidine gluconate, 2% iodine, Betadine, or benzalkonium chloride.
6. Follow the policy at your facility and current product directions to ensure that the site is cleansed properly.

Once the area is sterilized, it must not be touched, even with a glove. If touched, the site is considered contaminated and the entire cleaning procedure must be repeated. It is essential that the cleansing procedure be performed with great care. Patients requiring blood cultures are typically very sick, and

Cleaning the Blood Culture Site

As you are preparing a patient for blood culture collection, inform the patient about the procedure. If you plan to use iodine, ask about allergies and use another approved cleanser if the patient is allergic to iodine.

Explain the importance of a sterile puncture and why you are cleaning the puncture area. Sometimes patients have a tendency to touch a venipuncture site, and this must be avoided during blood culture collections. If you are collecting a blood culture and the patient touches the site, you have to clean the area again.

Butterfly Needles and Blood Cultures

The purpose of the anaerobic bottle is to allow bacteria that cannot survive in the presence of oxygen to grow in this medium. When using the butterfly assembly, DO NOT collect the anaerobic bottle first. Air from the tubing will be introduced into the anaerobic bottle, which may inhibit the growth of the anaerobic bacteria and cause inaccurate results.

preliminary results may take 24 to 48 hours. If the cleansing procedure is not done correctly, the patient can lose critical treatment time waiting for the procedure to be repeated.

In many facilities, the tops of the blood culture bottles are also cleaned with alcohol. Some bottles from the manufacturer have protective covers that do not require the tops to be cleansed because they are sterile when opened. Check what is appropriate for the blood culture system your facility uses and follow the manufacturer's recommendations.

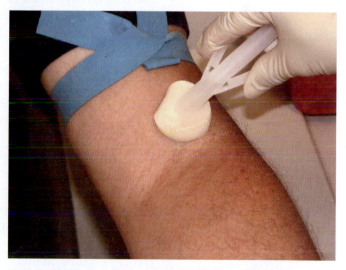

Figure 11-2 The blood culture site must be cleaned thoroughly using an approved cleanser, such as 0.5% chlorhexidine gluconate, to prevent a false-positive test result due to contamination by the bacteria normally found on the skin.

Blood Culture Volumes

The volume of blood collected for a blood culture is critical. Each manufacturer of blood culture bottles or tubes has determined the optimum amount of blood sample needed to increase the chance of growing the microorganisms in the laboratory. Usually, 8 to 10 milliliters (mL) per bottle or tube for an adult is sufficient, while lesser amounts are drawn on infants and children. (see Table 11-1). Special blood culture bottles are available for use with pediatric patients (see Figure 11-1C).

The amount of blood drawn can have an impact on the test. For example, some bacteria, such as *Escherichia coli*, can exist in the blood in very low amounts; this requires a larger volume of blood to be drawn. If the volume is too low, the bacteria may not be seen in the culture; this produces a **false-negative** result.

In addition to getting the correct amount in each blood culture container, phlebotomists must be certain to draw from the appropriate site and in the proper sequence. As mentioned earlier, a typical blood culture order requires two bottles (one aerobic and one anaerobic). These two bottles can be drawn

TABLE 11-1 Recommended Blood Culture Volumes

Type of Patient	Aerobic Bottle Amount	Anaerobic Bottle Amount
Adult	8 to 10 mL	8 to 10 mL
Adult—low volume*	All obtained	None
Pediatric (based on weight)	2.5 to 10 mL	2.5 to 10 mL
Infant	0.5 to 1 mL	0.5 to 1 mL

If 10 mL or less is obtained from an adult, place all the blood in the aerobic bottle.

from the same site. With some patients, however, the healthcare provider may order "blood cultures × 2." The blood for two separate collections can be collected at the same time but must be collected from two different sites. If two sites cannot be used, the phlebotomist must wait for a period of time— between 15 and 45 minutes, depending on the order—before collecting the second set of blood culture containers at the same site. Collecting "blood cultures × 2" from two different sites, or "blood cultures × 2 fifteen minutes apart," is frequently done to help prevent a false-negative result.

Collecting Blood Culture Specimens

Phlebotomists can perform the venipuncture procedure with an evacuated system, a syringe and transfer device, or a butterfly (winged) collection set. Special adapters may be used that accommodate both blood culture bottles and evacuated tubes (Figure 11-3). Once the site is selected and cleansed, the tourniquet is reapplied, taking extra care not to touch the clean site. If necessary, only touch at least an inch above and below the site.

When collecting blood for culture with a syringe, make sure to use one that will hold an adequate volume for both tubes and bottles (a 20-mL syringe for adults). Once enough blood is obtained, remove the needle from the patient and engage the safety mechanism. Remove the covered needle and attach the syringe to a transfer device. When using a syringe draw, fill the anaerobic bottle first to prevent air from entering the specimen. Next, fill the aerobic bottle and any other tubes required. If using an evacuated tube assembly, use the correct type of tube holder to prevent culture media from accidentally entering the patient's blood. Review the manufacturer's directions.

When using a butterfly assembly, draw the aerobic sample first to clear the air from the butterfly tubing before drawing the anaerobic culture sample. Competency Check 11-2 compares the procedures for blood culture collection using the syringe method and butterfly assembly method.

After the blood is collected in the culture containers, label each with patient identification information, date, time, and phlebotomist's initials or identification code. When collecting more than one set of cultures, label each set with the location of the draw and the order of draw—for example, #1 Lt hand and #2 Rt arm. This information is important because additional blood cultures may be ordered. If iodine was used, remove it from the patient's arm using a new alcohol prep pad to prevent absorption into the patient's skin. Use the competency checklist *Blood Culture Procedure* at the end of this chapter to review and practice the procedure.

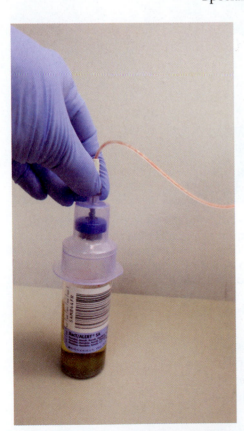

Figure 11-3 Blood culture transfer devices may be used with a butterfly needle to deliver blood directly into blood culture bottles.

Blood Culture Collection Comparison of Procedures	
Syringe Transfer Method	Butterfly Assembly Method
1. Greet the patient.	1. Greet the patient.
2. Properly identify the patient.	2. Properly identify the patient.
3. Explain the specimen collection procedure to the patient.	3. Explain the specimen collection procedure to the patient.
4. Wash your hands, put on gloves, and other PPE, if needed, and prepare the equipment.	4. Wash your hands, put on gloves, and other PPE, if needed, and prepare the equipment.
5. Select the venipuncture site and release the tourniquet.	5. Select the venipuncture site and release the tourniquet.
6. Cleanse the site using sterile technique and the appropriate antiseptic.	6. Cleanse the site using sterile technique and the appropriate antiseptic.
7. Allow the site to air-dry for 60 seconds.	7. Allow the site to air-dry for 60 seconds.
8. Sterilize the tops of the blood culture bottles (if required by facility policy).	8. Sterilize the tops of the blood culture bottles (if required by facility policy).
9. Reapply the tourniquet.	9. Reapply the tourniquet.
10. Perform the venipuncture.	10. Perform the venipuncture.
11. Fill syringe to the required volume.	11. Fill the aerobic bottle.
12. Release the tourniquet, withdraw the needle, engage the safety device, and apply pressure to the site.	12. Fill the anaerobic bottle.
13. Safely remove the needle and attach the syringe to the transfer device.	13. Release the tourniquet, withdraw the needle, engage the safety device, and apply pressure to the site.
14. Fill the anaerobic bottle.	14. Safely dispose of the used butterfly assembly.
15. Fill the aerobic bottle.	15. Label the bottles with patient and collection information.
16. Safely dispose of the used needle and syringe.	16. Complete postpuncture patient care.
17. Label the bottles with patient and collection information.	17. Thank the patient.
18. Complete postpuncture patient care.	
19. Thank the patient.	

Glucose Testing

Glucose testing is probably the most frequently ordered laboratory test and is used to diagnose disorders of carbohydrate metabolism. The most common carbohydrate metabolism disorders include

- **diabetes mellitus** (insufficient production of insulin)
- gestational diabetes (high blood sugar during pregnancy)
- hyperinsulinism (increased levels of insulin, resulting in low blood sugar)

If untreated, diabetes mellitus can lead to many complications, including blindness, kidney failure, and amputation due to problems in the lower limbs. Although an increase in blood glucose is an indicator of this disease, the patient's fasting glucose level may be within normal limits. A healthcare provider may order a glucose tolerance test, an insulin level, or a series of tests to determine the patient's medical problem. See Table 11-2 for the types of glucose tests. If diabetes is suspected, a hemoglobin A1C test—a test for glycosylated hemoglobin—may be ordered. According to the American Diabetes Association, an A1C value equal to or greater than 6.5 is one criterion for a diagnosis of diabetes.

Two-Hour Postprandial Glucose

A 2-hour postprandial glucose test is sometimes ordered to assist in diagnosing diabetes mellitus. Glucose levels obtained 2 hours after a meal can be elevated in diabetic patients but are generally within normal range for most of the population. Ideally, in 2 hours the glucose level will have returned to normal. Correct timing is important because, if the sample is collected too early, the glucose level may still be elevated and may lead to misinterpretation of the test results by the healthcare provider. A 2-hour postprandial glucose test result of 200 or over as part of the oral glucose tolerance test (OGTT) is another criterion for a diagnosis of diabetes.

Glucose Challenge

A glucose challenge screening test is frequently done to test for **gestational diabetes.** Gestational diabetes is elevated glucose that occurs during pregnancy. The cause for gestational diabetes is not well understood, but it may be influenced by a hormone from the placenta that makes the mother resistant to insulin. During a glucose challenge test, the patient receives a dose of 50 grams or 75 grams of oral glucose in the form of a sugary drink (Glucola). A blood sample is drawn 1 hour later. If this test is positive, then a complete OGTT is done.

TABLE 11-2 Glucose Tests

Name	Purpose	Test and Timing
Fasting blood sugar (FBS)	To identify risk for diabetes	Single blood sample after no intake of food or drink for 8 to 12 hours
2-hour postprandial blood sugar (2-hour PP)	To identify risk for diabetes	Taken exactly 2 hours after a meal; used less frequently because of inconsistent results
Random blood sugar (RBS)	To identify risk for diabetes or hypoglycemia	Taken randomly throughout the day; a wide variety of results indicates possible problem
2- or 3-hour oral glucose tolerance test (OGTT)	To diagnose gestational diabetes, diabetes mellitus, hypothalamic obesity, and reactive hypoglycemia	Fasting blood sugar, 30 minutes, 1 hour, 2 hours, and 3 hours after oral glucose
Glucose challenge screening test	To identify risk for gestational diabetes (1-hour) or polycystic ovary syndrome (2-hour)	Blood sample 1 hour or 2 hours after oral glucose
Intravenous glucose tolerance test (IVGTT)	To evaluate insulin secretion in prediabetics	Blood samples after glucose is administered directly into the bloodstream

High Fasting Glucose Levels

It is unsafe to give a patient with elevated glucose additional glucose, as this can cause nausea or extremely elevated blood glucose. If the glucose level is over 200 mg/dL (some facilities use a cutoff of 126 mg/dL), the glucose tolerance test (GTT) must be discontinued immediately and the patient's healthcare provider notified of the fasting result. Additionally, according to the American Diabetes Association (ADA), if the fasting blood glucose is 126 mg/dL or over, a GTT should not be utilized.

Safety & Infection Control

Oral Glucose Tolerance Test (OGTT)

An oral glucose tolerance test measures a patient's ability to metabolize a large oral dose of glucose (75 grams in liquid form, about ½ cup of glucose dissolved in water). A classic oral glucose tolerance test measures blood glucose levels five times over a period of 3 hours. Some healthcare providers order a shorter version of the OGTT that includes a baseline blood sample followed by a sample 2 hours after drinking the glucose solution. This is similar to the 2-hour postprandial and is used as a screening test rather than a diagnostic procedure.

Patient Restrictions During the GTT

During the GTT procedure, the consumption of food, drinks (even those without sugar), or alcohol is not allowed. Smoking and gum chewing are also not allowed for the duration of the tolerance test. All of these affect the way the body metabolizes glucose and can alter test results. The patient may consume sips of water during the test if he or she is feeling thirsty.

Patient Education & Communication

Children and Glucose Tolerance Tests

If a GTT is to be performed on a child, follow glucose manufacturer instructions on the side of the bottle and the facility's protocol for the amount of glucose to administer. Children are typically given a certain number of ounces of glucose solution according to their body weight.

Life Span Considerations

To perform a complete OGTT, ensure that the patient has been fasting for at least 12 hours. Once this is confirmed, a fasting blood specimen is collected and tested for glucose. If the blood glucose level is over 200 milligrams per deciliter (mg/dL), no further testing is required.

If the screening blood glucose level is less than 200 mg/dL, the OGTT procedure may continue. The patient receives a loading dose of glucose, taken orally as a drink purchased by laboratories (see Figure 11-4). These drinks may be available in a variety of flavors such as orange, grape, and lemon-lime. Commercially available glucose drinks contain a known amount of dissolved glucose, and the proper amount must be measured out according to the dose required. For example, if the bottle of glucose drink contains 100 grams of glucose in a 100-milliliter bottle and the required dose is 75 grams, measure out 75 milliliters to give to

Safety & Infection Control

Glucose Tolerance Test

Patients who arrive for a glucose tolerance test must be fasting. During this visit, they receive a large dose of glucose (sugar), which makes them prone to syncope (fainting). It is imperative that these patients not leave the facility during the test. The phlebotomist must go out to the waiting area to meet patients and walk with them to the blood drawing area. The phlebotomist should not just call a patient's name and wait for him or her to come to the drawing area. The phlebotomist should also escort patients back to the waiting area after the draw and make sure they are settled and feeling stable. Additionally, the phlebotomist should be ready to steady the patient if needed and to react appropriately should the patient faint. Patients can fall and hurt themselves, putting the phlebotomist at risk for a lawsuit. It is also recommended that the phlebotomist have a large container close by in case the patient becomes nauseated and vomits. Due to the high load of glucose on an empty stomach, this is a very common occurrence. Patients should be monitored to ensure that they do not snack, drink, smoke a cigarette, or chew gum during the testing time, which can interfere with the results.

the patient. The phlebotomist must ensure that the patient swallows all of the glucose solution within 5 minutes and that no vomiting occurs. If the patient vomits, the test is stopped and the primary care provider is notified.

Figure 11-4 Commercial glucose drinks are available in several flavors and glucose doses.

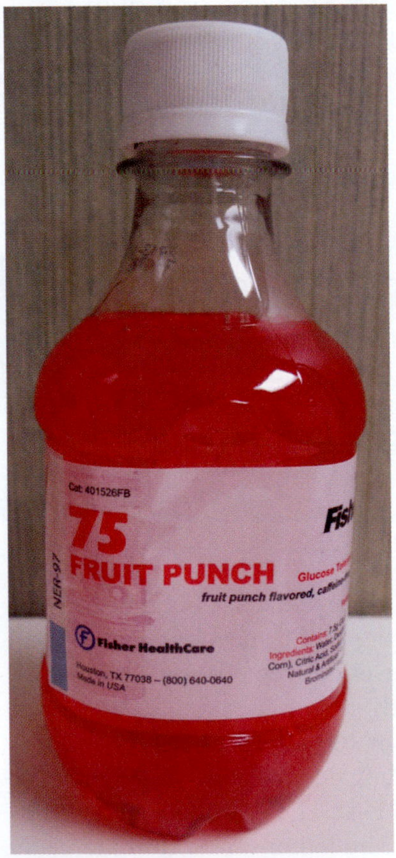

Next, collect blood and urine (if required) at specific time intervals of 30 minutes, 1 hour, 2 hours, and 3 hours. Be careful to label each sample (blood and urine) with both the time collected and the time interval (for example, 8:30 A.M., 30 minutes, 9:00 A.M., and so on). Also, make sure the patient understands what restrictions need to be followed during the course of the test.

A gray-topped tube is usually used for GTT specimens. As explained in the chapter *Blood Collection Equipment*, the sodium fluoride in this tube prevents **glycolysis** (the breakdown of glucose into an acid). Glucose testing should be performed as soon after collection as possible. If the test is performed immediately, a gold or light green tube may be used for collection. The laboratory sends the ordering healthcare provider the GTT results, which assists the healthcare provider in determining the presence and type of diabetes, as well as the appropriate treatment.

Neonatal Screening

In the United States, blood testing of newborns for the presence of various metabolic and genetic disorders is performed. Blood is drawn after the baby reaches the

Glucose Testing

1. Identify the patient.

2. Explain the specimen collection procedure to the patient.

3. Ensure that the patient has been fasting for at least 12 hours.

4. Wash your hands, put on gloves, and prepare the equipment.

5. Collect a fasting blood specimen using proper venipuncture technique.

6. Perform a POCT glucose test or obtain a glucose level of the specimen from the chemistry department.

7. Verify that the screening blood glucose level is less than 200 mg/dL.

8. Prepare the glucose drink according to the requirements of the type of glucose test.

9. Observe the patient consume it within 5 minutes and confirm no vomiting has occurred.

10. Collect blood at specific time intervals.

11. Properly label each sample with both the time collected and the time interval.

minimum age of 24 hours. If the infant's blood is collected before he or she is at least 24 hours old, the infant's blood will need to be redrawn. All states have mandatory screening, although the number of tests varies by state. Common screening tests include

- **biotinidase**—deficiency of the enzyme that breaks down the vitamin biotin
- **cystic fibrosis**—mucous secretions accumulating in various organs
- **galactosemia**—the inability to break down the milk sugar galactose
- **hypothyroidism**—a decrease in thyroid function
- **phenylketonuria (PKU)**—a buildup of phenylketone due to decreased metabolism of phenylalanine
- **sickle cell disease**—abnormal hemoglobin structure

Testing may also be performed for the infectious diseases of toxoplasmosis and human immunodeficiency virus (HIV) as well as other less common metabolic disorders. A phlebotomist should know the tests performed within his or her state and the procedures for obtaining the blood specimens.

Biotinidase Deficiency

A deficiency in the enzyme biotinidase impairs the activity of other enzymes that depend on the vitamin biotin. Biotin assists other enzymes in many functions, such as the synthesis of fatty acids and breakdown of amino acids. If not diagnosed or if left untreated, this disorder can result in neurological damage, such as hearing and vision loss, and problems with movement and balance. Biotinidase deficiency is treatable with biotin supplements.

Cystic Fibrosis

Cystic fibrosis (CF) affects many body systems, particularly causing damage to the respiratory system and producing digestive system problems. The mucus normally lining many body systems accumulates abnormally in people with cystic fibrosis. If not diagnosed or if left untreated, cystic fibrosis can be fatal at an early age. Treatments for cystic fibrosis do exist, and new treatments are currently under development that may help these patients reach adulthood and live fairly normal lives.

Neonate screening for CF includes performing a dermal puncture and collecting blood on a special card called a Guthrie card. If this screening test is positive, a chloride sweat test may be performed to confirm the diagnosis. The chloride sweat test measures the amount of salt in a newborn's sweat and is not performed by a phlebotomist. As newer genetic blood tests are developed, the procedure for collecting specimens for cystic fibrosis tests may change.

Galactosemia

The sugar galactose (part of a larger sugar, lactose) is present in small amounts in many foods, especially dairy products such as milk, cheese, and ice cream. Galactosemia is a disorder in which the body lacks the ability to use galactose as an energy source. Infants with galactosemia fail to gain weight, develop improperly, and have liver damage and bleeding problems. This disorder can be life threatening to infants if undiagnosed or left untreated. A diet low in lactose may help minimize the effects of this disorder.

Hypothyroidism

Hypothyroidism is a partial or complete loss of thyroid function. Hypothyroidism can be acquired but also can be **congenital** (existing at birth). The thyroid is responsible for making many iodine-containing hormones needed for growth, brain development, and the regulation of metabolism (chemical reactions in the body). If undiagnosed or left untreated, congenital hypothyroidism can delay normal growth and cause intellectual disabilities. Treatment for hypothyroidism is an oral dose of thyroxine (thyroid hormone).

Phenylketonuria (PKU)

PKU occurs due to a buildup of phenylketone in the blood when the body is deficient in the enzyme that breaks it down. If metabolized to a point where they are water soluble, phenylketones can be found in the urine, hence the word *phenylketonuria*. Phenylalanine, which is one of the amino acids found in many foods (proteins and artificial sweeteners), can cause damage to brain tissue if left untreated. Children with PKU may also have heart problems, have microcephaly (small head size), and be prone to skin disorders such as eczema. In addition to the first blood collection for neonatal screening, PKU should be retested when the infant is 10 to 15 days old. If diagnosed early, PKU is treatable with a diet low in phenylalanine.

Sickle Cell Disease

Sickle cell disease is a group of disorders in which hemoglobin has an abnormal structure due to a genetic mutation. In some forms of sickle cell disease, this abnormal structure causes the hemoglobin molecules to distort into a sickle, or crescent, shape (see Figure 11-5). These distorted cells can block small blood vessels and create organ pain. As these cells are removed from circulation, the red blood cell count decreases, resulting in anemia. Treatment for sickle cell disease includes closely monitoring the symptoms, staying well hydrated, and avoiding exposure to low-oxygen environments, such as high altitudes and anesthesia during surgery.

State Testing Specimen Collection

State-required blood tests are collected onto special forms that include an absorbent area for collecting specimens (see Figure 11-6). Be sure to check the expiration date on the form and provide all the required information. Follow the facility's protocol for gowning, handwashing,

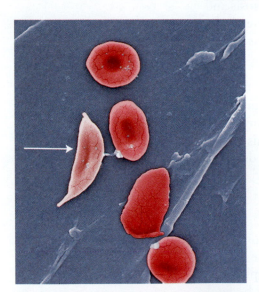

Figure 11-5 Cells containing sickle cell hemoglobin will deform to take on this characteristic shape (at arrow) when the cell loses oxygen.

and donning of PPE prior to entering the neonatal nursery and for patient identification. Be certain to use the correct form for the test to be collected.

Competency Check 11-4

Dermal Puncture State Testing on Infants

1. Check the patient identification band (usually on the infant's ankle) and verify the patient's identity with nursing staff.

2. Wash your hands, put on gloves, and prepare the equipment.

3. Select the appropriate area for dermal puncture on the infant's heel.

4. Sterilize and dry the skin.

5. Puncture the heel with a sterile lancet.

6. Allow a large blood droplet to form.

7. Touch filter paper to the blood and allow to soak through completely in each circle. Total saturation of the circles must be evident when the paper is viewed on both sides. DO NOT APPLY BLOOD TO BOTH SIDES.

8. Allow blood spots to air-dry thoroughly for 3 hours at room temperature. Keep away from direct sunlight and heat. Never superimpose one wet filter paper onto another before thoroughly drying.

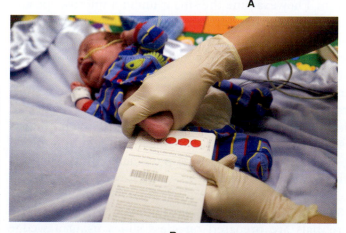

A

B

Figure 11-6 (A) Each state has its own form designed to screen newborns for various inherited disorders. (B) Blood must saturate all of the circles during collection.

Specimens may be unsatisfactory if

- all circles are not completely filled
- a circle is oversaturated
- the specimen is not allowed to dry thoroughly
- the specimen is contaminated with a foreign substance
- an expired form is used
- the form is not received within 14 days of collection

Most states use similar collection forms for their mandated testing of newborns. Once collected, these forms are mailed to the appropriate state laboratory for testing. Use the competency checklist *Neonatal Testing* at the end of this chapter to review and practice the procedure.

Critical Thinking

Handle with Care

The forms used for state-required newborn screening tests are made from a delicate material and must be treated gently. DO NOT use a capillary tube to collect and transfer a baby's blood to the form. Touching the tube to the form will scratch the surface and render the sample useless for testing. Strictly follow the directions on the form. States have their own requirements for how designated areas on the form should be filled. Always refer to your institution's procedure manual for the required protocol.

Peripheral Blood Smears

A blood smear (a thin film of blood spread onto a glass slide) is used for the microscopic examination of blood. Either venous blood (blood from a vein collected in a tube) or capillary blood (blood collected by dermal puncture) may be used to prepare a blood smear. A blood smear may also be prepared by applying blood directly from the finger to the slide. Some of the most valuable information about a patient's health can be obtained through a well-made peripheral blood smear.

A **differential** is a hematology test performed by technicians and scientists using a stained blood smear. They examine the smear under a microscope and count the types of white blood cells. In addition, they note any abnormalities in the morphology (size, shape, and color) of red blood cells and platelets as well as any abnormalities in the appearance of white blood cells.

The information obtained from blood smears, along with CBC results, is used to diagnose hematological disorders, such as anemia and leukemia. Screening for blood parasites, such as *Plasmodium* species that cause malaria, is also performed using blood smears. Some facilities may require phlebotomists to assist laboratory personnel by preparing blood smears. In addition, blood smears may need to be made at facilities such as physicians' offices when a smear is needed to confirm abnormal findings.

Thin Blood Smears

Blood smears for differentials are prepared on glass slides using a wedge method (two slides touching each other at an angle to form a wedge shape) and are referred to as *thin smears*. The blood smear should be made from fresh, noncoagulated drops of blood. To perform this procedure, first assemble the equipment needed for a dermal puncture or obtain a tube of uncoagulated blood, usually collected into EDTA. Select clean glass slides, ensuring that there are no chipped edges, and handle them so as not to leave fingerprints. Frosted slides may be labeled prior to making the blood smear; however, this may lead to the same specimen identification problems as labeling tubes before blood collection. Most facilities require slides to be labeled AFTER a blood film is made. In the case of slides that do not have frosted ends, you must wait until the smear has dried and write the name on the thick end of the smear. Always check with your facility's protocol for the required procedure. At least two clean glass microscope slides are needed to perform a blood smear. If performing a dermal puncture, wipe away the first drop of blood using a piece of gauze. Squeeze the punctured area to create a free-flowing drop of blood. Allow the drop of blood to fall onto the glass slide toward one end.

When preparing smears from tubes of blood, check the specimen for proper labeling. Use a safety device to access the blood without removing the cap (see Figure 11-7A). If these devices are not available, carefully uncap the specimen tube behind a safety shield; use a wooden applicator stick or capillary tube to remove some of the blood and place a drop on the slide toward one end (see Figure 11-7B and C). A disposable pipet/plastic dropper may be used in some cases. Follow the steps in Competency Check 11-5 to master the thin blood smear.

Competency Check 11-5

Thin Blood Smear

1. Wash your hands and put on gloves. Wear a face shield or work behind a table top shield.

2. Verify the identity of the specimen requiring a blood smear.

3. With the slide on the work surface, hold the capillary tube or applicator stick in one hand and the frosted end of the slide against the work surface with the other.

4. Apply a drop of blood to the slide, about ½ inch from the frosted end.

5. Place the applicator stick or capillary tube in the sharps container.

6. Pick up the spreader slide with your dominant hand and hold it at a 30- to 35-degree angle.

7. Place the edge of the spreader slide on the smear slide close to the unfrosted end.

8. Pull or back up the spreader slide toward the frosted end until the spreader slide touches the blood drop. Capillary action will spread the droplet along the edge of the spreader slide.

9. Allow the blood drop to spread almost to the edges of the spreader slide.

10. With one light, smooth, fluid motion, push the spreader slide toward the other, clear end of the slide until you come off the end, maintaining the 30- to 35-degree angle.

11. Immediately label the frosted end with two patient identifiers, the date, and the accession number of the specimen (if available).

12. Allow the smear to air-dry before staining.

Figure 11-8 shows the steps in the thin blood smear procedure. Most of the drop should be spread out onto the glass slide. The smear will be thick at the drop end and thin at the opposite end. A properly made blood film will have a thick portion, a thin portion, a critical area used for performing the differential, and a tail with a feathered edge that is straight to slightly rounded (see Figures 11-9 and 11-10).

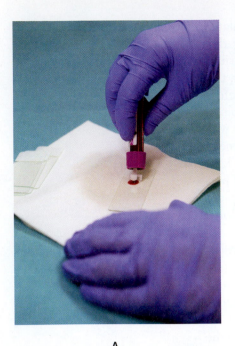
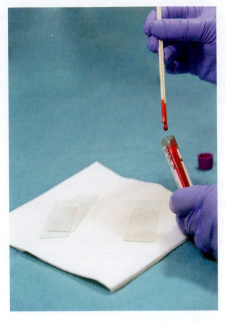
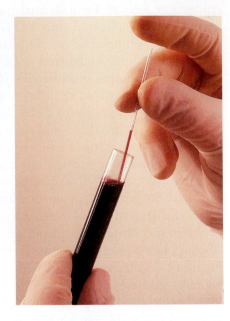

A   B   C

Figure 11-7 Methods for delivering a drop of blood to a slide. (A) A safety device is the preferred method to deliver a drop of blood to a glass slide for smear making. If unavailable, (B) a wooden applicator stick or (C) a capillary tube can be used to obtain the drop of blood.

Critical Thinking

Making Blood Smears Using Frosted-End Slides

If you are preparing smears using slides with a frosted end, be sure the frosted side is facing upward. Place the drop of blood near, but not on, the frosted end.

This frosted area is used to write the patient's information or affix an aliquot label. Labeling is performed after the blood smear is made; however, some facilities' protocols may have you label slides before the smear is made. Follow the protocol at your facility, taking care to avoid slide identification problems.

Life Span Considerations

Blood Smears for Newborns

When preparing blood smears from newborns, remember that their hematocrits may be high, which will result in smears that are too short. Using a normal to slightly large drop of blood with a decreased angle and pushing the spreader slide slowly will allow you to make a longer blood smear. At facilities that require blood smears to be made directly from the heelstick, prepare the smears first; then collect the blood into microcollection containers.

The blood smear should not touch the edges of the glass slide and should appear smooth, with no irregularities, streaks, or holes. When the smear is held up to light, it will display a rainbow in the feathered edge. Table 11-3 lists the criteria to ensure quality blood smears.

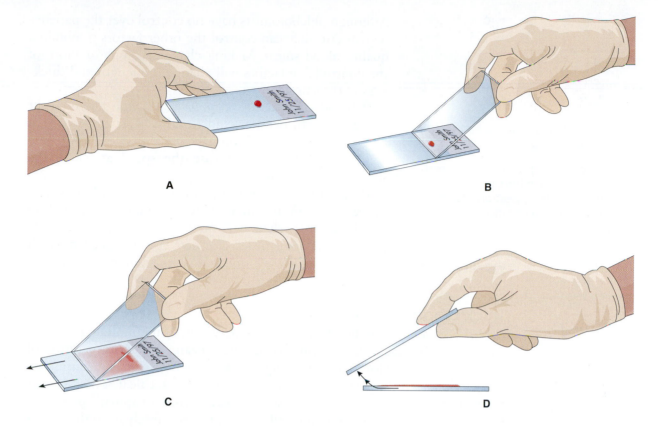

Figure 11-8 Making a blood smear. (A) Apply a drop of blood to the slide about ½ inch from the frosted end. (B) Hold the spreader slide at a 30- to 35-degree angle. Pull the spreader slide toward the frosted end until it touches the drop of blood. (C) When the drop finishes flowing along the edge of the spreader slide, push the spreader slide toward the unfrosted end of the smear slide. (D) Continue the steady motion past the edge of the smear slide and lift the spreader slide away from the smear slide, maintaining a 30- to 35-degree angle. The smear should be thicker at the frosted end of the slide.

Obtaining a Good Wedge Smear

Several factors affect the quality of a blood smear, including

- the angle of the spreader slide
- the size of the blood drop
- the speed of pushing the spreader slide
- the patient's hematocrit

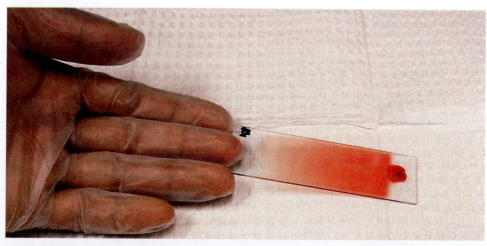

Figure 11-9 A correctly prepared blood smear should appear smooth, without irregularities, and should have a feathered edge.

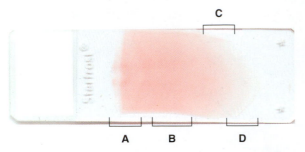

Figure 11-10 Portions of a properly prepared blood smear include (A) the head, or thick, portion; (B) the body, or thin, portion; (C) the critical area; and (D) the tail portion with a feathered edge.

Although phlebotomists have no control over the patient's hematocrit, they can control the other factors to obtain a quality blood smear. Making changes to one or more of the controllable factors will change the length and thickness of the smear.

If blood smears are too long, repeat the blood smear procedure with two new slides and use a smaller drop of blood or a steeper angle on the spreader slide (a 45-degree angle or greater), or increase the speed at which the spreader slide is pushed.

If blood smears are too short, repeat the blood smear procedure with two new slides and use a larger drop of blood or a shallower angle on the spreader slide (a 25-degree angle or less), or decrease the speed at which the spreader slide is pushed. Table 11-4 provides an explanation for causes of poorly prepared blood smears.

Thick Blood Smears

Malarial parasites may be present in peripheral blood in amounts too small to be detected easily on a routine blood smear examination. Preparation of thick smears allows for quick screening to detect the presence of malarial parasites, which can then be further examined using a thin smear. Thick smears for malaria screening are best prepared directly from a capillary puncture. Collect one large drop of blood by allowing it to drop freely onto the center of a clean glass slide. Place the corner of another glass slide or the tip of an applicator stick into the center of the drop. Prepare the smear by drawing a spiral from the center outward, spreading the blood into a thick circle. The resulting smear should be thick and circular to oval (see Figure 11-11).

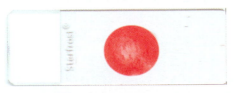

Figure 11-11 A thick smear, used for malaria parasite screening, should be circular to oval and be thin enough to visualize newsprint through it when still wet.

Label the frosted end with patient information. Protocols may state to label slides prior to making the blood smear. Always check with your facility's protocol for the required procedure. A well-prepared thick smear is dense yet allows newsprint to be seen through it when still wet. If a smear is too thick, it may peel away from the slide during drying or staining. Allow the smear to air-dry for at least 30 minutes. If preparing thick smears from an EDTA specimen, prepare them no more than 1 hour after collection. Use the competency checklist *Preparation of Blood Smears* at the end of this chapter to review and practice the procedure.

TABLE 11-3 Criteria to Ensure Quality Blood Smears

- Glass slides must be clean and free of chipped edges.
- The drop of blood should be about 2 millimeters (mm) in diameter.
- The smear should be made immediately after placing the blood on the slide.
- The spreader slide angle should be correct, normally at a 30- to 35-degree angle.
- The pushing motion should be smooth and fluid.
- The smear should be allowed to air-dry.
- The smear should cover two-thirds to three-fourths of the length of the slide (approximately 1½ inches).
- The smear should have a "rainbow" in the feathered edge.
- The smear should not touch any edge of the slide.

TABLE 11-4 Causes for Various Appearances of Blood Smears

Smear	Description	Cause
A	Good blood smear has a straight feathered edge.	Proper control was used over the blood drop size, angle of spreader slide, and speed at which the spreader slide was pushed.
B	Good blood smear has a slightly rounded feathered edge.	
C	Blood smear is too rounded.	The drop of blood was not allowed to form a uniform line along the spreader slide before it was pushed.
D	Blood smear has a sharp angle on one side.	Uneven pressure was used when pushing the spreader slide.
E	Blood smear is too short.	The spreader slide was used at too steep an angle, was pushed too quickly, or both.
F	Blood smear is too long.	The spreader slide was used at too shallow an angle, was pushed too slowly, or both.
G	Blood smear does not have a critical area or feathered edge.	The spreader slide was not pushed all the way off the bottom slide; it was lifted off midway during pushing.
H	Blood smear has a back-and-forth, wavy appearance and is too long.	A stop-and-start movement was used during pushing.
I	Blood smear has areas where no blood is on the slide.	A stop-and-start, shaky movement was used during pushing.
J	Blood smear has a jagged edge and a large amount of blood remaining at the head.	The entire drop of blood was not allowed to flow along the spreader slide edge and the spreader slide edge was not clean.
K	Blood smear has holes in it.	The slide has fingerprints on it. Slides should be clean and handled only by the edges.

Blood Collection for Blood Bank

Patients who require a blood transfusion or blood products must have certain tests to prepare for receiving blood. Blood collection for the transfusion services of the immunohematology department includes specimens for transfusion as well as antibody screening. The order may read *type and cross-match* or *type and screen*. Special procedures must be followed when collecting blood from these patients.

Type and Cross-Match/Type and Screen Blood Specimens

For all blood tests, phlebotomists must follow a standard procedure for patient identification and documentation on specimen tubes and requisitions. However, more complete identification is required for specimens from patients who may receive blood products. Hospital transfusion services and blood banks have strict protocols for patient identification prior to blood collection for transfusion testing and immediately prior to transfusing a blood product. A special identification wristband, in addition to the hospital admission band, and tube labeling systems may be used. Because these systems vary by hospital, phlebotomists must become familiar with the system used by their facility. Both the patient wristband and the tubes must display special transfusion numbers. For example, the requisition shown in Figure 11-12 displays the number R 165146. This number is on the patient's blood bank wristband, on the patient's blood sample, on the requisition, and on the blood product tag. It is a number used only once, for only one patient.

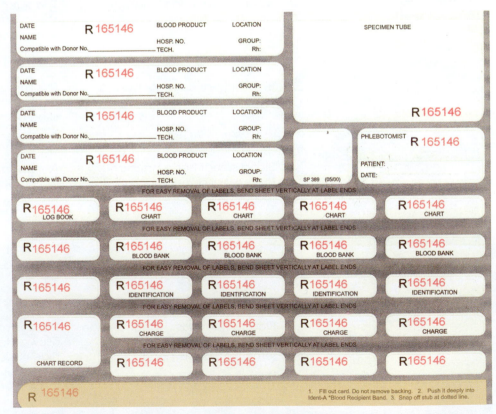

Figure 11-12 Labels with unique numbers are used to identify patients, their blood specimens, and the units of blood that have been cross-matched for them. The highlighted area becomes an arm band that the phlebotomist must put on the patient.

Facilities using barcodes for patient identification may use a blood bank identification system similar to that shown in Figure 11-13. An armband that displays the order for type and screen or type and cross-match is placed on the patient's arm by the phlebotomist. This special blood bank armband must also display the transfusion number and its barcode. The same transfusion number and corresponding barcode must appear on the specimen tube; additional stickers are available for labeling units of blood and/or accompanying paperwork. This type of bar code identification system helps to reduce errors in blood transfusion administration.

A sample drawn for type and cross-match or type and screen is usable for 72 hours. Once the sample expires, if additional products are required for the patient, a new sample must be drawn. Generally, a new unique number is assigned at that time, although some protocols allow patients to maintain the same number for the length of their hospital stay.

The following steps, seen in Competency Check 11-6, help ensure that this procedure is performed correctly. However, procedures vary from facility to facility, so always follow the policy at the facility where you are employed.

Competency
Check 11-6

Type and Cross-Match

1. Identify the patient as you would for routine blood draws by asking the patient his or her name and date of birth.

2. Compare this information with that on the blood bank requisition and labels.

3. Compare this information with that on the hospital wristband. If they are different, contact the patient's nurse immediately for clarification of the patient's identity. Discrepancies must be resolved before blood is drawn.

4. Attach the identification bracelet to the patient's wrist above or below the hospital band.

5. Wash your hands, put on gloves, and prepare the equipment.

6. Perform the venipuncture procedure and collect the appropriate tubes (usually one or two pink-topped EDTA tubes).

7. Label the specimens with the special blood bank labels and recheck information by comparing the labels on the tubes with the blood bank identification band. Be sure to complete all of the information required on the blood bank labels.

8. Carry out postvenipuncture patient care.

9. Deliver the specimens and blood bank requisition to the blood bank or transfusion service at your facility.

Use the competency checklist *Specimen Collection for Type and Cross-Match* at the end of this chapter to review and practice the procedure.

Donor Blood Collection

Another aspect of blood bank phlebotomy is collecting blood from donors. Certified phlebotomists can obtain training to perform blood collection in donor collection centers, where blood is donated for patient use. Donations can occur at a blood collection center, such as the American Red Cross or LifeSource; at the blood bank section of a hospital laboratory; or at community drives arranged by hospitals or blood centers. Blood donor vans travel to many locations, such as schools, civic organizations, places of worship, and places of employment.

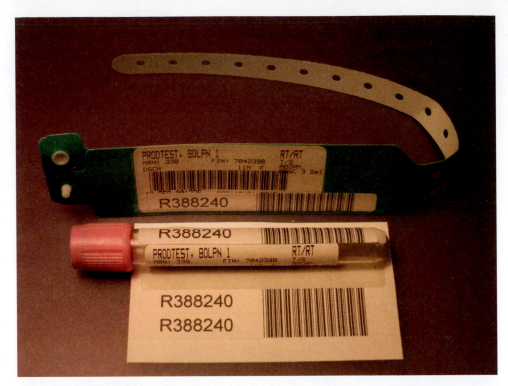

Figure 11-13 Barcode systems are available for blood bank identification. The reference number "R" on the unit of blood must match the one on the patient's armband as well as the one on the tube used for the type and crossmatch specimen.

The process of making and processing blood components is usually performed at the donor center's testing laboratory or facility. Collected units of blood may be processed to provide any of the following products:

- Red blood cells (see Figure 11-14A)
- Plasma (see Figure 11-14B)
- Platelets

Blood products such as platelets, plasma, and granulocytes can be collected using *apheresis* techniques, in which one or more of these blood products is removed during blood collection through a special apparatus. For example, plasmapheresis removes blood plasma. All blood products require meticulous labeling so that each unit is identified correctly and can be traced back to the blood donor.

Patient Education & Communication

Donor Communication

People who volunteer to donate blood are screened both orally and using a detailed questionnaire. The information they provide helps screen for diseases such as malaria, hepatitis C virus, and variant Creutzfeldt-Jakob disease (vCJD), which may have been picked up during travel to Europe. Questions about sexual activity are necessary to screen for sexually transmitted infections (STIs), such as human immunodeficiency virus (HIV) infection and syphilis. Donors may be surprised at the depth of these questions and need to be assured that their information is maintained with the strictest confidence.

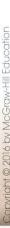

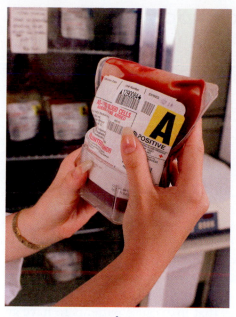
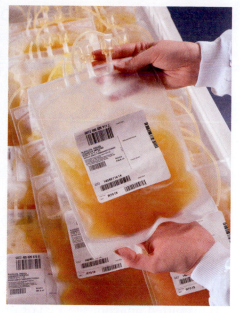

A   B

Figure 11-14 Donated blood can be processed into a number of products, such as (A) red blood cells and (B) plasma.

Blood donation candidates must meet strict guidelines and requirements for blood donation, which have been developed by the FDA and other regulatory bodies. Donor collection facilities are periodically subjected to unannounced inspections to ensure compliance with guidelines and regulations.

To qualify for blood donation, a person must

- be at least 16 years old (written parental consent is required for minors)
- weigh at least 110 pounds
- be in good general health
- have eaten within 4 hours prior to donation
- *not* have donated blood in the past 8 weeks

In addition, a mini-physical is given. The donor's temperature, blood pressure, and pulse are taken. The donor's hematocrit or hemoglobin is often determined by using a fingerstick technique (explained in the *Waived Testing and Collection of Non-Blood Specimens* chapter). The donor must be healthy enough to donate, and the donor unit must be of the highest quality.

Donor Well-Being

During and following any type of blood donation, donors must be monitored for potential side effects, such as dizziness and nausea. If dizziness occurs, keep the donor in a reclining position, preferably with the head lower than the heart. Do not allow the donor to stand or walk, as this may lead to injury as a result of falling or fainting. After the donation, a small snack and fruit juice usually prevent these common side effects. The donor's blood glucose level might be lower than normal, and the snack and fruit juice help increase glucose level quickly before the donor leaves the area.

Safety & Infection Control

Donors must also complete a health history form that includes questions about recent travel out of the country, sexual activity, and the medications they are taking. These questions are asked to screen for diseases that may have been acquired in a foreign land and to screen for the possibility of transfusing sexually transmitted infections (STIs) or drugs that may cause patients to have an adverse reaction. The donor then signs a consent, which gives permission for the blood bank to use the blood.

Once the initial screenings are completed, donors are placed in a comfortable sitting or reclining position. It takes several minutes to collect one donor unit of 450 to 500 milliliters. The preferred site of venipuncture is from a large vein in the antecubital area, such as the median cubital vein. A two-step skin cleansing process, similar to the process for blood culture collection, is followed. Blood units are collected in a sterile, closed collection system consisting of the blood collection bag to collect the blood, tubing, and a 16-gauge needle. Once the vein is accessed, blood flows via gravity into the collection bag, which is placed lower than the donor's arm. An anticoagulant—citrate phosphate dextrose (CPD or CPDA1)—is present in the blood collection bag. The amount of CPD present anticoagulates and preserves 450 milliliters (about a pint) of blood for 21 days. During the collection process, the phlebotomist can place the bag on a mixing unit next to the donor. The mixing unit agitates the contents, which ensures that the blood is being mixed properly with the anticoagulant. In some facilities, the phlebotomist performs manual mixing by gently manipulating the bag as the blood flows into it. This sterile, closed blood collection unit must be used only once. If for some reason the bag does not fill with blood, the needle and the blood collection bag must be discarded because it will be affected by the presence of too much CPD for the amount of blood collected. If this occurs, the entire process will have to be repeated, using another blood donor collection setup. This is done to maintain the sterility of the donor unit.

Some blood collection centers, especially those collecting blood at community blood draws, provide a final opportunity for donors to disclose any possibility that their donation is not safe for transfusion. One method is self-exclusion, in which the donor places a phone call the next day to voluntarily remove his or her unit from usage.

Autologous Blood Collection

In addition to donating blood to help others, individuals can donate blood for their own future use. Their blood may be drawn at outpatient settings so that it can be stored in a blood bank to be used later. When this pre-drawn, donated blood is given back to the patient, this is referred to as **autologous** blood donation. Autologous donations became popular primarily because of the increased concern about the transmission of bloodborne pathogens, such as HIV.

Autologous blood can be placed on reserve for the individual to use within a certain amount of time. If, however, the patient is donating blood prior to a surgical procedure, certain prerequisites must be met. First, the patient must have a written order from a healthcare provider and be capable of regenerating red blood cells. In other words, the patient must be in good enough health to replace the blood donation. In addition, the individual's hemoglobin must be at least 11 grams and the surgical procedure must be scheduled for more than 72 hours from the time of autologous donation. The collection process for an autologous unit of blood is the same as for donor blood collection.

Another form of autologous blood transfusion can occur during surgical procedures where extensive blood may be lost. Patients can be readministered some of the blood lost during the surgery. A patient's blood is collected from body cavities into special reservoirs on an instrument called a Cell Saver. Blood is delivered to the Cell Saver through tubing. The blood is then cleaned by washing with a saline solution and removing impurities by spinning the blood-saline mixture to separate the cleaned blood from the impurities. The blood is then infused back into the patient. Similar to the Cell Saver, but smaller, an OrthoPAT is used to collect blood lost primarily during knee surgery. Highly trained surgical staff or blood transfusion specialists perform these procedures.

Therapeutic Phlebotomy

Therapeutic phlebotomy is the intentional removal of a large amount of blood to lower the red blood cell concentration. Unlike blood donation, which benefits the recipient, therapeutic phlebotomy is performed for that person's benefit. Therapeutic phlebotomies are performed for many medical reasons, including overproduction of iron or red blood cells or an abnormal storage mechanism of iron. Therapeutic phlebotomy is most commonly used as a method of treatment for **polycythemia vera** (a disease that causes an overproduction of red blood cells) and **hemochromatosis** (a disease in which the body stores iron in abnormal amounts). Patients undergoing therapeutic phlebotomy may not be as healthy as normal blood donors, so they require closer monitoring (see Figure 11-15). The blood from patients with polycythemia is not suitable for use in a blood transfusion, so it is discarded. However, some patients with hemochromatosis are eligible to have their units crossed over for patient use.

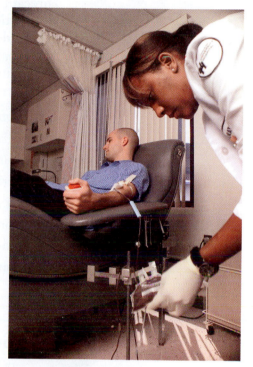

Figure 11-15 Collecting large amounts of blood requires careful monitoring of donors, especially patients undergoing therapeutic blood collection.

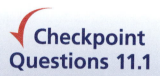

Checkpoint Questions 11.1

1. Explain why the procedure for blood culture site cleansing is different from that for routine venipuncture.

2. Why are blood culture bottles filled in different orders depending on the method used?

3. What is the purpose of the oral glucose tolerance test (OGTT)?

4. When collecting blood from a neonate for state-required tests, why is it important not to touch the paper to the skin or capillary tube?

5. What is the purpose of the extensive screening process for voluntary blood donors?

6. How is autologous blood donation different from regular blood donation?

11.2 Arterial Blood Collection

Arterial blood is collected directly from an artery for special tests that determine the ability of the lungs to exchange oxygen and carbon dioxide. An **arterial puncture** (procedure used to collect arterial blood) is usually performed to test arterial blood gases (ABGs). ABGs measure the ability of the lungs to exchange oxygen and carbon dioxide. They are commonly used to test the partial pressure of oxygen (PO_2) and carbon dioxide (PCO_2) present in arterial blood, along with the pH level. Phlebotomists do not normally perform arterial punctures; special training is required for any medical personnel who perform this procedure. Arterial puncture training must cover the complications associated with arterial puncture, precautions for patient safety, and specimen handling procedures. In many institutions, the respiratory therapy department is responsible for collecting and performing arterial punctures. Other licensed professionals (physicians, nurses, and medical laboratory scientists) may also be trained to perform this procedure.

Several conditions require the measurement of arterial blood gases, including:

- chronic obstructive pulmonary disease (COPD)
- cardiac failure
- respiratory failure
- severe shock
- lung cancer
- coronary bypass
- open-heart surgery
- respiratory distress syndrome

Law & Ethics

Scope of Practice

Phlebotomists do not normally perform an arterial puncture because it is outside a phlebotomist's scope of practice. An arterial puncture should never be attempted without proper training. If performed improperly, a nerve can be accidentally damaged. In addition, the risk of infection is greater in arterial punctures. A sterile cleansing procedure similar to blood culture collection must be used. Compared with venipuncture, an arterial puncture is far more dangerous to the patient. Many complications can occur, such as hematoma formation, thrombosis, hemorrhage, infection, and permanent nerve damage. A phlebotomist should never attempt an arterial puncture until professionally trained.

Usually, patients who have arterial blood gases drawn are critically ill. Therefore, when an arterial specimen is drawn, it must be tested immediately. A phlebotomist may be asked to transport an arterial specimen to the laboratory for testing and must handle this specimen as a STAT.

Arterial Puncture Procedure

Phlebotomists receive specialized training for the performance of an arterial puncture. Before an arterial puncture is performed, an Allen test is done to ensure that the blood supply to the wrist is adequate for the puncture. After making positive patient identification, the arterial puncture is explained to the patient and equipment is prepared. Arterial blood for blood gas analysis is collected with a short needle into a heparinized syringe and placed immediately into an ice bath. The syringe and ice bath should be prepared ahead of time. In order to properly perform an arterial procedure, the steps in Competency Check 11-7 need to be followed in order.

Competency Check 11-7

Arterial Puncture

1. Identify the patient and perform the Allen test. If the Allen test is positive, proceed with the arterial puncture.

2. Wash your hands, put on gloves, and prepare the equipment.

3. Position the patient comfortably, with his or her arm resting on a flat surface, and hyperextend the wrist over a rolled towel or an armboard.

4. Select a site by palpating the path of the radial artery. Note that a tourniquet is not used.

5. Cleanse the site according to facility policy and procedure. Special cleansing may be required.

6. Palpate the artery again using both the index and middle fingers separated by a space of approximately 2 to 4 cm. Leave fingers in place.

7. Hold the syringe near the needle hub end of the syringe barrel at a 45-degree angle or slightly steeper.

8. Puncture the artery midway between the fingers with a smooth, forward motion.

9. A flash of blood will appear in the hub of the needle when the artery is punctured. Do not advance the needle any farther.

10. Do not pull on the syringe plunger; the syringe will fill automatically in a pulsating fashion. Allow the syringe to fill to the required level.

11. Withdraw the needle and immediately apply pressure directly to the puncture site with a clean gauze pad. Direct pressure must be applied for a minimum of 5 minutes.

12. While still applying pressure, quickly complete the specimen handling procedure.

13. Follow the facility's procedure for removing any air from the syringe, removing and discarding the needle, and capping the syringe.

14. Gently roll or invert the syringe to mix the blood with the heparin coating the syringe.

15. Label the syringe with the specimen label and place the syringe immediately into the ice bath (see Figure 11-16).

16. After bleeding stops, cover the puncture site with a sterile bandage.

17. Before leaving the patient, label the syringe with any additional information required by the facility.

18. Thank the patient and transport the specimen to the laboratory immediately.

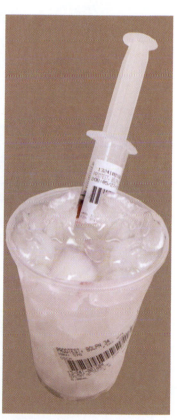

Figure 11-16 Specimens for arterial blood gases are drawn by syringe and immediately placed on ice for delivery to the laboratory.

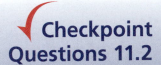

Specimen Labeling

Specimens—whether evacuated tubes, microcollection containers, or syringes—must be labeled with all the required information explained in the chapter *Patient and Specimen Requirements*. Placing specimens into an ice bath, as required for arterial blood gas specimens, may cause the label to get wet and detach from the syringe. To avoid this, the specimen may be placed into a plastic biohazard bag and then into the ice bath. In addition, it is a good idea to label the cup of ice with the same patient information as on the specimen. Doing so will allow laboratory personnel to see the information without removing the specimen from the ice bath. However, always refer to the information on the actual specimen during processing.

Addressing Anxiety

Patients may be uneasy or nervous when anticipating an arterial puncture procedure. Instill confidence by answering questions appropriately. Pay close attention to see if the patient is excessively anxious. Anxious patients have the tendency to hyperventilate, grit their teeth, or hold their breath. These actions will alter blood gas values and therefore not give a true assessment of a patient's cardiopulmonary status. Keeping calm and confident will help relax the patient.

Outpatient Arterial Punctures

Although an arterial puncture is rarely performed on an outpatient, if you do, you must be careful to ensure that bleeding has stopped before allowing the patient to leave. Because blood flow is more forceful in arteries than veins, pressure must be applied to the arterial puncture site for a minimum of 5 minutes. The patient should remain in the outpatient drawing area with strict instructions not to leave until the site is rechecked to ensure that bleeding has completely stopped. The patient should remain in the area for at least 30 minutes. After 30 minutes, check the site for any abnormalities, such as continued bleeding, swelling, hematoma formation, and redness. Once all bleeding has completely stopped, the patient is allowed to leave the area.

✓ Checkpoint Questions 11.2

1. What equipment preparations must be made before collecting arterial blood?
2. At what angle should the needle be inserted to draw arterial blood?

11.3 Venous Access Devices

A venous access device is typically a hollow tube, known as a **cannula,** inserted and left in a vein. Saline locks and heparin locks are venous access devices that are commonly used for obtaining blood samples. A saline or **heparin lock** is a special winged needle set (similar to the butterfly assembly) that may remain in a patient's vein for 48 to 72 hours, depending on institutional policy. A saline or heparin lock is inserted into a patient's vein when obtaining blood is difficult or when a patient must have multiple draws in a short period of time (Figure 11-17). Licensed practitioners may also use this device to administer certain medications. The cannula must be flushed periodically with heparin or normal saline to keep the lock from clotting.

Although drawing blood through venous access lines is not a procedure normally performed by phlebotomists, a phlebotomist may be present during this collection process and may need to provide evacuated tubes for the procedure and transport the specimens to the laboratory. Only specially trained personnel should draw blood from a heparin or saline lock assembly, as determined by each facility. Facility-specific procedures must be followed when collecting blood for blood cultures (ensuring sterility of the collection procedure). The first 5 milliliters (mL) of blood must be discarded before specimens are collected to reduce contamination with heparin or saline.

Other types of venous access devices used to collect a specimen include central venous therapy lines and shunts (see Figure 11-18). Central venous therapy is the introduction of a cannula into a vein other than a peripheral vein. An arterial venous **fistula** is a surgically inserted shunt (usually a U-shaped tube) connecting an artery and a vein, usually in the forearm, to allow for hemodialysis (a procedure for removing waste products from the blood). In hemodialysis (typically done for patients with severe kidney disease), the shunt is connected to a machine that filters the blood. It is important to note that a phlebotomist NEVER accesses shunts or central venous lines or collects blood from arms that have venous access devices installed.

Even with proper care, the potential for hemolysis increases when blood is collected through a venous access device. Blood is collected using a syringe and must be transferred to tubes immediately and mixed adequately. Being pulled into the syringe and then pulled into an evacuated tube may cause enough turbulence to hemolyze the blood. Blood should NEVER be forced out of the syringe by pushing hard on the plunger during the transfer procedure.

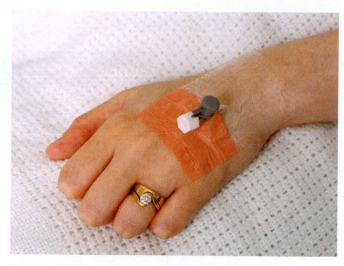

Figure 11-17 A cannula left in place must be flushed with normal saline between blood collections to ensure an accurate specimen.

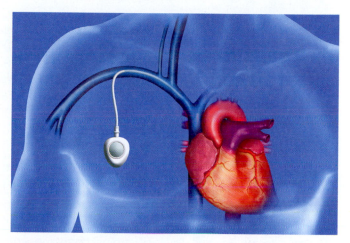

Figure 11-18 A central line is a port that allows for easy venous delivery of medication or collection of blood samples.

1. For what reasons might a venous access device be ordered for a patient?
2. Explain the purpose of a heparin lock.

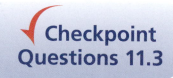

✓ **Checkpoint Questions 11.3**

Chapter Summary

Learning Outcomes	Key Concepts/Examples	Related NAACLS Competency
11.1 Recognize the requirements of special collection procedures. Pages 290–313.	• Blood cultures must be drawn under strict aseptic technique to prevent false-positives. A set of cultures may include one aerobic and one anaerobic specimen, and more than one set of cultures are frequently taken to ensure against false-negatives. • Various types of glucose tests include fasting blood glucose, 2-hour postprandial blood glucose, random blood glucose, 2- or 3-hour oral glucose tolerance test; glucose challenge screening test, and intravenous glucose tolerance test. • Newborns are screened for many disorders, including cystic fibrosis, galactosemia, hypothyroidism, phenylketonuria, biotinidase deficiency, and sickle cell disease. Testing varies among states; however, the blood must be drawn after the infant is 24 hours old. • Peripheral blood smears require a drop of blood on a slide that is spread across the slide using a spreader slide. A thin smear (used for differentials) has a straight or slightly rounded, feathered edge. A thick smear (used for malaria screening) is circular and requires a long time to dry. • Collecting blood for cross-matching units required for transfusion must follow a special patient identification procedure. • Only specially trained personnel may perform donor collection procedures. Donors must meet strict criteria to be eligible to donate. • Patients may donate blood for their own future use (autologous donation) or may have blood drawn to treat a disease or disorder of the blood (therapeutic phlebotomy).	2.00, 2.2, 4.00, 4.3, 4.4, 5.00, 5.3, 6.00, 6.3, 6.7, 7.00, 9.7
11.2 Identify steps to competent and effective arterial puncture. Pages 314–316.	Specially trained personnel may perform arterial punctures using the radial artery and specific arterial puncture procedures.	4.2, 4.3
11.3 Classify venous access sites and their uses. Page 317.	Although not accessed by phlebotomists, other sites for blood specimen collection include heparin lock, arterial venous shunt, and central venous therapy lines.	6.7, 7.00, 7.3

Chapter Review

A: Labeling

Label the parts of a well-made blood smear.

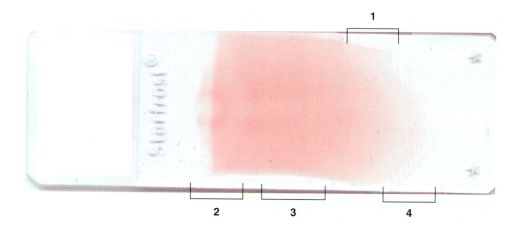

1. [LO 11.1] _____

2. [LO 11.1] _____

3. [LO 11.1] _____

4. [LO 11.1] _____

B: Matching

Match the disorders on the right to their descriptions.

_____ **5.** [LO 11.1] failure to break down milk sugars

_____ **6.** [LO 11.1] deficiency that causes hearing and vision loss

_____ **7.** [LO 11.1] symptoms include respiratory problems

_____ **8.** [LO 11.1] cannot make iodine-containing hormones

_____ **9.** [LO 11.1] failure to break down an amino acid, which spills into the urine

_____ **10.** [LO 11.1] abnormal structure of hemoglobin molecule

a. biotinidase deficiency
b. cystic fibrosis
c. galactosemia
d. hypothyroidism
e. phenylketonuria
f. sickle cell disease

C: Fill in the Blank

Write in the word(s) to complete the statement or answer the question.

11. [LO 11.3] _____ devices may be used when the patient needs multiple blood collections in a short period of time.

12. [LO 11.1] Newborn screening tests required by all states include _____, _____, _____, and _____.

13. [LO 11.1] Qualities of a good blood smear slide include _____,
_____, and _____.

14. [LO 11.1] Components that can be obtained from a unit of donated blood include
_____, _____, and _____.

D: Sequencing

Place the following procedural steps in order for a blood culture collection using a butterfly assembly. Write the number for each step in the space provided.

15. [LO 11.1] _____ Allow the site to air-dry for 60 seconds.

16. [LO 11.1] _____ Cleanse the site using sterile technique and the appropriate antiseptic.

17. [LO 11.1] _____ Complete postpuncture patient care.

18. [LO 11.1] _____ Fill the aerobic bottle.

19. [LO 11.1] _____ Fill the anaerobic bottle.

20. [LO 11.1] _____ Identify the patient, wash your hands, and put on gloves.

21. [LO 11.1] _____ Label the bottles with patient and collection information.

22. [LO 11.1] _____ Perform the venipuncture.

23. [LO 11.1] _____ Reapply the tourniquet.

24. [LO 11.1] _____ Release the tourniquet and apply pressure to the site.

25. [LO 11.1] _____ Select the venipuncture site and release the tourniquet.

26. [LO 11.1] _____ Sterilize the tops of the blood culture bottles.

Place the steps for an oral glucose tolerance test in order. Write the number for each step in the space provided.

27. [LO 11.1] _____ Collect blood and have the patient provide a urine specimen (if required) at specific time intervals.

28. [LO 11.1] _____ Collect a fasting blood specimen using proper venipuncture technique.

29. [LO 11.1] _____ Ensure that the patient has been fasting for at least 12 hours.

30. [LO 11.1] _____ Explain the procedure to the patient.

31. [LO 11.1] _____ Identify the patient.

32. [LO 11.1] _____ Label each sample (blood and urine) with both the time collected and the time interval.

33. [LO 11.1] _____ Observe the patient drinking the glucose dose within 5 minutes.

34. [LO 11.1] _____ Perform a POCT glucose test or obtain a glucose level on the specimen from the chemistry department.

35. [LO 11.1] _____ Prepare the glucose drink according to procedure requirements.

36. [LO 11.1] _____ Verify that the screening blood glucose level is less than 200 mg/dL.

E: Case Study/Critical Thinking

37. [LO 11.2] As a phlebotomist, you're asked to perform arterial blood gases on your first official day as a phlebotomist. You have not had any further training and development. How would you handle this situation?

38. [LO 11.1] You have orders to obtain blood cultures × 2. You have finished the procedure for one site but cannot use the other arm for the second site. What should you do?

39. [LO 11.1] You are about to draw an outpatient's 2-hour postprandial glucose. He informs you that it has been only 1½ hours since he ate his lunch. You are on a tight schedule because, of the three phlebotomists scheduled to work today, you are the only one who showed up. What should you do?

40. [LO 11.1] When collecting blood on a newborn for state-required testing, the baby kicks the form, scraping the form with her heel and scraping the area where blood is being collected. What should you do?

41. [LO 11.1] When instructing a phlebotomy student who is preparing blood smears, you notice that his smears are too short. What should you ask him to do the next time he makes smears?

F: Exam Prep

Choose the best answer for each question.

42. [LO 11.1] A heparin lock is used when
   a. patients need blood drawn several times in a short period of time.
   b. phlebotomists collect blood into a green-stoppered tube.
   c. certain medications must be administered on a regular basis.
   d. all sites for blood collection have already been accessed.

43. [LO 11.2] Arterial puncture is used to assess (*Choose all that apply*)
   a. blood counts.
   b. blood gases.
   c. blood glucose.
   d. blood pH.

44. [LO 11.1] *Aerobic* means
   a. air loving.
   b. nothing to eat.
   c. room air.
   d. without air.

45. [LO 11.1] The aseptic collection of blood cultures requires that the skin be cleaned with
   a. soap and water.
   b. 70% alcohol and then 95% alcohol.
   c. 70%–90% alcohol and then 2% iodine.
   d. 95% alcohol only.

46. [LO 11.1] Specimen collection containers that are appropriate for blood cultures include (*Choose all that apply*)
   a. anaerobic ARD bottles.
   b. non-ARD aerobic bottles.
   c. yellow-stoppered SPS tubes.
   d. yellow-stoppered ACD tubes.

47. [LO 11.1] Glucose testing includes (*Choose all that apply*)
   a. fasting blood draw.
   b. 3-hour tolerance.
   c. 2-hour postprandial.
   d. 1-hour challenge.

48. [LO 11.1] Specimens for glucose testing that may be delayed is BEST collected in
   a. a gold serum separator tube.
   b. a mint plasma separator tube.
   c. a gray-stoppered tube.
   d. none of these.

49. [LO 11.1] When outpatients are having a glucose tolerance performed, they may (*Choose all that apply*)
   a. smoke.
   b. drink black coffee.
   c. chew gum.
   d. drink sips of water.

50. [LO 11.1] All states in the United States require which of the following tests to be performed on neonates? *(Choose all that apply.)*
   a. Cystic fibrosis
   b. Galactosemia
   c. Hypothyroidism
   d. Phenylketonuria

51. [LO 11.1] Galactosemia results from the body's inability to metabolize
   a. fatty acids.
   b. milk sugar.
   c. proteins.
   d. vitamins.

52. [LO 11.1] A common defect in hemoglobin structure is screened for by which test?
   a. Phenylketonuria
   b. Biotinidase
   c. Galactosemia
   d. Sickle cell

53. [LO 11.1] Which of the following procedures would help diagnose an infection caused by a blood parasite?
   a. Blood cultures
   b. Blood smear
   c. Bleeding time
   d. Cold agglutinins

54. [LO 11.1] The most common angle used to make a blood smear is
   a. 10 degrees.
   b. 20 degrees.
   c. 30 degrees.
   d. 45 degrees.

55. [LO 11.1] What factors can a phlebotomist control when preparing blood smears? *(Choose all that apply.)*
   a. Drop size
   b. Hematocrit
   c. Spreading angle
   d. Spreading speed

56. [LO 11.1] Blood collection for type and screen requires *(Choose all that apply)*
   a. sterile blood collection technique.
   b. special consideration for specimen temperature.
   c. special patient identification and banding.
   d. special capillary blood collection procedure.

57. [LO 11.1] Removal of large amounts of blood is required for *(Choose all that apply)*
   a. autologous blood donation and transfusion to self.
   b. donation of red blood cells for use by other patients.
   c. donation of a component of blood other than red blood cells.
   d. removal of blood for therapeutic treatments.

58. [LO 11.1] Sterile blood collection procedures are required for *(Choose all that apply)*
   a. arterial punctures.
   b. blood cultures.
   c. blood donor draws.
   d. neonatal screening.

59. [LO 11.2] Performing an arterial puncture is a procedure requiring specialized training because arteries
   a. are not easily palpated.
   b. lie close to nerves, which may be accidentally damaged.
   c. are not found in the antecubital area.
   d. have lower pressures than veins.

60. [LO 11.1] An antibiotic removal device is
   a. a resin found in some blood culture bottles.
   b. any antiseptic used for cleansing the venipuncture site.
   c. given to a patient who has a bacterial infection.
   d. used to clean a surface after a biohazard spill.

61. [LO 11.1] Special blood collection procedures for which most phlebotomists are trained include all of these EXCEPT
   a. collection of blood cultures.
   b. glucose tolerance collections.
   c. neonatal blood screening collection.
   d. collection of units from blood bank donors.

connect

Enhance your learning by completing these exercises and more at connect.mheducation.com

References

American Diabetes Association. (2011). *Diabetes care.* Retrieved September 2, 2011, from http://care.diabetesjournals.org/content/34/Supplement_1/S11.full

American Red Cross. (2011). *Donating blood.* Retrieved April 29, 2011, from www.redcrossblood.org/donating-blood

Centers for Disease Control and Prevention. (n.d.). *Laboratory identification of parasites of public health concern: Diagnostic procedures, specimen collection.* Retrieved May 1, 2011, from www.dpd.cdc.gov/dpdx/HTML/DiagnosticProcedures.htm

National Accrediting Agency for Clinical Laboratory Sciences. (2010). *NAACLS entry-level phlebotomist competencies.* Rosemont, IL. NAACLS.

State of Illinois Department of Public Health neonatal screening instructions. (n.d.). Greenville, SC: ID Biological Systems.

U.S. National Library of Medicine. (2011). *Genetics home reference: Cystic fibrosis.* Retrieved April 26, 2011, from http://ghr.nlm.nih.gov/condition/

U.S. National Library of Medicine. (2011). *Genetics home reference: Sickle cell disease.* Retrieved April 26, 2011, from http://ghr.nlm.nih.gov/condition/

COMPETENCY CHECKLIST: BLOOD CULTURE PROCEDURE

Procedure Steps	Practice			Performed		
	1	2	3	Yes	No	Master
Preprocedure						
1. Examines the requisition.						
2. Verifies the timing of blood cultures (two sites same time, etc.).						
3. Greets the patient; introduces self.						
4. Identifies the patient verbally using two identifiers, including comparing the identification band with the requisition.						
5. Explains the procedure to the patient.						
6. Washes hands and puts on gloves.						
7. Correctly selects and assembles the equipment.						
8. Applies a tourniquet, identifies the venipuncture site, and releases the tourniquet.						
9. Performs site sterilization using friction scrub.						
10. Allows the site to air-dry (does not blot or wipe dry).						
11. Marks the minimum and maximum fill levels on the culture bottles.						
12. If recommended by the manufacturer, cleanses the culture bottle stoppers while the site is drying.						
Procedure						
13. Reapplies the tourniquet without touching the site.						
14. Performs venipuncture without touching or palpating the site.						
15. Inoculates the blood culture media as required (yellow-stoppered SPS tubes or blood culture bottles).						
16. Inoculates the blood culture bottles in the correct sequence (aerobic first if using winged-infusion butterfly assembly).						
17. Releases the tourniquet.						
18. Covers the puncture site with gauze.						
19. Withdraws the needle smoothly.						
20. Activates the safety engineering control device.						
21. Applies pressure to the venipuncture site.						
22. Disposes of the collection unit (vacuum or butterfly assembly) in the correct container.						
23. Mixes the blood culture bottles as recommended by the manufacturer.						

Procedure Steps	Practice			Performed		Master
	1	2	3	Yes	No	
Procedure						
24. Properly labels the blood culture bottles (including the date, time, site of collection, and phlebotomist identification).						
25. Cleans the patient's skin.						
26. Checks the venipuncture site.						
27. Applies a bandage.						
28. Thanks the patient.						
29. Disposes of used supplies appropriately.						
30. Removes gloves and washes hands.						
31. Transports the specimens to the laboratory.						
32. Documents the specimen collection.						

COMMENTS: _____
_____
_____
_____

SIGNED

EVALUATOR: _____

STUDENT: _____

COMPETENCY CHECKLIST: NEONATAL TESTING

Procedure Steps	Practice			Performed		
	1	2	3	Yes	No	Master
Preprocedure						
1. Examines the requisition.						
2. Obtains state neonatal blood collection form.						
3. Follows facility's procedure for access to neonatal unit (in the case of outpatients, performs proper handwashing and donning of PPEs).						
4. Identifies the patient verbally using two identifiers, including comparing the identification band with the requisition.						
5. Washes hands and puts on gloves.						
6. Selects appropriate site for dermal puncture on heel.						
7. Properly prepares the puncture site.						
Procedure						
8. Correctly performs a dermal puncture on the heel.						
9. Follows the instructions on the state form for properly filling the specimen circles.						
Postprocedure						
10. Correctly performs post-puncture care.						
11. Correctly maintains specimen integrity while drying (air-dry 3 hours, room temperature, out of direct sunlight, NOT overlapping another form).						

COMMENTS: _____
_____
_____
_____

SIGNED

EVALUATOR: _____

STUDENT: _____

COMPETENCY CHECKLIST: PREPARATION OF BLOOD SMEARS

Procedure Steps	Practice			Performed		
	1	2	3	Yes	No	Master
Preprocedure						
1. Washes hands and wears protective clothing.						
2. Inspects the slides for chips, cracks, fingerprints, etc.						
3. Uses the equipment correctly (Diff Safe, hematocrit tubes, applicator sticks, etc.).						
4. Prepares slides behind a safety shield.						
5. Uses EDTA blood to prepare smears.						
6. Inspects the specimen for clots.						
Procedure						
7. Places the correct size drop on slide.						
8. Prepares the smears, using the slide wedge technique.						
9. Uses the appropriate angle of the spreader slide.						
10. Uses the appropriate speed of the spreader slide.						
11. Inspects the smear for acceptability.						
12. Repeats, if necessary, adjusting the technique to create an acceptable smear.						
Postprocedure						
13. Labels the smear from the patient information off the tube.						
14. Allows the smear to air-dry.						
15. Removes protective gear and washes hands as needed.						

COMMENTS: _____
_____
_____
_____

SIGNED

EVALUATOR: _____

STUDENT: _____

NAME: _____ DATE: _____

COMPETENCY CHECKLIST: SPECIMEN COLLECTION FOR TYPE AND CROSS-MATCH

Procedure Steps	Practice			Performed		Master
	1	2	3	Yes	No	
Preprocedure						
1. Examines the requisition.						
2. Greets the patient; introduces self.						
3. Identifies the patient verbally using two identifiers, including comparing the identification band with the requisition.						
4. Explains the procedure to the patient.						
5. Properly attaches the blood bank identification bracelet to the patient's wrist alongside the hospital identification band.						
6. Washes hands and puts on gloves.						
7. Properly performs the equipment selection and assembly process.						
8. Correctly performs the site selection and preparation procedures.						
9. Reassures the patient.						
Procedure						
10. Reapplies the tourniquet.						
11. Correctly performs the venipuncture procedure.						
12. Properly performs the tube filling procedure.						
13. Releases the tourniquet and safely performs the needle withdrawal procedure.						
Postprocedure						
14. Properly performs postprocedure patient care.						
15. Labels the specimens with the special blood bank labels.						
16. Rechecks the information by comparing the labels on the tubes with the blood bank identification band.						
17. Properly performs postprocedure supply disposal.						
18. Transports the specimens to the laboratory.						
19. Documents the specimen collection.						

COMMENTS: _____
_____
_____
_____

SIGNED

EVALUATOR: _____

STUDENT: _____

12

Quality Essentials

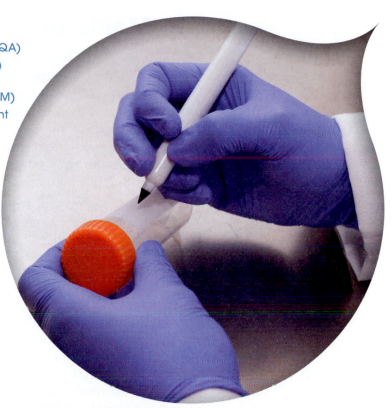

Learning Outcomes

12.1 Identify policies and procedures used in phlebotomy and in the clinical laboratory to assure quality in obtaining blood specimens.

12.2 Carry out documentation of quality control.

12.3 Identify corrective actions for failures of quality control.

Related NAACLS Competencies

8.00 Demonstrate understanding of quality assurance in phlebotomy.

8.1 Describe the system for monitoring quality assurance in the collection of blood specimens.

8.2 Identify policies and procedures used in the clinical laboratory to assure quality in the obtaining of blood specimens.

Introduction

Assuring quality when obtaining and processing specimens is essential to the practice of phlebotomy. This chapter presents the concepts and systems put in place, starting with the phlebotomist and the lab, to ensure quality in the delivery of healthcare.

12.1 Maintaining Quality

The word *quality* implies a state of excellence (free from defects or deficiencies) that earns the confidence and trust of consumers. Quality is accomplished by adherence to a set of measurable standards adopted by an industry, such as healthcare. Quality in the delivery of healthcare, including laboratory results, ensures patient safety and customer satisfaction. Laboratory tests are a vital link that assists healthcare providers in identifying a patient's medical diagnosis. Quality performance—starting with the healthcare provider's order and the work of the phlebotomist and continuing until the specimen results are reported—is imperative to quality patient care. A consistent level of quality must exist at all stages of the process—from the completed lab requisition to specimen processing—in order for test results to be accurate.

Accuracy is how close a result is to the actual value. For example, if the true result for a glucose control or patient value is 125 mg/dL, an accurate result measured by a chemistry test is as close as possible to that value. The **precision** of a test is its ability to give nearly the same result when performed repeatedly. Using the same example, if repeated glucose measurements fall within a close range of 120 to 130 mg/dL, the results are precise. A result can still be precise even if it is not accurate. If the true value of a glucose measurement is 125 mg/dL but repeated measurements fall within the range of 90 to 105 mg/dL, the results are precise but not accurate. This is why controls must be performed and verified to be accurate, and any errors corrected, before tests can be run on patient samples. Controls and errors are discussed later in this chapter. Figure 12-1 and Table 12-1 demonstrate the concepts of accuracy and precision.

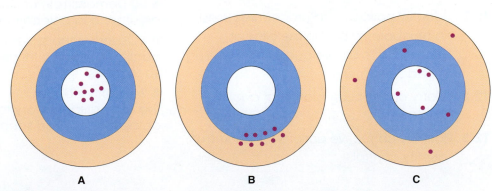

Figure 12-1 Target values. The desired test value falls in the area that is represented by the bull's-eye in the target's center. The points of impact on the target (red dots) represent glucose measurements. (A) These measurements show both accuracy and precision; they repeatedly fall inside the expected range of results. (B) These measurements are precise because they fall close together; however, they are not accurate because they do not fall within the range of expected results. (C) These measurements are neither precise nor accurate because they are not close together and very few fall within the expected range of results.

TABLE 12-1 Glucose Quality Control Measurements with a True Value of 125 mg/dL*

Results Accurate AND Precise (a)	Results Precise but NOT Accurate (b)	Results NOT Accurate or Precise (c)
122 mg/dL	100 mg/dL	122 mg/dL
127 mg/dL	102 mg/dL	162 mg/dL
125 mg/dL	90 mg/dL	135 mg/dL
126 mg/dL	95 mg/dL	126 mg/dL
122 mg/dL	101 mg/dL	102 mg/dL
124 mg/dL	98 mg/dL	124 mg/dL
125 mg/dL	95 mg/dL	85 mg/dL
120 mg/dL	103 mg/dL	150 mg/dL
127 mg/dL	100 mg/dL	117 mg/dL

*The results in each column represent the points charted on Figure 12-1 (A) to (C).

Column (a) in Table 12-1 lists a series of glucose control measurements that are very near the actual value provided by the control manufacturer (accurate) and that are also statistically close to one another (precise). Target (A) in Figure 12-1 represents this dual accuracy and precision as a tight group of points in the center of the target.

Column (b) in Table 12-1 lists a series of glucose control measurements that are far from the actual value provided by the control manufacturer (not accurate) but that are statistically close to one another (precise). Target (B) in Figure 12-1 represents this precision but lack of accuracy as a tight group of points outside of the center of the target.

Column (c) in Table 12-1 lists a series of glucose control measurements, some of which are near and some are far from the actual value provided by the control manufacturer (may not be accurate). These glucose values are statistically far apart from one another (not precise). Target (C) in Figure 12-1 represents lack of both accuracy and precision as points around the target, some in the center and others not.

A high level of quality must be present throughout the process. Physicians and patients rely on laboratory team members for quality performance. The Clinical and Laboratory Standards Institute (CLSI) recognizes a hierarchy of **processes** (step-by-step events that include procedures performed on patients, documentation into the EHR, and all associated quality activities) that lead to the achievement of quality. These processes include total quality management (TQM), quality cost management (QCM), quality management system (QMS), quality assurance (QA), and quality control (QC). Sometimes the terms QA and QC are used interchangeably in the laboratory even though they are different processes. Another term associated with processes for assuring quality includes quality assessment and process improvement (QAPI), which may also be called continuous quality improvement (CQI). Even though the terminology used when describing the quality process changes from time to time, the goal is still the same—improved quality of care for patients. Although phlebotomists may not be involved at every level of quality management, they are the people from whom the patient forms his perception of laboratory quality. Understanding the similarities and differences among these quality processes will help phlebotomists be more knowledgeable during communications about quality. The functions of the quality hierarchy are intertwined as shown in Figure 12-2.

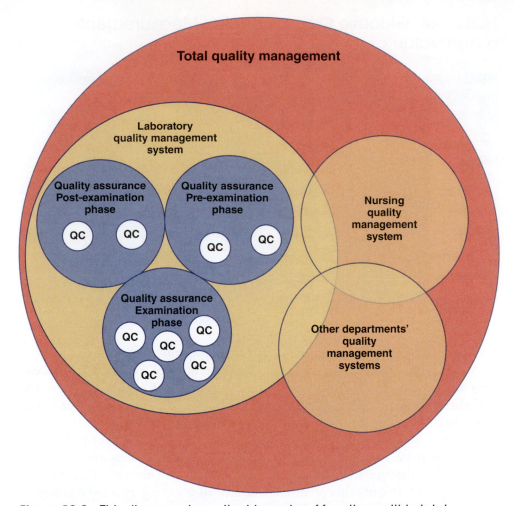

Figure 12-2 This diagram shows the hierarchy of functions within total quality management for parts of a healthcare facility that are responsible for laboratory results. **Pink** represents oversight of the entire process. **Yellow** represents individual departments that have their own quality management systems. The yellow areas represented by nursing and other departments, such as respiratory care, overlap with the laboratory and each other because they are involved in laboratory specimen collection and testing and are inspected by laboratory accreditation agencies. **Blue** represents the QA systems that are in place for each phase of laboratory testing (they are not depicted in the other yellow areas but are performed by other departments as well): pre-examination, examination, and post-examination phases. **White** represents the individual tasks that are performed to maintain quality, which are contained within a particular phase of testing.

Total Quality Management

Total quality management (TQM) is the highest level of quality oversight and is managed at the organizational or institutional level. TQM governs the behavior of a set of individuals, in this case healthcare workers. The purpose of TQM is to identify an organization's internal and external customers and design operations that produce the highest customer satisfaction. TQM involves all members of the healthcare team creating quality processes to improve customer satisfaction. This satisfaction is achieved as a result of both the healthcare encounter and the *accuracy* (correctness) of the results. For example, as mentioned in the chapter *Phlebotomy and Healthcare*, a phlebotomist with an unprofessional appearance and demeanor may adversely or negatively affect the patient's satisfaction with the services he or she has received. Patients form opinions about the laboratory and healthcare facility based on how the phlebotomist appears or acts. Patient perception can be affected when the phlebotomist wears a dirty lab coat over a pair of jeans with frayed hems and sneakers with holes in them instead of maintaining a clean and neat appearance, or when the phlebotomist appears annoyed at having to help a patient or acts hurried.

Likewise, inaccurate test results may not only yield poor patient satisfaction but also result in medical liability and cause the patient to lose trust in the facility and healthcare system. Healthcare teams are empowered to do more than just the bare minimum. Team members' responsibilities include monitoring and documenting processes and ensuring patient satisfaction. Some healthcare facilities ask patients to complete surveys or other forms of rating systems to determine their level of satisfaction with the care they receive.

Patients requiring phlebotomy services evaluate the care they receive not just on their lab results but also on the following factors:

- How long they had to wait for the procedure
- The presence or absence of bruising to the site
- How many needlesticks or attempts were required
- Their perception of the phlebotomist (e.g., dress, communication skills)

Patients who have to wait a minimum amount of time for their blood to be drawn with only one needlestick and who encounter a well-groomed, professional phlebotomist generally rate their experience positively.

Quality Cost Management

Quality cost management (QCM) is a system used to measure and manage the cost of quality. Cost of quality is not simply the cost of a procedure or product; it includes the cost of delivering healthcare with the highest level of quality. In the laboratory, this includes the cost of repeating tests when results are in question, the cost of correcting errors in a process (at every phase of testing), and the cost of maintaining customer satisfaction. Quality cost management works closely with total quality management.

Quality Management System

A **quality management system (QMS)** is both a set of quality objectives established to achieve the goals identified by TQM as well as the methods used to monitor the achievement of those objectives. In the medical laboratory, QMS includes the organizational structure of the laboratory as well as the procedures, processes, and resources needed to develop and meet quality objectives. A QMS includes the functions that most directly involve laboratory personnel—quality assurance and quality control.

Quality Assurance

Since the 1980s, The Joint Commission has defined **quality assurance (QA)** as a system of planned activities that assess operational processes for the delivery of services or the quality of products provided to consumers, customers, or patients. This system is set forth to guarantee quality patient care by continued reassessment of all the processes. *Quality assurance* refers to examining the performance of a process to ensure that testing is being carried out correctly, results are accurate, and mistakes are found and corrected to avoid adverse outcomes. For example, the overall blood collection and handling process along with all of the individual tests these samples can undergo are frequently evaluated. Quality assurance involves looking at every step in the pre-examination, examination, and post-examination phases of a procedure.

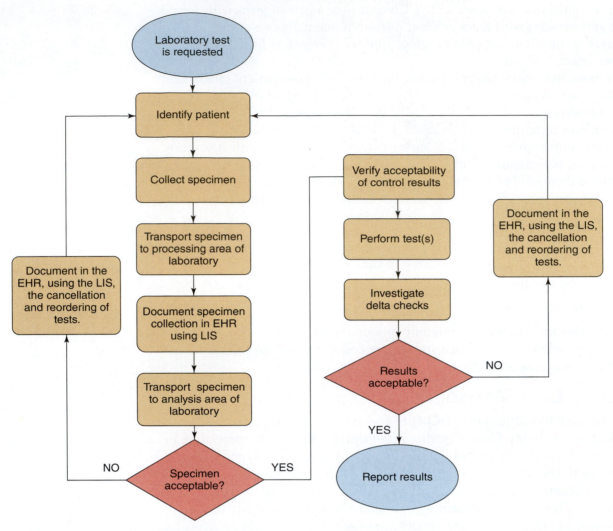

Figure 12-3 A laboratory process flowchart shows the steps followed in the process of laboratory testing.

Figure 12-3 shows an example of this ongoing, cyclical process. Quality assurance activities should be in place during the entire testing process—from initial contact with the patient until the results are documented and logged or charted on the patient's medical record. Each activity contributes to the overall assurance of quality. Any step in an activity can fail, so appropriate control measures are used constantly to minimize or eliminate failures.

When a QA program is put in place, **standards** (rules of practice) are defined and should be followed in order to meet customer safety and satisfaction requirements. Developing, evaluating, and modifying the processes, policies, and procedures used in the medical laboratory are the functions of a QA program.

Quality assurance focuses on the overall process used to measure patient **outcomes** (condition and length of hospital stay), which includes error detection activities (double-checking information) as well as corrective and preventive activities (documentation and training). In the medical laboratory setting, QA is applied to everything involved in producing a quality laboratory test result, including

- the ordering and requisitioning of tests
- positive patient identification
- collection processes

- the integrity of the specimen
- test analysis processes
- the reporting of results
- turnaround time (the time between placing the order and receiving the results)
- the training of lab personnel
- performance on proficiency testing
- performance on laboratory inspections
- documentation and follow-up on corrective action

In addition, the assessment of any process requires the establishment of a chain of accountability, as shown in Figure 12-4, and a series of **indicators** (observable events used as evidence) that are measurable, specific, well defined, and essential to the process. Indicators are designed to assess areas of care that tend to cause problems or negative outcomes (results). They measure quality, accuracy, timeliness, customer satisfaction, adequacy, and other factors. "Wristband identification errors will be less than 1%" is one common example. To evaluate such an indicator, specific, scheduled evaluations of various documents (such as patient records, incident reports, and lab reports) and direct patient observations may be used.

Informing Patients

Patient Education & Communication

Certain blood tests, such as plasma cortisol levels (used for detecting adrenal gland disorders), are affected by diurnal variations (meaning they yield different results based on the time of day they are drawn) and by whether the patient has been moving (walking or engaging in physical activity). Hospitalized patients and outpatients must have such lab tests drawn at specific times to ensure quality results. Plasma cortisol levels drawn around 3:00 P.M. will be much lower—about half the value—than levels drawn between 7:00 A.M. and 9:00 A.M. This information should be shared with patients so that they will understand the importance of adhering to scheduled times for draws. Quality assurance programs ensure that policies and procedures are available to address instances such as this to guarantee quality results.

Using Quality Assurance Resources

Critical Thinking

The laboratory quality assurance policy and procedure manual should provide instructions for handling situations such as the following example. If a patient is scheduled to have a plasma cortisol level drawn at 9:00 A.M. but the patient does not arrive for the blood work until 3:00 P.M., the phlebotomist should notify the licensed practitioner immediately. It is very likely that the physician will request that the test be rescheduled for the following day because of the diurnal variations or changes that occur throughout the day associated with plasma cortisol levels. Other substances affected by diurnal variations are hormone levels, serum iron, and serum glucose levels. Always refer to the standard operating procedure (SOP) when making decisions about specimen collection procedures.

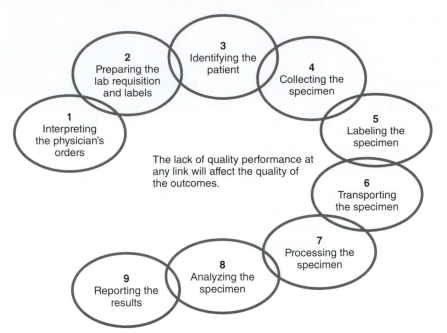

Figure 12-4 In the phlebotomy chain of accountability for laboratory tests, the phlebotomist is always responsible for 3, 4, 5, and 6 of the nine chain links listed, and perhaps all nine, depending on the place of employment.

The purpose of **evaluation** (examining the evidence found when measuring the indicators) is to determine the acceptability of both outcomes and processes. Using the sample indicator just mentioned, if the number of wristband identification errors were to exceed 1%, the outcome would be unacceptable. Knowing the number of errors has exceeded 1% does not solve the problem, but it does trigger a review to evaluate each step of the process for flaws. Most patients would assume that the cause of such a problem is the phlebotomist's failure to check the wristband. However, the hospital admitting clerk, the healthcare personnel caring for the patient, and the phlebotomist drawing the blood are all vital checkpoints that might cause this unwanted outcome. The process of evaluating each procedural step for accuracy is another component of quality assurance commonly referred to as *quality control (QC)*.

Quality Control

Quality control (QC) is defined as activities that ensure specific steps in a process meet acceptable standards or **parameters** (limitations). QC checks are essential to ensuring reliable results and are mandated by accrediting agencies. Accreditation inspectors periodically review QC documents. Activities such as verifying patient identity, checking reagent expiration dates, testing control material prior to patient samples, and reviewing data recording for errors are all part of quality control. Normal parameters are established for all laboratory tests in order to evaluate the outcomes. Basically, quality control measures

Critical Thinking

Quality Control in Phlebotomy

Practicing quality control as part of phlebotomy service includes checking equipment and supplies for defects that may contribute to erroneous results or poor service. One example is examining the needle for defects (which can cause undue pain for the patient) before performing the venipuncture. Another example is checking the expiration dates on evacuated tubes prior to use.

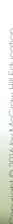

ensure that procedural steps are followed and yield consistent results. Quality control focuses on detecting the defects in a process, which are indicated by the presence of **variances** (deviations from the procedure, such as blood collection from an arm with an IV or controls that are out of range).

Once variances are identified, corrective action plans can be implemented and monitored for improvement. Evaluating the whole process is essential, especially with laboratory tests. These tests require appropriate preparation of both the equipment and the patient prior to specimen collection, and different tests require different types of preparation.

Healthcare facilities have instruction manuals that describe these special and often mandatory preparations and collection procedures. The laboratory user or procedure manual contains the **standard operating procedure (SOP)** for each test performed in the laboratory. Each procedure's SOP explains its purpose, specimen requirements, step-by-step instructions, limitations, normal and critical values, and interpretation. Each procedure is developed using guidelines from The Joint Commission, Clinical and Laboratory Standards Institute (CLSI), Food and Drug Administration (FDA) and other regulatory agencies. This manual must be an available reference for all healthcare personnel involved in the specimen collection process.

Procedures performed at laboratories that are accredited by the College of American Pathologists (CAP) are observed during inspections to ensure compliance with the laboratory's SOP. Failure to adhere to the SOP can adversely affect the quality of the specimen obtained and may therefore alter the results. Quality control activities help to ensure that

- tests are performed on the correct patient
- specimen collection procedures are performed correctly and safely
- specimens are handled, transported, and processed properly
- tests are performed accurately
- **reliable** (believable and dependable) results are reported

Table 12-2 lists some of the processes in the medical laboratory setting to which QC may be applied.

Controls

A **control material** is a liquid, a serum, or freeze-dried material that has been prepared and tested by the manufacturer and that has a known value such as a serum with a known glucose value of 125 mg/dL. This substance is used on a device when doing a system check. If the readings from the control checks are not within the acceptable parameters, the equipment will not yield accurate results. For example, a glucometer test system may have both a high control and a low control with an acceptable range for each. Values obtained during a system check of the glucometer that fall outside the established parameters indicate that corrective action is required.

Expiration dates on control materials and reagent strips should be double-checked; if out of date, they should be replaced and the control check repeated. If expiration dates are current, the control may be repeated. However, a repeat failure warrants immediate calibration, repair, or replacement of the system.

Calibration

Calibration is a procedure used to ensure that equipment is providing accurate results. In most cases, a control sample is run to validate accuracy. For example, if the control sample results yield 80 mg/dL, but the correct concentration is known to be 90 mg/dL, the equipment may not be reading accurately. A second control sample may be run to make sure that the equipment, rather than the

TABLE 12-2 Examples of Quality Control in the Medical Laboratory

Phase of Laboratory Testing	Quality Control Target	Quality Control Activity and Purpose
Pre-examination	Patient identification	Using a two-identifier system to ensure that the correct patient is being drawn
Pre-examination	Specimen labeling	Reviewing specimen labels to determine if the required information is on the tube to ensure correct patient identification
Pre-examination	Specimen labeling	Labeling evacuated tubes only AFTER collection PRIOR to leaving the patient
Pre-examination	Specimen collection	Checking the quality of phlebotomy equipment prior to use for specimen collection
Pre-examination	Refrigerators and freezers	Recording minimum and maximum (low and high) temperatures on a daily basis to determine if stored items are maintained at the correct temperature
Pre-examination	Centrifuges	Checking the speed calibration with a tachometer to determine if the centrifuge setting and timer reflect accurate rotations per minute (RPMs) and elapsed time
Examination	Incubators and water baths	Recording temperatures to determine if the instrument is at the correct temperature prior to use
Examination	Analytic instruments	Testing samples with known concentrations of an analyte to determine if the instrument is functioning correctly
Examination	Analytic instruments	Checking internal instrument temperatures, pressures, and other parameters needing monitoring during testing
Post-examination	Patient results	Retesting sample when results are critical or flagged with delta check error
Post-examination	Patient results	Re-collection of specimen to confirm questionable results
Post-examination	Patient results	Having phoned results read back by staff accepting results by phone
Post-examination	Patient results	Supervisor review of results for accuracy

sample, was the reason for the inaccuracy. If the results are the same, the equipment must be adjusted to provide an accurate reading. Although some adjustments are made manually, newer systems calibrate themselves automatically without operator assistance.

Validation

Another important quality control activity is **validation** (ensuring accuracy and precision). Validation ensures that the results obtained will yield the same or similar results if the test is repeated. In other words, if you were to obtain a glucose result of 107 mg/dL, the same or a similar value must be obtained on the same specimen if the test is repeated several times by different healthcare personnel or with a different instrument. Validation is required when adopting a new procedure or method for a test, when purchasing a new instrument, and when putting a new lot of controls or reagents to use. Both accuracy and precision must be validated to ensure reliable results.

Another check of validity, called a **delta check**, occurs prior to reporting patient results. Delta checks are used to confirm the validity of unexpected variation in patient test results from one collection time to another, before reporting.

If results do not match previous results, expected results, or the patient's clinical symptoms, the test should be repeated, and re-collection of the specimen may be required.

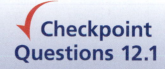

Checkpoint Questions 12.1

1. What is the difference between quality assurance and quality control?
2. List three types of quality control measures that are routinely used in laboratories.

12.2 Documenting Quality Control Activities

Documentation of testing and all related quality control activities is essential to ensuring reliable results. All quality control tests for each analyte tested on each instrument are documented on quality control log sheets (either in paper or electronic form). Figure 12-5 shows a log sheet for monitoring the performance of a point-of-care glucose monitor. The operators of the equipment enter the results of QC performed daily and compare this to acceptable limits prior to testing patient samples. Figure 12-5 also shows a **Levey-Jennings chart** (a graph showing acceptable limits), which is used to visualize whether results fall within the acceptable parameters or if there is a **trend** (results showing an upward or downward progression) or **shift** (a sudden jump in results that continue at the higher or lower level). These log records are usually maintained for at least two years. Trends and shifts are known as **systematic errors** and may be due to aging reagents or control material, deterioration of light sources, or changes in temperature. Errors that occur with no predictable pattern are **random errors** and may have several causes, such as the following:

- Operator procedural error
- Equipment failure
- Outdated reagents
- Clerical errors

Quality Control Errors

Critical Thinking

When performing quality control checks on multiple instruments of the same type, be sure to record data on the appropriate log sheet. Each instrument may measure the same control material differently and must have its own log sheet. If control values are outside acceptable limits, you must investigate and correct the source of the error. For example, imagine that you are testing two glucose meters. After testing the first one, you notice that the result is much lower than those of the previous several days. You first must double-check that you are recording the control data on the correct log sheet. Double-check the expiration dates on the control material and test strips. Finally, review your SOP to ensure that you are performing the procedure correctly. Was the reagent prepared properly and stored at the appropriate temperature? If no apparent cause for the error is revealed, repeat the control test; if the meter still reads out of control, do not use it for patient testing. Consult the manufacturer's information for the appropriate action in correcting the readings on the meter.

QUALITY CONTROL RECORD

PRACTICE NAME
PRECISION HEALTH CARE INC.

DEPARTMENT	Glucose Monitor-Institution #55		NAME/LEVEL
CONTROL LOT #	H542A	EXPIRATION DATE 01/29/XX	
DIRECTOR SIGNATURE DATE:			

TEST		**UNITS**
LOWER LIMIT **91**	MEAN **100**	UPPER LIMIT **109**

DATE	No.	VALUE	TECH	COMMENT	DATE	No.	VALUE	TECH	COMMENT
12/8/XX	1	99	KBH			17			
12/9/XX	2	103	KBH	prev. maintenance		18			
12/10/XX	3	100	KBH			19			
12/11/XX	4	100	KBH			20			
12/14/XX	5	105	KBH			21			
12/15/XX	6	97	KBH			22			
12/16/XX	7	95	KBH			23			
12/17/XX	8	96	KBH	new battery		24			
12/18/XX	9	103	KBH			25			
12/19/XX	10	100	KBH			26			
12/20/XX	11	103	KBH			27			
12/21/XX	12	97	KBH			28			
	13					29			
	14					30			
	15					31			
	16								

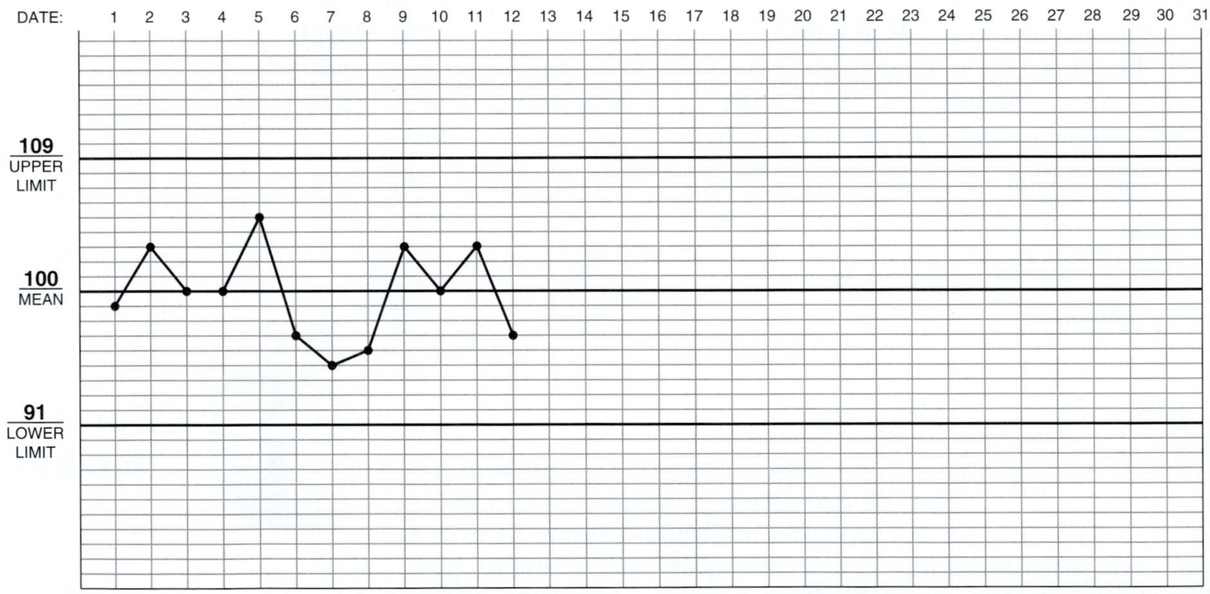

Figure 12-5 Quality control records are maintained on equipment to ensure accuracy of test results. Results are recorded on log sheets and graphed on Levey-Jennings charts that provide a visual assessment of result acceptability.

Figure 12-6 shows a Levey-Jennings chart that exhibits random and systematic errors. Levey-Jennings charts are developed using statistical calculations, which are beyond the scope of this text. Phlebotomists should know how to complete and interpret Levey-Jennings charts if they find themselves in a position that requires them to record control data.

Quality control documentation also includes activities such as recording the temperatures of refrigerators, incubators, water baths, and even the room. Specimens and reagents have ideal storage requirements, as do testing procedures,

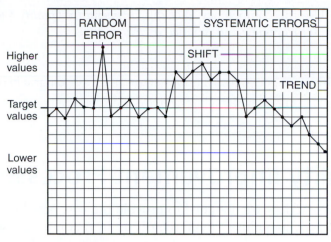

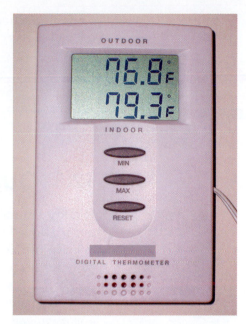

Figure 12-6 Levey-Jennings charts can help identify errors in testing such as random errors, where one or more values are outside of acceptable limits; shifts, where the values show a sudden jump to higher or lower numbers; and trends, where values gradually move farther away from the target value.

Figure 12-7 Minimum/maximum thermometers record the lowest and highest temperatures detected.

and laboratories must demonstrate that these requirements are being met. Daily log sheets must be maintained for documenting temperatures. Some situations require the use of a minimum/maximum thermometer (see Figure 12-7) for recording the daily variation in temperatures. Figure 12-8 shows samples of temperature log sheets. Corrective actions (adjusting settings or defrosting freezers) must be performed when temperatures exceed minimum or maximum acceptable limits. Follow the facility's SOP for documenting temperatures and taking

Refrigerator Make: Westinghouse				**Location:** Phlebotomy Processing #1																	
Record for the year: 2015				**Acceptable Range:** 2–6°C				**Note:** reset thermometer on the first of the month													
January	1	2	3	4	5	6	7	8	9	10	11	12	13	14	15	16	17	18	19	20	21
min	3.0	3.0	3.0	2.8	2.7	2.7	2.5	2.5	2.5	2.4	2.4										
max	3.5	3.6	3.9	4.0	4.0	6.8 / 4.2	4.5	4.6	4.7	4.7	4.7										
tech	lm	lm	lm	lm	lm	lm	lm	lm	lm	lm	lm										
February																					
min																					
max																					
tech																					
March																					
min																					
max																					
tech																					

Corrective Actions Taken	
Date 1/6/2015	Action: Door found ajar, reset thermometer and ensured door is closed tightly. Rechecked temp in range KB.
Date	Action
Date	Action

Reviewed by _____ Date _____

Figure 12-8 Temperature logs are used to record either single daily temperature, or, as illustrated in this figure, the minimum and maximum temperatures on a daily basis. An important feature of the temperature log is the notes section that documents corrective action taken when temperatures fall out of range.

corrective action. Use the competency checklist *Temperature Quality Control* at the end of this chapter to review and practice the procedure.

> ## ✓ Checkpoint Questions 12.2
>
> 1. What is the difference between a random error and a systematic error?
> 2. What document should you consult if you are not sure how to perform a procedure?

12.3 Quality Improvement Processes

Quality assurance practices are designed to provide the best possible care for our patients. However, sometimes circumstances occur that interfere with the delivery of this quality care and may even threaten patient safety. It is vital that laboratories have a system in place that both looks at laboratory processes and events that result in decreased quality care and determines how to improve the process to eliminate these errors. This system is usually referred to as *quality assessment and process improvement.*

Quality Assessment and Process Improvement

Quality assessment and process improvement (QAPI) is the review of documentation to discover weaknesses in a process, so that they can be eliminated and the quality of patient outcomes improved. This process is also called **continuous quality improvement (CQI)**. An assessment, or **audit** (review of records), is performed to discover any weaknesses in a process. Improvements to the process are implemented and the results are monitored to see if process problems are eliminated and future errors are prevented. QAPI is also used to make a process easier to perform. Table 12-3 summarizes the steps in quality assessment and process improvement. Each of these steps helps ensure that a laboratory is providing quality patient care.

Not only are QC records reviewed, but **incident forms** (documents recording procedural or process errors) are also examined to determine if a process problem exists. Figures 12-9 and 12-10 show examples of quality

TABLE 12-3 Quality Assessment and Process Improvement

Step	Activity
Quality assurance	Examining processes to determine if they are functioning correctly
Quality control	Performing and documenting activities that ensure that specific steps in a process meet acceptable standards
Corrective action	Fixing problems that have occurred
Preventive action	Determining ways to prevent errors from happening in the future
Training	Educating employees about new processes and procedures
Competency assessment	Observing staff performing activities and determining adherence to policies and procedures
Proficiency testing	Testing of personnel by an external agency such as CAP (College of American Pathologists)
Audit	Examining records for processes and procedures that were performed and the presence, frequency, and resolution of any errors
Evaluation	Determining the acceptability of both outcomes and processes
Process improvement	Developing and implementing ways to make processes and procedures better

QUALITY ASSESSMENT: OCCURRENCE OF VARIANCE

(a) _____

      Patient name   Medical record #   Date

(b) _____

      Patient location   Form completed by

_____

    Specimen accession #   Specimen type   Tests affected

(c) Complaint: [ ] Patient Issue   [ ] Safety Issue   [ ] Armband Issue   [ ] Employee Issue

(d)

Pre-examination-Specimen Related	[ ] Laboratory collect	[ ] Nurse collect
[ ] Clotted	[ ] Mislabeled	[ ] Wrong patient
[ ] Hemolyzed	[ ] Missing specimen	[ ] Wrong specimen type
[ ] Insufficient specimen	[ ] Missed test / wrong order	[ ] Wrong time collected

(e)

Examination Results Questionable	[ ] Laboratory collect	[ ] Nurse collect
[ ] Delta check	[ ] Specimen integrity issue	[ ] Other concern _____

(f)

Post-Examination Results Invalid	[ ] Laboratory collect	[ ] Nurse collect
[ ] Reported on wrong patient	[ ] Erroneous results reported	[ ] Other _____

(g) Licensed caregiver notified _____ Date and time _____

Investigation Summary

_____

(h)

Severity [ ] Caused healthcare provider to take wrong action	[ ] Caused delay in patient care

(i)   [ ] Training issue   [ ] Non-compliance issue   [ ] Other

(j)

Follow-up

[ ] Discussed variance with employee

[ ] Reviewed SOP with employee   Supervisor _____ Date _____

[ ] Modified procedure

[ ] Re-training scheduled   Employee _____ Date _____

[ ] Other _____

Figure 12-9 This quality assessment form documents the occurrence of a variance in the delivery of quality healthcare. Documentation includes (A) patient information; (B) specimen information; (C) type of complaint; (D,E,F) phase of the procedure and the cause; (G) the person notified and an investigation summary, including the corrective action; (H) the severity of the incident; (I) classification of the issue; and (J) the preventive action.

QUALITY ASSURANCE VARIANCE FORM

Patient name _____ Medical Number _____ Date of Service _____

Accession # _____ Specimen Type _____ Test(s) Affected _____

Physician _____ Form Completed by _____ Date and Time _____

Missing information

[ ] Insurance information: (Responsible Party, SSN, Address, Diagnosis, etc.)_____

[ ] Test(s) Requested _____

[ ] Correct Spelling of Name _____

[ ] Name on Specimen _____ [ ] Name on Requisition _____

[ ] Source _____

[ ] Date and Time of collection _____

[ ] Other _____

Specimen Rejection

[ ] Reason

[ ] Specimen to be recollected

[ ] Requested by _____ Date and Time _____

Mislabeled / Unlabeled Specimen

[ ] Mislabeled
Specimen labeled as: _____ Specimen actually Collected from _____

Date of birth _____

[ ] Unlabeled specimen
Patient Name _____ Date of birth _____

Accountability
I attest that the specimen sent to the laboratory was collected from the above patient.

_____   _____
Print Name   Job Title

_____   _____
Signature   Date

Figure 12-10 A form used to document variance in quality care.

assessment forms used to identify problems and document corrective actions. These forms may reveal problems with specimen collection and handling, testing procedures, equipment that affects patient safety, and the reporting of laboratory test results. Laboratory managers and QAPI committees review these forms and implement changes to processes to eliminate particular problematic patterns. Documentation of problems is never meant to be used as a punitive measure but rather to identify areas where improvements need to be made.

A **corrective action** is an activity that helps eliminate the cause of an error or undesirable situation. Examples of corrective actions include turning up the setting on a refrigerator that is too cold, discarding outdated reagents, and calling the manufacturer to correct an instrument problem. An example of corrective action in phlebotomy is re-collecting blood from a patient whose specimen produced invalid results or was clotted, hemolyzed, or insufficient. A **preventive action** is an activity that helps ensure that a problem does not occur or does not occur again. An example is the modification of a technique, such as counting the number of tube inversions during specimen mixing to prevent clotting of anticoagulated specimens. Another form of preventive action is employee **training**, providing staff with the knowledge to perform their job correctly and accurately. Part of the training process may include observation of an employee by a supervisor to determine the level of competence the employee has in performing a procedure.

QAPI committees summarize their findings in monthly, quarterly, and yearly reports or as requested by their healthcare facility. Figure 12-11 is an example of a form that may be used by QAPI committees to document progress concerning the number of rejected phlebotomy blood collections.

Competency and Proficiency

Competency assessment is a method of documenting an employee's ability to perform assigned tasks correctly. These tasks can include any step in the laboratory testing process, from patient identification all the way through to the reporting of test results (pre-examination, examination, and post-examination processes). Competency assessment documents are kept in employee files and may reveal the need for additional training. Also, documentation of individual competency is often required of laboratories during institutional or laboratory-specific inspections.

Proficiency testing (PT) is a means of evaluating the performance of a laboratory and its personnel in comparison with that of other, similar laboratories. External agencies, such as the College of American Pathologists (CAP), Department of Public Health (DPH), and Centers for Disease Control and Prevention (CDC), provide samples to be tested, such as cell identification, chemistry analysis, or other routine and specialized tests a lab may perform. Laboratories perform the required tests and return the results to the agency. An analysis of the results is given to the laboratory, along with suggestions for improving performance if the results are out of range. Laboratory inspectors require documentation of proficiency testing, along with documentation of corrective actions taken if performance deficiencies are identified. Continued errors on proficiency testing may result in a laboratory no longer being able to provide the affected test or service.

LABORATORY QUALITY ASSESSMENT AND PERFORMANCE IMPROVEMENT FORM

[ ] Initial Assessment   [ ] Scheduled Study   [ ] Unscheduled Study   [ ] Mandatory Report

| Indicator Description | | | | Specimen Rejections | | | | | | | | |

I. RESULTS

Quarter	1ST			2ND			3RD			4TH		
Month	Jan	Feb	Mar	Apr	May	Jun	Jul	Aug	Sep	Oct	Nov	Dec
TOTAL												
Mislabeled												
Hemolyzed												
Clotted												
QNS												
Contaminated												

BENCHMARK / GOAL:

Less than 1 mislabeled specimen per month; less than 5 specimen rejections in all other categories

II. ATTACH GRAPHED DATA

III. INDICATOR DEFINITION

Numerator: number of rejected blood specimens	Denominator: total number of blood specimens processed.
Exclusions if any:	Exclusions if any:

IV. RESULT SUMMARY   V. WAS GOAL MET? [ ] YES   [ ] NO

V. PLAN OF ACTION

REVIEWED BY: _____   _____

Figure 12-11 Reports such as this one are generated by **QAPI** committees to monitor progress with a particular measure of quality.

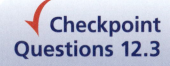 **Checkpoint Questions 12.3**

1. How does a corrective action differ from a preventive action?
2. Explain the purpose of filling out a variance form when errors in phlebotomy procedures occur.

Chapter Summary

Learning Outcome	Key Concepts/Examples	Related NAACLS Competency
12.1 Identify policies and procedures used in phlebotomy and in the clinical laboratory to assure quality in obtaining blood specimens. Pages 330–339.	• Systems exist for monitoring the quality of laboratory procedures, including blood collection. • Quality assurance processes include assessment and evaluation of all steps in a procedure. • Quality control is the activity that ensures specific steps in a procedure meet performance standards.	8.00, 8.1, 8.2
12.2 Carry out documentation of quality control. Pages 339–342.	Accurate documentation of all quality assurance and quality control activities is essential for monitoring quality.	8.00, 8.1, 8.2
12.3 Identify corrective actions for failures of quality control. Pages 243–346.	Quality assessment and process improvement (QAPI) provides a system for error detection and correction to ensure patient safety and satisfaction, valid test results, and accurate reporting of results.	8.00, 8.1, 8.2

Chapter Review

A: Labeling

For the following form, indicate what is recorded in each numbered section.

QUALITY ASSESSMENT: OCCURRENCE OF VARIANCE

(1) _____

    Patient name   Medical record #   Date

    Patient location   Form completed by

(2) _____

    Specimen accession #   Specimen type   Tests affected

(3) Complaint: [ ] Patient Issue   [ ] Safety Issue   [ ] Armband Issue   [ ] Employee Issue

(4)

Pre-examination-Specimen Related   [ ] Laboratory collect   [ ] Nurse collect

[ ] Clotted   [ ] Mislabeled   [ ] Wrong patient
[ ] Hemolyzed   [ ] Missing specimen   [ ] Wrong specimen type
[ ] Insufficient specimen   [ ] Missed test / wrong order   [ ] Wrong time collected

(5)

Examination Results Questionable   [ ] Laboratory collect   [ ] Nurse collect
[ ] Delta check   [ ] Specimen integrity issue   [ ] Other concern _____

(6)

Post-Examination Results Invalid   [ ] Laboratory collect   [ ] Nurse collect
[ ] Reported on wrong patient   [ ] Erroneous results reported   [ ] Other _____

(7) Licensed caregiver notified _____ Date and time _____
    Investigation Summary

_____

(8)

Severity   [ ] Caused healthcare provider to take wrong action   [ ] Caused delay in patient care

(9)   [ ] Training issue   [ ] Non-compliance issue   [ ] Other

(10)

Follow-up
[ ] Discussed variance with employee
[ ] Reviewed SOP with employee   Supervisor _____ Date _____
[ ] Modified procedure
[ ] Re-training scheduled   Employee _____ Date _____
[ ] Other _____

---

1. [LO 12.3] _____

2. [LO 12.3] _____

3. [LO 12.3] _____

4. [LO 12.3] _____

5. [LO 12.3] _____

6. [LO 12.3] _____

7. [LO 12.3] _____

8. [LO 12.3] _____

9. [LO 12.3] _____

10. [LO 12.3] _____

B: Matching

Match these terms with their definitions.

____11. [LO 12.3] audit

____12. [LO 12.3] competency assessment

____13. [LO 12.3] corrective action

____14. [LO 12.3] preventive action

____15. [LO 12.3] process improvement

____16. [LO 12.3] proficiency testing

____17. [LO 12.1] quality assurance

____18. [LO 12.2] quality control

____19. [LO 12.2] random errors

____20. [LO 12.2] systematic errors

____21. [LO 12.3] training

a. examining process functionality

b. ensuring acceptability of a specific procedural step

c. fixing problems that have occurred

d. ensuring that errors do not reoccur

e. educating employees

f. testing and documenting an employee's ability to perform tasks correctly

g. external agency evaluation of a testing procedure or process

h. examination of records

i. making processes and procedures better

j. can cause a shift or trend in test results

k. have no predictable pattern

C: Fill in the Blank

Write in the word(s) to complete the statement or answer the question.

22. [LO 12.1] The terms quality _____ and quality _____ are often used interchangeably.

23. [LO 12.1] A(n) _____ is the procedure performed on a patient.

24. [LO 12.1] How close a test result is to being correct is its _____.

25. [LO 12.1] Rules of practice are commonly called _____.

26. [LO 12.3] _____ is the examination of a process or procedure for acceptability of outcomes.

27. [LO 12.1] A laboratory procedure manual contains the _____ for every test performed in the laboratory.

28. [LO 12.1] Reliable test results are both _____ and _____.

29. [LO 12.1] _____ is the procedure used to check and adjust settings on instruments.

30. [LO 12.2] Serum that is specially prepared for use in testing the reliability of instruments is a(n) _____.

31. [LO 12.2] A graph that shows if control results are within acceptable limits is a(n) _____.

32. [LO 12.2] A jump in the values of control results is a(n) _____, whereas a gradual change in one direction is a(n) _____.

D: Sequencing

Place the links of quality performance in their order of occurrence for the laboratory testing process.

33. [LO 12.1] _____ Analyze the results.

34. [LO 12.1] _____ Collect the specimen.

35. [LO 12.1] _____ Identify the patient.

36. [LO 12.1] _____ Interpret the physician's orders.

37. [LO 12.1] _____ Label the specimen.

38. [LO 12.1] _____ Prepare the lab requisition.

39. [LO 12.1] _____ Process the specimen.

40. [LO 12.1] _____ Report the results.

41. [LO 12.1] _____ Transport the specimen.

E: Case Study/Critical Thinking

42. [LO 12.1] You are about to perform a venipuncture procedure. Upon examining the expiration dates on the evacuated tubes, you notice that the EDTA tube has been expired for 2 months. What is your course of action? How is this action part of quality assurance? What would be the consequences if you had not checked the expiration dates?

43. [LO 12.2] You are performing a routine quality control check on the glucometer machine prior to using it. The machine function check is fine with the low control check, and the high control check reading is 90. The machine you are using has a high control value of 110 mg/dL with an acceptable range of 105–115 mg/dL and a low control value of 75 mg/dL with an acceptable range of 70–80 mg/dL. Determine what actions, if any, are required.

44. [LO 12.3] As an experienced phlebotomist, you have been asked to serve on the laboratory's QAPI committee. What may be some of your responsibilities as a member of this committee?

45. [LO 12.3] A phlebotomy supervisor has received a complaint that the turnaround times for STAT tests ordered by the emergency department are too long. The complaint was communicated through the laboratory manager, who was informed by laboratory personnel that the specimens were not delivered to them for over 30 minutes after the collection time on the tubes. What should be put in place and what are some possible scenarios for this variance in quality care?

F: Exam Prep

Choose the best answer for each question.

46. [LO 12.1] Surveying patient satisfaction with the healthcare delivery system at a facility is an example of

    a. quality assurance.

    b. quality control.

    c. quality documentation.

    d. quality management.

47. [LO 12.1] Which event will most likely negatively affect patient satisfaction with the laboratory?

    a. One attempt was needed to obtain a blood specimen.

    b. No hematoma formed after the venipuncture procedure.

    c. The patient's breakfast was delayed because the phlebotomist was late in arriving to collect the fasting specimen.

    d. The phlebotomist wore a lab coat during the procedure.

48. [LO 12.1] A system for evaluating the delivery of a healthcare service, such as specimen collection, is

    a. quality assurance.

    b. quality control.

    c. quality documentation.

    d. quality management.

49. [LO 12.1] An ongoing set of activities used to monitor turnaround times is an example of

    a. quality assurance.

    b. quality control.

    c. quality documentation.

    d. quality management

50. [LO 12.1] The focus of quality assurance is on processes that involve all of these EXCEPT

    a. requisitioning of tests.

    b. integrity of the specimen.

    c. performance on lab inspections.

    d. laboratory staff salaries.

51. [LO 12.1] Achieving complete correctness or acceptable measures as close as possible to the true value is known as

    a. accuracy.

    b. calibration.

    c. process.

    d. none of the above.

52. [LO 12.1] Liquid or freeze-dried sera that have a known value and have been prepared and tested by the manufacturer are

    a. analytes.

    b. control materials.

    c. reagents.

    d. testing agents.

53. [LO 12.1] When should quality assurance activities be in place?

    a. The pre-evaluation phase of testing

    b. The evaluation phase of testing

    c. The post-evaluation phase of testing

    d. All of these

54. [LO 12.1] Rules of practice for performing a procedure are referred to as

    a. standards.

    b. codes of ethics.

    c. parameters.

    d. none of these.

55. [LO 12.1] Determining the turnaround time for STAT tests ordered for patients in the emergency department is a function of

    a. quality assurance.

    b. quality control.

    c. competency assessment.

    d. proficiency testing.

56. [LO 12.1] Acceptable limits for quality control results are referred to as

    a. standards.

    b. variances.

    c. parameters.

    d. none of these.

57. [LO 12.1] Deviations from the standard operating procedure are referred to as

   a. standards.

   b. variances.

   c. parameters.

   d. none of these.

58. [LO 12.1] An individual's ability to perform a procedure, such as blood collection, is documented in the

   a. quality assessment form.

   b. standard operating procedures.

   c. competency assessment form.

   d. proficiency testing materials.

59. [LO 12.2] Recording the temperatures of the refrigerators used to store blood for testing is an activity of

   a. quality assurance.

   b. quality control.

   c. competency assessment.

   d. proficiency testing.

60. [LO 12.3] Reviewing the temperature logs for variances in blood storage temperatures is an activity of

   a. quality assessment and process improvement.

   b. quality control.

   c. competency assessment.

   d. proficiency testing.

61. [LO 12.3] Questioning the accuracy of test results may occur if

   a. the results are significantly different than the last time the test was performed on the same patient.

   b. the results are consistent with the medical provider's diagnosis or expectations.

   c. the results are consistent with the patient's clinical symptoms.

   d. all of these apply.

62. [LO 12.2] Quality control activities include recording temperatures for *(Choose all that apply)*

   a. freezers.

   b. incubators.

   c. refrigerators.

   d. patients.

63. [LO 12.3] Problems with any step in a process may be discovered when reviewing *(Choose all that apply)*

   a. incident report forms.

   b. competency assessments.

   c. proficiency testing results.

   d. continuing education records.

64. [LO 12.3] Educating employees about the use of a new piece of phlebotomy equipment is an example of

   a. audit and evaluation.

   b. corrective action.

   c. competency assessment.

   d. training.

65. [LO 12.3] Developing and implementing ways to make processes and procedures better is the purpose of

   a. audit and evaluation.

   b. corrective action.

   c. preventive action.

   d. process improvement.

connect

Enhance your learning by completing these exercises and more at connect.mheducation.com

References

Clinical and Laboratory Standards Institute. (2011). *Quality management system: A model for laboratory services; Approved guidelines.* (4th ed.). GP26-A4. Wayne, PA. CLSI.

Cox, P., & Wilken, D. (2011). *Palko's medical laboratory procedures* (3rd ed.). New York, McGraw-Hill.

Harmening, D. (2007). *Laboratory management principles and processes* (2nd ed.). St. Petersburg, FL. D. H. Publishing & Consulting.

U.S. Department of Health & Human Services. (2011). *Hospital compare.* Retrieved August 8, 2011, from www.hospitalcompare.hhs.gov/

Kurec, A. S., Schofield, S., & Walters, M. C. [Eds]. (2000). *The CLMA guide to managing a clinical laboratory* (3rd ed.). Wayne, PA. Clinical Laboratory Management Association.

National Accrediting Agency for Clinical Laboratory Sciences. (2010). *NAACLS entry-level phlebotomist competencies.* Rosemont, IL. NAACLS.

NAME: _____ DATE: _____

COMPETENCY CHECKLIST: TEMPERATURE QUALITY CONTROL

Procedure Steps	Practice			Performed		
	1	2	3	Yes	No	Master
Preprocedure						
1. Locates the appropriate temperature log for the instrument to be checked.						
Procedure						
2. Correctly reads the minimum temperature.						
3. Correctly reads the maximum temperature.						
4. Correctly records temperatures on the temperature log.						
5. Compares temperatures with acceptable range.						
6. Applies corrective action (according to facility policy).						
7. Correctly documents corrective action.						
8. Properly signs and dates the temperature log.						
Postprocedure						
9. Returns thermometer and temperature log to the correct location.						

COMMENTS: _____

_____

_____

_____

SIGNED

EVALUATOR: _____

STUDENT: _____

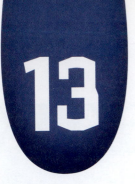

13

Waived Testing and Collection of Non-Blood Specimens

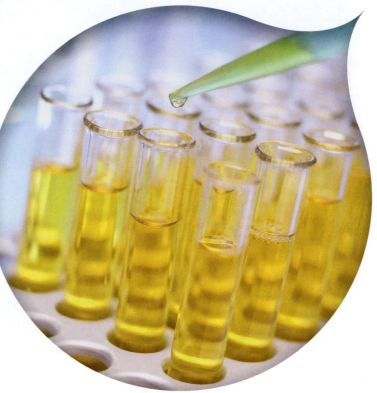

Learning Outcomes

13.1 Explain how to collect various non-blood specimens.

13.2 Differentiate among waived tests, moderately complex tests, and high complexity testing.

13.3 Describe procedures for various waived and point-of-care tests that a phlebotomist may be asked to perform, including quality controls.

Related NAACLS Competencies

4.00 Demonstrate understanding of the importance of specimen collection in the overall patient care system.

4.2 Describe the types of patient specimens that are analyzed in the clinical laboratory and the phlebotomist's role in collecting and/or transporting these specimens to the laboratory.

4.3 Define the phlebotomist's role in collecting and/or transporting these specimens to the laboratory.

4.5 Explain the importance of timed, fasting, and stat specimens, as related to specimen integrity and patient care.

Introduction

At some facilities, the phlebotomist's role may include collecting specimens other than blood, instructing patients in the collection of certain specimens, and performing simple laboratory tests. This chapter presents collection procedures for non-blood specimens, an overview of laboratory test classification, as well as procedures for other tests phlebotomists may be asked to perform.

13.1 Collection of Non-Blood Specimens

Although phlebotomists primarily collect blood specimens, they may also be required to collect non-blood specimens or to instruct patients on how to collect these specimens. Non-blood specimens include throat swabs, sputum specimens, stool specimens, semen specimens, and urine specimens.

Sterile swabs (Figure 13-1) are used for collection of many types of non-blood specimens requiring a culture or rapid methods of detecting the presence of microorganisms. Swabs are comprised of synthetic materials such as

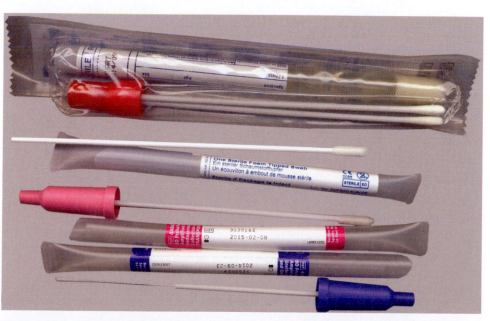

Figure 13-1   Disposable sterile swabs come in sterile plastic containers that have a transport medium to help keep microorganisms viable (alive).

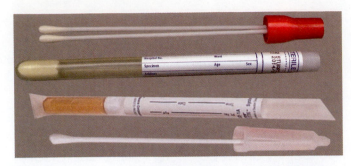

Figure 13-2 Swabs for throat culture may be single swabs or double swabs for collecting specimens used to run both a culture and rapid testing at the same time.

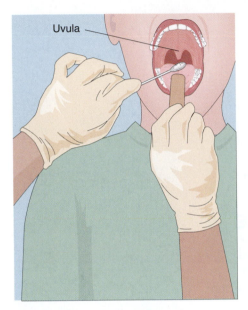

Uvula

Figure 13-3 Collecting and processing a throat culture. Swab the throat area and any white patches on the tonsils. Do not touch the uvula.

calcium alginate, Dacron, or rayon. Cotton swabs are not used. The type of swab used varies depending on the specific area being cultured. Always refer to your facility's protocol when selecting swabs for specimen collection. Before beginning any procedure, check the expiration dates on the swab container. An expired swab may no longer be sterile or the transport medium present with some swabs may no longer be effective.

Throat Swabs

Throat swabs are samples taken from the back of the throat. These samples are collected for use in screening tests for Group A *Streptococcus*, the microorganism that causes strep throat. In addition, throat swabs are used for growing cultures of throat microorganisms to identify other pathogens that may be present, such as *Haemophilus influenzae* and *Neisseria gonorrhoeae*.

Sterile swabs with spongelike tips made of Dacron or calcium alginate are used for collecting throat culture specimens (see Figure 13-2). Most culture swabs have an ampule of growth medium located at the bottom of the swab container. This ampule must be crushed to release the medium after the swab has been reinserted into the container. Keeping the swab in contact with the medium ensures that any microorganisms present remain viable (alive). Do not use cotton-tipped swabs for throat cultures as they may inhibit bacterial growth.

Throat Swab Collection Procedure

Ensure that the room in which throat swab collection will occur has sufficient lighting and all equipment needed. Use the competency checklist *Throat Swab Collection* at the end of this chapter to review and practice the procedure.

Competency Check 13-1

Throat Swab Collection
1. Identify the patient.
2. Explain the procedure. Determine if the patient has used an antiseptic mouthwash to gargle recently or is taking antibiotics. These actions could affect the results of the test.
3. Put on PPE including gloves, mask, and eye protection.
4. Obtain a tongue depressor.
5. Remove the sterile swab from its container (do not set it down).
6. Have the patient tilt his or her head back and stick out the tongue.
7. Hold the tongue down with the tongue depressor.
8. Rub the back of the throat and each tonsil with the swab using a rolling action (see Figure 13-3). To minimize the gag reflex, avoid touching the uvula (the tissue that hangs between the oral cavity and the throat). Do not touch the sides of the mouth or teeth because these contain bacteria normally present and can make interpreting culture results confusing.
9. Withdraw the swab, then the tongue depressor.

10. Place the swab back into its sterile container and crush the media ampule, if applicable.

11. Discard the tongue depressor.

12. While the patient is still present, label the specimen with all required patient and collection information, which is the same as for blood specimens.

13. Remove your PPE and wash your hands.

14. Thank the patient.

The Gag Reflex

Some patients may be afraid of having a gag reflex during a throat swab collection. To help prevent this reaction, be sure to instruct patients to breathe through their nose. Breathing through the nose will help minimize movement of the patient's uvula and make it easier for you to collect the specimen quickly.

Patient Education & Communication

Two Is Better Than One

Often, two throat swabs must be collected. One is used for the strep screen test and the other is sent to the microbiology laboratory for throat culture. Some throat swabs come in pairs and should be used together to collect the specimen. If swabs are separate, it is still a good idea to use two at the same time to eliminate having to do the procedure twice.

Critical Thinking

Throat Swabs and PPEs

Gloves must always be worn when performing procedures on patients. Wearing a mask and eye protection when collecting throat cultures is desirable since the patient may cough. Wearing all appropriate PPE is especially important to prevent the spread of pathogens.

Safety & Infection Control

Nasal Swabs

Nasal swabs are samples taken from the nares (the cavity just inside the nasal opening). These samples are collected for the detection of microorganisms such as *Staphylococcus aureus (S. aureus)*. As discussed in the chapter *Infection Control and Safety*, *S. aureus*'s antibiotic-resistant strain (MRSA) is the most common cause of skin and soft tissue infection in both the healthcare and community settings.

Similar to throat culture swabs, nasal swabs have an applicator stick and a rayon tip. The swab container has a transport medium into which the swab applicator is placed after sampling. Microorganisms in the sample are kept moist in the transport medium. Use the competency checklist *Nasal Swab Collection* at the end of this chapter to review and practice the procedure.

Nasal Swab Collection

1. Identify the patient.

2. Explain the procedure.

3. Put on PPE including gloves, mask, and eye protection.

4. Remove swab from its container (do not set it down).

5. While seated, have the patient tilt his or her head back. Support the back of the head by placing the hand without the swab against the back of the patient's head. Patients have a tendency to pull away during this procedure.

6. Insert the swab approximately 2 cm (about ¾ inch) into a naris. See Figure 13-4.

7. Rotate the swab against the anterior nasal mucosa for 3 seconds.

8. Using the same swab, repeat for other naris.

9. Place the swab back into the transport tube and crush the media ampule, if applicable.

10. Before leaving the patient, label the specimen with all required patient and collection information.

11. Remove PPE and wash your hands.

12. Thank the patient.

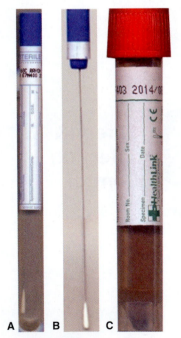

Figure 13-5
Nasopharyngeal swab (A) in original sterile container and (B) removed from sterile container to show Dacron-tipped thin wire. Have a container of (C) viral transport medium available before beginning the nasopharyngeal swab collection procedure.

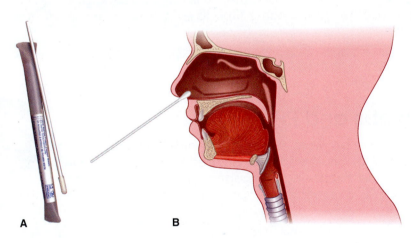

Figure 13-4 (A) A nasal swab is used to collect a specimen (B) from the nares.

Nasopharyngeal Swabs

Nasopharyngeal swabs are samples taken from the nasopharynx (the upper part of the throat behind the nose). These samples are collected for the detection of influenza and respiratory virus infections. Nasopharyngeal specimens are collected using only Dacron-tipped swabs on a very thin wire (Figure 13-5A and B). Cotton or calcium alginate swabs are not acceptable because they may introduce residues into the transport medium and cause false results, especially when molecular testing is performed. Dry swabs are not acceptable for testing. Nasopharyngeal swabs must be kept moist in a special viral transport medium (Figure 13-5C). Use the competency checklist *Nasopharyngeal Swab Collection* at the end of this chapter to review and practice the procedure.

Competency Check 13-3

Nasopharyngeal Swab Collection

1. Identify the patient.

2. Explain the procedure.

3. Put on PPE including gloves, mask, and eye protection.

4. Obtain nasopharyngeal swab, transport medium, and scissors.

5. Remove swab from its container (do not set it down).

6. While seated, have the patient tilt his or her head back. Support the back of the head by placing your hand (not holding the swab) against the back of the patient's head. Patients have a tendency to pull away during this procedure.

7. Insert swab into one nostril straight back (not upwards) and continue along the floor of the nasal passage for several centimeters until reaching the nasopharynx (you will feel a resistance). See Figure 13-6. Do not force the swab if obstruction is encountered before reaching the nasopharynx. Remove the swab and try the other side.

8. Rotate the swab gently for 5–10 seconds to loosen cells from the epithelial lining.

9. Remove swab, open the viral transport medium, and immediately place it into the container. Use scissors to cut the wire enough below the swab handle to fit the transport medium container. Reattach the cap securely. See Figure 13-7.

10. Before leaving the patient, label the specimen with all required patient and collection information.

11. Remove PPE and wash your hands.

12. Thank the patient.

13. Transport to the laboratory immediately. If immediate transport is not possible, the specimen must be refrigerated and kept refrigerated during transport.

Nasal Discharge

Critical Thinking

A patient needing collection of a nasal swab or nasopharyngeal swab may have nasal discharge. Provide the patient with a non-scented tissue and ask him/her to attempt to clear the discharge by "blowing the nose" into the tissue. Children may need assistance with this. Do not try to clear the nasal discharge with swabs. Attempting to do so might be excessively traumatic, especially for children.

Other Swabs

Other types of swabs are used for collection of specimens that the phlebotomist normally does not collect. However, you may be asked to provide a nursing unit with a swab from laboratory stock or handle the specimen after collection. Specimens such as wound cultures, vaginal cultures, and urethral cultures require specific swabs and may also have special transport and handling requirements. Follow the protocols at your facility and your scope of practice.

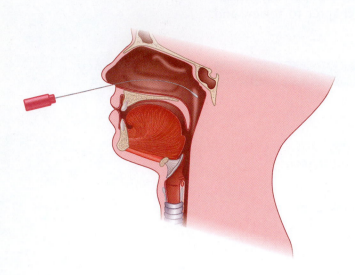

Figure 13-6 A nasopharyngeal swab is used to collect specimens from the nasopharynx.

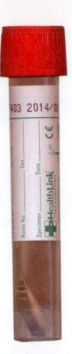

Figure 13-7 Nasopharyngeal swab in viral transport medium. Remember to cut off the swab handle before capping the container.

Sputum Specimens

Sputum is mucus that collects in the air passages of the respiratory system. Sputum specimens are used in diagnosing various disorders of the respiratory tract as well as for sputum culture to identify pathogenic microorganisms. Have patients rinse their mouth with water before collecting the specimen. This will minimize contamination by bacteria. Then instruct patients to **expectorate** (generate a cough from deep within the lungs and bronchi) sputum and spit it into a sterile container. Label the container with patient and collection information and then deliver it to the microbiology laboratory for testing. The laboratory will examine the sample for squamous epithelial cells (SECs) and white blood cells (WBCs) to determine whether the specimen is acceptable. If the specimen is to be sent to a reference laboratory, follow the specific preservation and transport requirements for that facility.

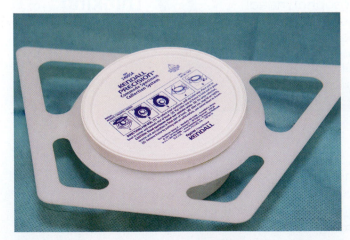

Figure 13-8 Some stool specimen containers are designed to fit over toilet seat openings.

Stool Specimens

Stool specimens are used in diagnosing various disorders of the digestive tract. Examples of tests include stool culture, fecal fat analysis, fecal hemoglobin screening, and ova and parasite identification. The phlebotomist may need to instruct patients on how to collect this specimen. Containers may be provided as part of a collection kit, but these need to be clean, dry, sealable, and leakproof. Container type and size depend on the ordered tests (see Figure 13-8). In addition, patients may need to be instructed in how to transfer a specimen to another container.

Stool specimens for the detection of pathogenic microorganisms must be transferred immediately to special vials containing a medium to preserve

Stool Collection

The phlebotomist must instruct the patient not to contaminate the stool specimen with urine or water. Urine can destroy some parasites, and toilet water often contains strong cleaners that interfere with laboratory testing. If a special diet is prescribed, not adhering to it can affect the stool sample and alter laboratory test results. Enemas or barium sulfate for radiologic examinations can also affect stool samples and laboratory tests by altering the morphology of parasites or by interfering with the stain used for identifying parasites. If any of these conditions are present, be sure to note it in the documentation that accompanies the specimen to the lab. Recording this additional information is critical for correct interpretation of stool specimen laboratory test results.

them (Figure 13-9C). Specimens for immunochemical fecal occult blood may also need to be transferred by the patient, a nurse, or the laboratory staff to special vials used for this test (Figure 13-10). The specimen and any samples taken from it must be labeled with all patient and specimen collection information.

Semen Specimens

Semen is produced by males and contains sperm and some substances necessary for fertilization to occur, such as fructose and acids. Semen may be analyzed to evaluate infertility problems or to verify that a vasectomy is

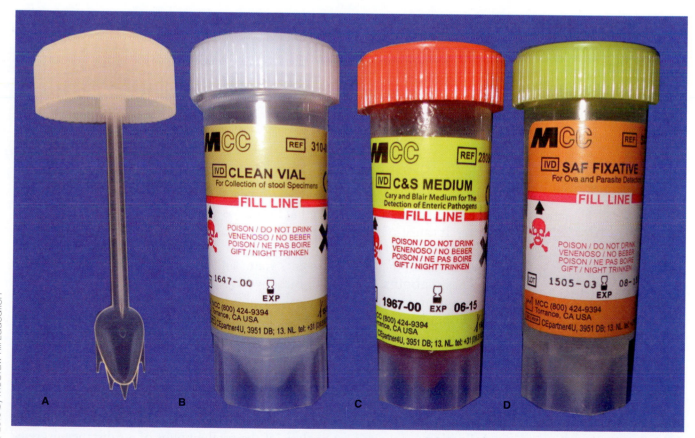

Figure 13-9 (A) A "scoop" attached to each container lid is used to sample a portion of the stool specimen and place it directly into the appropriate container: (B) clean vial for various tests, (C) vial with special medium to preserve bacteria for culture and microbial sensitivity testing, and (D) vial with special fixative for detecting ova and parasites.

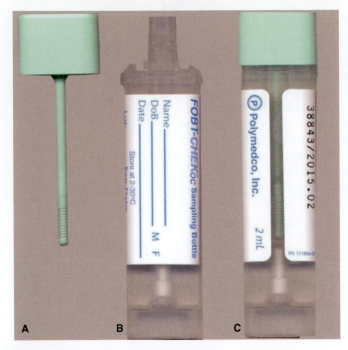

Figure 13-10 Stool samples for some brands of immunochemical fecal occult blood tests (iFOBT) are collected by "poking" the (A) applicator stick, which is attached to the container cap, into the stool specimen and then inserting it into (B) a special container. (C) A properly filled and capped iFOBT container.

successful. A vasectomy is a surgical procedure done as a method of male birth control. The vas deferens is clipped, preventing sperm from being released into semen. A semen specimen is checked for sperm after this procedure. Although the patient receives written instructions for providing a semen specimen, phlebotomists may be required to instruct patients in this process.

Semen for testing is best obtained by masturbation and must include the entire ejaculate. The most accurate results are obtained on specimens collected after a 48- to 72-hour **continence** (abstinence from sexual activity). Most facilities provide patients with a private, comfortable room in which to collect the specimen to allow for quick delivery to the laboratory. If the specimen is collected at home or at a facility that is not close to the laboratory, it should be kept near body temperature and delivered within 30 minutes of collection, or as soon as possible. Semen analysis test results can be affected by delayed delivery.

Specimen collection containers for semen should be clean, wide-mouthed glass or plastic jars with secure lids. Specimens must be labeled with all patient and collection information.

Patient Education & Communication

Semen Collection

Patients should be informed not to use a condom for semen collection, as many condoms contain spermicidal (sperm-killing) compounds. They may also contain lubricants that can interfere with laboratory tests.

Urine Specimens

Urine is a convenient body fluid to collect and can be used for many types of laboratory analysis, such as screening for glucose, drugs, alcohol, and general well-being. It can also be used to measure the total amount of substances excreted in a 24-hour period, such as urine protein. Additionally, urine specimens can be used to assess the urinary system's status and to screen for metabolic diseases such as **diabetes mellitus** (a carbohydrate metabolism disorder), amino acid overflow, and proteinuria (the leakage of glucose, amino acids, and protein into the urine). Table 13-1 summarizes the types of urine specimen collection.

A **first morning void** is the best specimen for routine testing and evaluation of general well-being because it is the most concentrated, containing the highest levels of the chemicals present in the urine. However, a specimen collected at a *random* time may be acceptable. Another type of specimen is the **clean-catch midstream specimen,** which is used for urine culture collection. It requires skin cleansing and collection of the mid-portion of the urine stream. A **24-hour collection** is required for analysis of the total amount of a substance excreted in a day. Nursing staff may collect urine from a **catheter** (tube inserted into the bladder), or a physician may perform a **suprapubic puncture** or **aspirate** (rarely performed insertion of a needle directly into the bladder). Catheterization

TABLE 13-1 Types of Urine Specimen Collection

First morning void	Best specimen to use for general health assessment, hormone levels such as hCG testing, and other chemicals such as glucose and protein
Random void	Specimen of convenience; acceptable for routine assessment
Clean-catch midstream	Required for urine culture specimens
24-hour collection	Used for quantitation of proteins and other substances
Legal specimens	Drug screening to be used in a court of law
Catheterization	Used for urine collection on patients unable to void
Suprapubic puncture	Performed by physicians to collect urine directly from the bladder

and suprapubic puncture collections may be used to collect urine on patients who cannot void urine normally. Urine may also be collected from a catheter if a sterile specimen is needed for culture or to determine if blood cells are present as a result of bleeding into the kidneys or bladder instead of from urethral or vaginal bleeding. In addition, urine specimens may need to be collected for testing submitted as evidence in a court of law (**legal specimens**). The chain-of-custody requirements, as explained in the chapter *Blood Specimen Handling* apply to all specimens collected for legal reasons, including urine.

If the urine is not tested within 1 hour after it has been collected, it must be refrigerated. If urine is kept at room temperature for more than 1 hour, it can alter the test results of the chemical and microscopic components. Changes that occur to urine specimens left at room temperature over time include

- changes in urine color and clarity
- bacterial growth
- increase in pH and nitrites (due to bacterial growth)
- decomposition of casts and cellular elements
- decrease in several substances, if initially present (such as glucose, bilirubin, ketones, and urobilinogen)

Depending on the policies at your facility, the urine may be sent to the laboratory in the initial container or may need to be transferred to the appropriate tube for testing. Routine urine tests are performed on specimens in the initial container (see Figure 13-11A) or those stored in urine analysis tubes, whereas urine for culture requires collection into sterile cups and may need to

Urine Collection Tubes

Phlebotomists must be aware that evacuated tubes, similar to those used for blood specimen collection, are used as urine preservative tubes. The yellow- and red-topped urine preservative tubes contain the chemicals chlorhexidine, ethyl paraben, and sodium propionate to preserve urine for testing. Care must be taken not to confuse this urine tube with similarly colored gray and red or gray and yellow blood collection tubes. The gray-topped urine culture tube contains sodium formate, sodium borate, and boric acid, which maintain the quality of the specimen for urine cultures. Care must be taken not to confuse this urine tube with gray-topped tubes containing sodium fluoride used for blood collection.

Critical Thinking

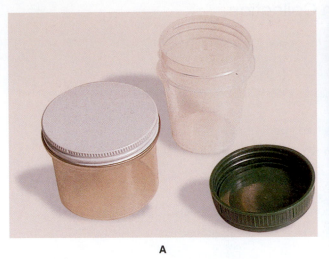 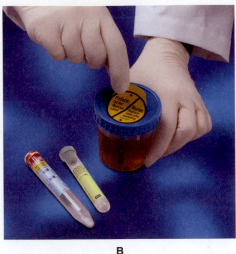

| A | B |

Figure 13-11 (A) Examples of routine urine collection cups. (B) Sterile urine collection containers may have an opening on their lids through which urine can be transferred into specialized tubes, such as a urine preservative tube (yellow- and red-topped) or a urine culture tube (gray-topped).

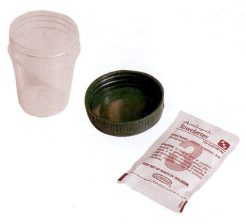

Figure 13-12 A special kit for urine collection for culture includes a sterile container and three cleansing towelettes.

be transferred to a tube containing a preservative (see Figure 13-11B).

Obtaining Urine Specimens

Random void is a urine specimen that is collected at any time of the day. However, the best urine specimen for routine testing is the first morning void, which is the most concentrated. Patients collect urine directly into a container, which should then be labeled immediately with the required information.

The clean-catch midstream procedure for collecting urine is required for urine culture specimens. Special instructions for collecting urine for culture must be explained to the patient in order to obtain a quality specimen. Urine that has been contaminated by normal flora (bacteria) of the skin may produce false results. A special sterile kit, as shown in Figure 13-12, is used during the clean-catch procedure.

The directions for obtaining a clean-catch specimen are as follows.

Competency Check 13-4

Female Clean-Catch Urine Specimen Collection

1. Instruct the patient to follow these steps to clean the perineum.

   a. Separate the skin folds (labia) and keep them separated throughout the cleaning and collection process. With one antiseptic towelette, wipe from front to back down one side of the skin folds and then discard the towelette.

   b. With a second towelette, wipe down the other side of the skin folds from front to back; discard the towelette.

   c. With a third towelette, wipe down the middle of the labia front to back and discard the towelette while keeping the skin folds open with the other hand.

2. Instruct the patient to follow these steps to obtain the specimen.

    a. Keeping the skin folds spread apart to avoid contamination, start to urinate into the toilet.

    b. Place the cup under the flow of urine after it has begun and remove the cup before it has finished. *Do not* collect the first or last part of the stream of urine. Instead, collect the urine at midstream; this is why the phrase "clean-catch midstream" is used.

3. Once the patient is finished, place the lid on the cup. Ideally, the cup should be about three-fourths full.

4. Label the specimen (name, date of collection). Remember, your facility might require other identification on the specimen, so check with your supervisor.

Infant Specimens

Life Span Considerations

Special equipment is used when collecting urine from an infant or a small child (see Figure 13-13). This equipment consists of a sterile plastic bag that has an opening to fit around genitalia and is secured with an adhesive backing. The diaper is placed over the bag during collection. Once collected, the specimen may be transferred to a urine collection cup or tube. However, if the specimen is for urine culture, it may be better to leave it in the collection bag and transport it to the laboratory immediately. Always use the established procedure at your facility.

Competency Check 13-5

Male Clean-Catch Urine Specimen Collection

1. Instruct the patient to follow these steps to clean the penis.

    a. Use an antiseptic towelette to clean the head of the penis.

    b. Take a second towelette and wipe across the head of the penis. If uncircumcised, retract the foreskin before cleaning the penis.

2. Instruct the patient to follow these steps to obtain the specimen.

    a. If uncircumcised, keep the foreskin retracted and urinate into the toilet. Place the cup under the flow of urine after it has begun and remove the cup before it has finished. Do not collect the first or last part of the stream of urine. Instead, collect the urine at midstream.

3. Once the patient is finished, place the lid on the cup. Ideally, the cup should be about three-fourths full.

4. Label the specimen (name, date of collection). Remember, your facility might require other identification on the specimen, so check with your supervisor or procedure manual for further instructions.

24-Hour Urine Collection

A 24-hour collection of urine is required to measure the total amount of substances, such as protein, sodium, and hormones, that are excreted in the urine over a 24-hour time period. When tests such as total aldosterone, cortisol, creatinine, potassium, protein, sodium, or urea nitrogen are ordered, a phlebotomist may need to prepare specimen collection containers (see Figure 13-14) and instruct patients in the correct method of collecting the 24-hour specimen. Not all 24-urine collections require preservatives, but for those that do, care must be taken when adding preservatives to containers. Wear appropriate PPE (gloves, goggles or face shield, rubber apron) and use a chemical fume hood, as described

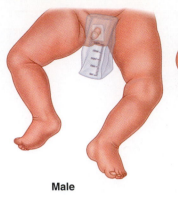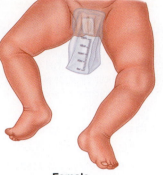

Male   **Female**

Figure 13-13 A pediatric collection unit consists of a clear, sterile plastic bag with adhesive for attaching to the child.

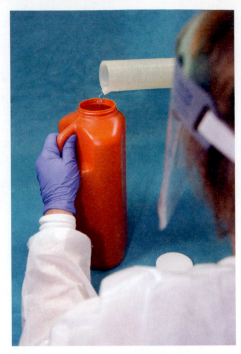

Figure 13-14 A container for 24-hour urine collection may require the addition of a preservative.

in the chapter *Infection Control and Safety.* Preservatives may include acids or chloroform. Add acids slowly, and if diluting with water is required, add the acid to the water. The container must have a lid that closes tightly and should be labeled with caution information. Also note that 24-hour urine specimens may require refrigeration or need to be placed on ice during the time of collection.

Patient Education & Communication

Patient Safety and 24-Hour Urine Collection

Patients should be made aware of the hazardous chemicals used as urine preservatives in 24-hour urine collection containers. Make sure patients understand the risks associated with these chemicals and that they should add urine to the container slowly, close the container, and mix gently but thoroughly. Patients must also be informed about the need to refrigerate the container, if required.

The 24-hour urine collection procedure begins and ends with an empty bladder. Follow the directions in Competency Check 13-6 to properly obtain this type of specimen.

Competency Check 13-6

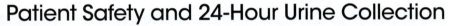

Twenty-Four-Hour Urine Specimen Collection
1. Upon waking the morning of the collection, empty the bladder. Do not collect this urine. Record the time at which this urination occurs.
2. Collect all urine voided throughout the next 24 hours directly into the preservative container or into a urine collection cup and add to the container.
3. Use caution when adding the urine to the container because it contains an acid that may splash.
4. Be sure to add all urine into the container; do not spill; do not contaminate the inside of the container.
5. Refrigerate the container, or keep it on ice, for the entire time of collection.
6. On the second morning, at exactly the same time as the previous day, collect a final void and add it to the container. Record this time.
7. Keep the specimen refrigerated or on ice, if necessary, until transported to the laboratory.

Urine Specimens as Legal Specimens

Legal specimens require chain-of-custody procedures, as discussed in the chapter *Blood Specimen Handling*. Specifically, urine specimens may be needed for everything from drug or alcohol testing in criminal cases or in employee physical examinations to insurance company screenings. Phlebotomists must fill out paperwork showing specific identification, who obtained and processed the specimen, the date, the location, and the signature of the patient documenting that the specimen in the container is the one that was obtained from the person identified on the label. The specimen must be placed in a specimen transfer bag that permanently seals the specimen bag until it is cut open for analysis. The seal ensures that there has been no tampering with the bag's contents prior to reaching the lab for testing.

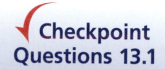

Checkpoint Questions 13.1

1. Why should the sides of the mouth NOT be touched during collection of a swab for throat culture?
2. Why is it important to instruct patients not to allow urine to contaminate a stool specimen?
3. List the tests performed on urine collected from a clean-catch midstream specimen and explain why this type of sample is the best for each test.
4. What risks should be explained to patients collecting a 24-hour urine specimen at home?

13.2 Levels of Laboratory Testing

The **Clinical Laboratory Improvement Amendments** of 1988 (**CLIA '88**) identified three levels of complexity for medical laboratory tests: waived tests, moderate complexity tests, and high complexity tests. A fourth level, provider-performed microscopy, was recognized and added to this law in 1997.

Testing Levels

High complexity tests are tests that require close attention to detail. These difficult tests have numerous steps and present challenges during the pre-examination, examination, and/or post-examination phases. Medical laboratory personnel are required to have specialized training and "substantial experience" to perform these procedures.

High complexity tests include those that require manual manipulation of highly complex equipment and **reagents** (lab test chemicals) and that require interpretation and troubleshooting skills. Manual DNA extraction procedures, intricate special staining procedures, and operation of complex analyzers that require detailed setup or operator interaction are included in this category.

Moderate complexity tests fall between waived (low complexity) and high complexity tests with respect to the difficulty of the test and the training required. Moderate complexity tests have a few procedural steps that are not highly complex but do require some formal training to perform. In some cases, medical laboratory personnel require direct supervision while performing these tests.

Moderate complexity tests include running automated instruments. These tests also require little manual manipulation of the sample or reagents, with minimal interpretation and troubleshooting skills.

Provider-performed microscopy procedures (PPMP) is a subcategory of moderate complexity testing. Healthcare providers perform these tests only for their own patients. PPMPs include the following:

- Direct wet mounts
- Potassium hydroxide (KOH) preparations
- Pinworm examinations
- Fern tests
- Post-coital qualitative
- Urine sediment examinations
- Nasal smears for granulocytes
- Fecal leukocyte examinations
- Qualitative semen evaluation

Waived tests are procedures that the Food and Drug Administration (FDA) has cleared for home use and for the laboratory that are simple to use, are easy to interpret, and produce accurate results. These tests usually do not produce false results. Other tests categorized as waived tests are those that "pose no reasonable risk of harm" if the test is performed incorrectly.

Performing waived testing does not require as much training as higher complexity tests and learning how to perform these tests can be done through on-the-job instruction. Learning to perform waived tests in an educational setting such as a phlebotomy or medical assisting training program ensures the personnel possess at least minimal knowledge about these tests along with the skills to perform them.

The following waived tests are explained later in this chapter:

- Blood glucose by glucose monitoring devices cleared by the FDA specifically for home use
- Erythrocyte sedimentation rate—nonautomated
- Fecal occult blood
- Spun microhematocrit
- Urine chemical screening
- Urine pregnancy tests—visual color comparison tests

Regulatory Compliance

All laboratories, including hospitals, physician offices, and reference laboratories, must comply with CLIA '88 and apply for certification to perform tests of varying complexity. The different levels of certification include those listed below.

- A Certificate of Accreditation (COA) is awarded to laboratories that perform moderate and/or high complexity testing that meet the standards of a private not-for-profit accreditation program. These laboratories must be surveyed every other year.
- A Certificate of Compliance (COC) is awarded to laboratories that perform moderate and/or high complexity testing after inspectors find that the laboratory is in compliance with all applicable CLIA requirements. These laboratories are required to be surveyed every other year.
- A Certificate of Registration (COR) is granted to a laboratory that has applied for either COA or COC. COR enables the laboratory to perform moderate and/or high complexity testing until it has been inspected and verified to meet all requirements for COA or COC.

- A Certificate for Provider-Performed Microscopy Procedures may be granted to laboratories at facilities where physicians, midlevel practitioners, or dentists perform only certain microscopy procedures as described earlier in the section *Testing Levels*.

- A **Certificate of Waiver** may be granted to a laboratory that only performs waived tests. Inspections are not required unless there is a complaint about the laboratory.

Laboratories performing waived tests must apply to the Department of Health and Human Services, Centers for Medicare and Medicaid Services (CMS), and be approved for a Certificate of Waiver. Waived testing is performed at various types of healthcare facilities. At inpatient facilities, the clinical laboratory professionals provide oversight for quality of testing, regulatory compliance, method validation, accuracy checks, testing procedures, staff training, and technical support to areas or units performing testing. Laboratories that function under a Certificate of Waiver must submit to random inspections and investigation, if indicated. Though waived tests are simple to perform and interpret, care must still be taken when performing them. Patient care decisions are often made based on the outcome of waived tests.

In order to help ensure quality testing procedures and reduce patient error, the **Clinical Laboratory Improvement Advisory Committee (CLIAC)** has made several recommendations for good practice in a Certificate of Waiver laboratory. These recommendations include laboratory management considerations and testing procedures before, during, and after the test.

Laboratory Management and Personnel

Facilities performing laboratory testing must designate the person who will be responsible for laboratory supervision. This is usually a physician or someone with enough laboratory experience to make decisions about testing. In addition, it is important that all laboratory personnel adhere to the established laboratory guidelines, regulations, and requirements. These include the following:

- Follow all applicable federal, state, and local regulations.
- Perform waived tests only.
- Follow the manufacturer's instructions in the package insert.
- Do not make modifications to the instructions.
- Allow random inspections by authorized agencies, such as the CMS.
- Establish a laboratory safety plan that follows OSHA guidelines.
- Have a designated area that has adequate space and conditions.
- Have enough personnel in the lab and train them appropriately.
- Have written documentation of each test performed.

The person who is performing waived testing must follow **standard operating procedures (SOP)** for each test performed. The testing personnel must pay close attention to pre-examination, examination, or post-examination steps in the testing process.

Before the Test—Pre-Examination

- Confirm written test orders.
- Establish a procedure for patient identification.
- Give patients pre-test instructions and determine whether they have followed these instructions.

- Collect specimens according to package insert instructions.
- Label specimens appropriately.
- Never use expired reagents or test kits.

During the Test—Examination

- Perform quality control testing as indicated in the package insert.
- Correct any problem discovered during quality control testing before testing patient samples.
- Establish a policy for frequency of control testing.
- Carefully follow all test-timing instructions.
- Interpret test results as instructed in product inserts.
- Record test results according to your office policy.

After the Test—Post-Examination

- Report test results to the physician in a timely manner.
- Follow package insert recommendations for follow-up or confirmatory testing.
- Follow OSHA regulations for disposing of biohazardous waste.

To ensure the quality of testing, laboratories are also required to participate in quality assurance/assessment programs for each test they perform. Quality assurance and assessment are discussed in the chapter *Quality Essentials*.

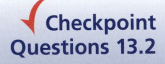

Checkpoint Questions 13.2

1. What is a Certificate of Waiver and when is it needed?
2. What are PPMP tests? Who is allowed to perform them? Within what level of testing do PPMP tests fall?

13.3 Waived Testing

With appropriate training, phlebotomists may perform waived testing in states that do not restrict them. Many tests are included on the ever-changing list of waived tests. Phlebotomists should be aware of the level of testing that they may be asked to perform and only perform tests that are waived. Waived testing procedures can be performed using kits that are available from a number of manufacturers. These kits include easy-to-follow instructions and most come with built-in controls. Healthcare employees in various clinical settings may perform these tests, which include (but are not limited to)

- erythrocyte sedimentation rate
- fecal occult blood testing
- microhematocrit
- strep screening
- urine pregnancy testing
- urine chemical screening
- point-of-care testing (POCT)

Although phlebotomists do not typically perform these tests, in some settings, such as rural communities or where laboratory personnel shortages exist, phlebotomists may be instructed on the performance of these tests. Phlebotomists must be aware that, in some states, such as California, licensure laws regulate waived testing, so phlebotomists may not be allowed to perform them.

Erythrocyte Sedimentation Rate

The **erythrocyte sedimentation rate (ESR)** is the rate at which red blood cells (RBCs) settle in whole blood. What is actually measured is the distance, in millimeters, that they fall in 1 hour when allowed to settle in a calibrated tube. The ESR screens for the presence of any inflammatory process and is not diagnostic of any one condition. When inflammation is present, plasma proteins, such as albumin and globulin, are increased. An increase in these substances causes red blood cells to come closer together, which may result in **rouleaux formation** (RBCs sticking to each other). Several cells sticking together settle faster than a single RBC does. This results in an elevated sedimentation rate.

Several methods exist for performing the ESR, including Wintrobe, Westergren, and Modified Westergren. Manufacturers of kits for these methods have varying requirements for specimen tube type. Most require a lavender-topped EDTA tube, whereas others require a light-blue-topped tube or their own specialty tube, usually with a black stopper or top. ESR procedures are best performed on fresh specimens less than 4 hours old, but they may be performed on refrigerated blood up to 12 hours old, depending on the test method. Always check the procedures and policies at your facility before performing laboratory tests.

A simple method for performing an ESR requires the following equipment (see Figure 13-15):

- Specimen transfer pipets
- ESR kit
- ESR vials containing a premeasured amount of diluent (usually saline)

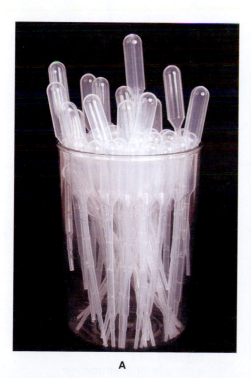
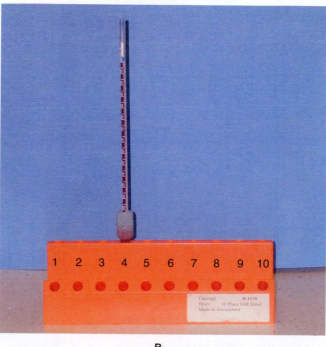

A   B

Figure 13-15 (A) Transfer pipets—plastic, disposable droppers for transferring liquids. (B) An example of a Westergren method for erythrocyte sedimentation rate. The setup includes a vial that holds the diluted sample, a tube calibrated in millimeters, and a testing rack.

- Calibrated ESR tubes
- ESR testing rack

ESR Procedure

To perform an ESR procedure properly, follow the steps in Competency Check 13-7.

See Figures 13-16 and 13-17 for an example of one such ESR procedure.

Competency Check 13-7

Erythrocyte Sedimentation Rate Testing

1. Transfer the blood from an appropriate specimen to the diluent vial and fill it to the mark on the vial (amounts vary by manufacturer).

2. Replace the vial cap and gently mix the blood with the diluent by inversion.

3. Insert a calibrated ESR tube through the vial cap and into the blood-diluent mixture; adjust the tube until the blood is even with the 0-mm mark.

4. Place the ESR tube in the testing rack (it should be absolutely level).

5. Label the ESR tube or vial with the patient's identification.

6. Allow the blood to settle for one hour.

7. After 1 hour, read the level to which the red blood cells have fallen and record this information as millimeters per hour.

8. Consult the manufacturer's instructions for proper interpretation of the results. Normal values vary by method and may vary by gender.

1 - Remove the stopper (pink cap) on the prefilled vial (0.2 mL of 3.8% sodium citrate is used as diluent). Using a transfer pipet, fill the vial to the indicated fill line with blood (0.8 mL) to make required 4:1 dilution. Replace pierceable stopper and gently invert several times to mix.

2 - Place vial in its rack on a level surface. Carefully insert the pipet (tube) through the pierceable stopper until the pipet comes in contact with the bottom of the vial. (The diaphragm of the pink stopper is calibrated to break under the light pressure made by inserting the pipet.) The pipet will autozero the blood and any excess will flow into the closed reservoir compartment.

3 - Let the sample stand for exactly 1 hour and then read the numerical results of erythrocyte sedimentation in millimeters. This is done by reading the plasma meniscus on the calibrated pipet. Dispose of properly after use.

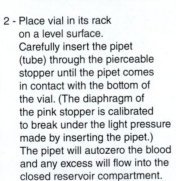
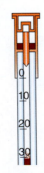

Figure 13-16 An example of one manufacturer's method for Westergren erythrocyte sedimentation rate (Sediplast ESR system).

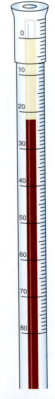

Figure 13-17 An example of erythrocyte sedimentation after 1 hour. The reading in this example is 22 millimeters.

Factors Affecting ESR Results

Several factors that may affect ESR results are time from collection to testing, testing time, temperature, tilting, and vibrations. If the specimen has been left at room temperature for more than 4 hours, it may have a lower-than-actual ESR result due to swelling of red blood cells over time. Reading the ESR result sooner than 1 hour may result in a falsely lower ESR, whereas reading the ESR sometime after 1 hour may result in a falsely higher ESR value. ESR tests can be affected by temperatures higher or lower than room temperature (20–25°C or 68–77°F) and by drafts or direct sunlight. Tilting the ESR tube, even slightly, will cause the red blood cells to settle faster, so it is important for the test rack to be absolutely level. Vibrations of the countertop on which the testing rack is placed will also cause the red blood cells to settle faster. To prevent this, the rack should not be placed on the same counter as centrifuges or other vibration-generating equipment.

Fecal Occult Blood Testing

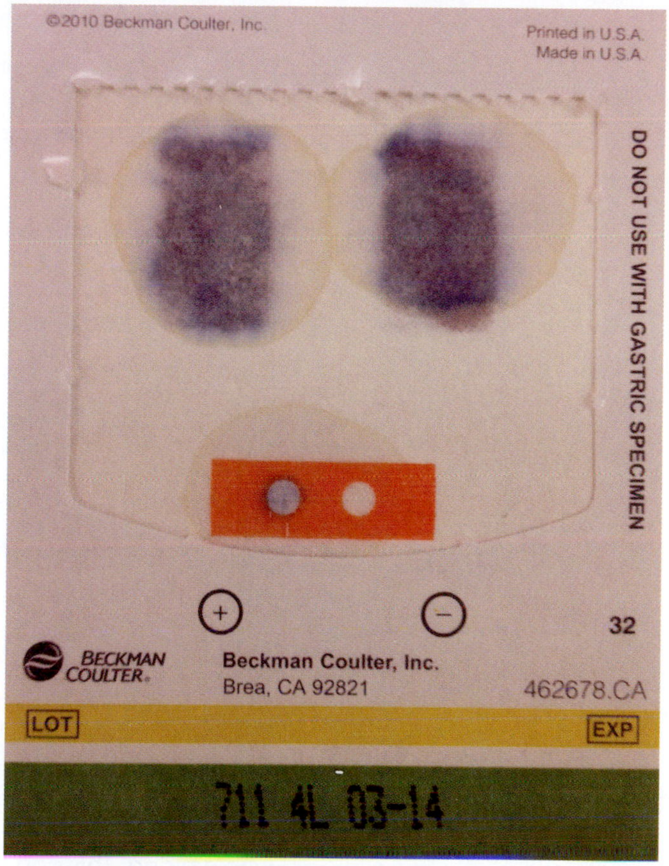

Fecal occult blood is blood that is found in the feces/stool and may not be visible, therefore *occult*. Fecal occult blood can be present in infections, inflammatory conditions, trauma, ulcers, hemorrhoids, and colorectal cancer. Although highly specific tests such as the fecal immunohistochemical test are available, common waived methods for fecal blood testing may still be used by some facilities. Testing stool for occult blood is done using a cardboard holder that contains a paper impregnated with guaiac, a chemical that will turn blue when blood is present (see Figure 13-18). Several portions of the stool specimen are sampled to maximize blood detection. For this test, apply a thin layer of stool to the front of the guaiac card as directed. Next, add a few drops of hydrogen peroxide developer to the back of the card (always follow manufacturer's procedure). If a sufficient amount of hemoglobin is present, the guaiac paper will turn blue. False-negative results may occur if a very small amount of hemoglobin is present or if not enough stool was applied. False-positive results may occur if another type of peroxidase or pseudoperoxidase (enzyme present in some foods) is present. In some cases, the physician will order fecal occult blood "times three," requiring that three stool specimens be collected.

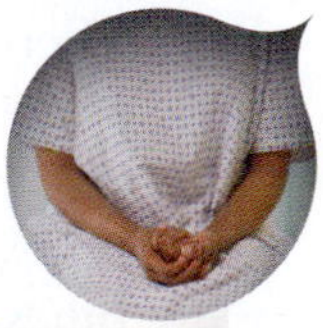

Figure 13-18 A small amount of stool is applied to the Hemoccult (Beckman Coulter, Inc.) guaiac test card, followed by a reagent containing peroxide. If occult blood is present, the card's test area will turn blue.

False-Positive Fecal Occult Blood

False-positive fecal occult blood results may occur if patients have ingested fish, meat that contains a high amount of heme (such as beef and lamb), or foods that contain peroxidase, including some fruits and vegetables. Fruits that may cause false-positive results include bananas, cantaloupe, pears, and plums. Vegetables that may cause false-positive results include broccoli, cauliflower, horseradish, and turnips. Patients should be instructed to avoid these foods for a few days prior to stool specimen collection. In addition, aspirin and vitamin C must also be avoided because they may interfere with the guaiac test.

Patient Education & Communication

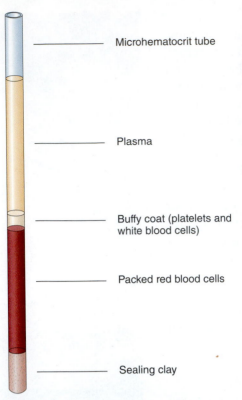

Microhematocrit tube

Plasma

Buffy coat (platelets and white blood cells)

Packed red blood cells

Sealing clay

Figure 13-19 Hematocrit is the percentage of red blood cells in whole blood. This can be determined by measuring the percentage of packed red blood cells in a capillary tube that has been centrifuged.

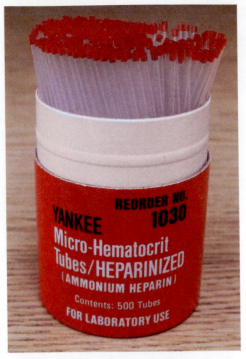

Figure 13-20 Heparinized capillary tubes are used as microhematocrit tubes.

Microhematocrit

A **hematocrit** (Hct or Crit) is used as a screening test for anemia and is measured as the **packed cell volume (PCV)** of red blood cells, or the percentage of red blood cells in whole blood. Figure 13-19 shows the separation of cells from plasma in a microhematocrit tube. A **microhematocrit** is a procedure for determining the hematocrit and requires only a small amount of blood. The microhematocrit procedure uses capillary tubes, which are narrow-diameter tubes with a red band around one end, indicating that they are coated with heparin (see Figure 13-20). Capillary tubes with a blue band do not contain any anticoagulant but may be used with EDTA specimens.

Microhematocrit Testing

Microhematocrit testing can be performed directly from dermal (capillary) puncture blood or blood that has been collected into a microcollection container or an evacuated tube. For tests performed directly from dermal punctures, wipe away the first drop of blood with gauze. Using red-tipped capillary tubes, touch the tube to the edge of the blood drop without touching the skin. When filling capillary tubes from pre-collected tubes, tilt the specimen tube slightly and insert one end of the capillary tube (see Figure 13-21A).

Capillary tubes fill by capillary action, which occurs when blood flows freely into the tube without suction. Avoid allowing air to enter the tube, which may cause erroneous results. Fill two capillary tubes three-quarters full. The rate of filling can be increased or decreased by tilting the tube. However, do not remove the tip of the tube from the blood source with the tube lower than the

Microhematocrit Tubes

Microhematocrit tubes/capillary tubes are very slender and usually made of glass, making them prone to breakage. A broken sharp edge can cause a break in the phlebotomist's glove and skin, and consequently exposure to blood. Phlebotomists must use caution when handling these tubes. For safety, some brands of capillary tubes are made of plastic or glass that is wrapped in plastic.

blood. This will allow air to enter. Keep the tube horizontal or tilted upward during the filling process. Wipe excess blood off the outside of the capillary tubes with gauze. Hold the tube horizontally to prevent blood from leaking out of the tube.

Once a microhematocrit sample has been obtained, place a gloved finger over the dry end (the end of the capillary tube that was not used to collect the specimen) and hold it horizontal so no blood can spill out. Remove your finger from the dry end and seal it by embedding the clean end in a clay sealant designated for this use. Be careful not to lose any blood from the tube (see Figure 13-21B). Improper sealing of the capillary tube can cause blood to leak out, which may result in a decreased hematocrit reading, or no blood remaining in the tube. Some microhematocrit tubes are self-sealing and do not require this puttylike sealant. Follow manufacturer's directions to avoid tube breakage or blood leakage during centrifugation.

If microhematocrit tubes must be transported to the laboratory, place them in a larger tube for labeling and transport (see Figure 13-22). This is done because microhematocrit capillary tubes are fragile and too small to attach patient labels. Attempts to label these small capillary tubes can result in tube breakage, loss of the sample, and potential injury to the phlebotomist.

A microhematocrit centrifuge (see Figure 13-23) is used to obtain packed red blood cells. To obtain these cells, balance the microhematocrit tubes in the microhematocrit centrifuge with the clay ends facing outward. Tighten

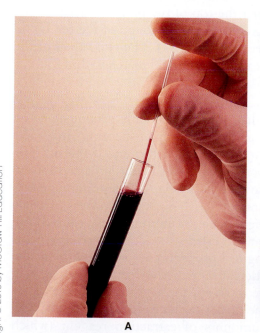
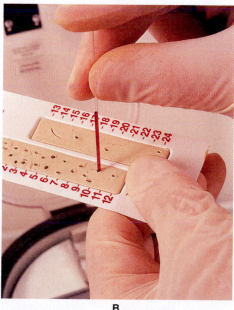

A   B

Figure 13-21 (A) A capillary tube may be filled from a pre-collected blood sample tube and (B) sealed with clay at the dry end.

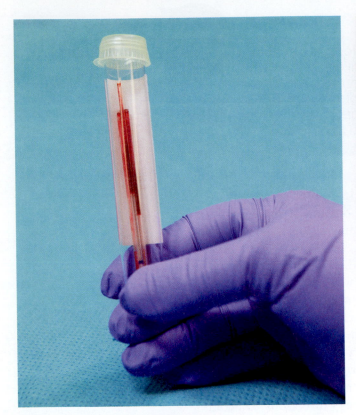

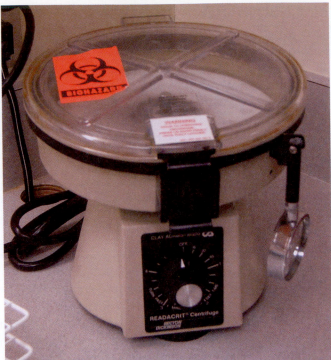

Figure 13-22 Filled capillary tubes may be transported in a larger tube with a label.

Figure 13-23 Microhematocrit centrifuge. When loading a microhematocrit centrifuge, make sure that the tubes are balanced by placing them directly across from each other, with the sealed ends pointing outward.

the head cover on the centrifuge and close the lid. Turn on the microhematocrit centrifuge for the appropriate time, according to manufacturer's instructions.

The hematocrit is determined by using a microhematocrit-reading device. Some microhematocrit centrifuges have this device built in. The bottom of the red blood cell layer is placed at the 0% mark and the scale is adjusted so that the top of the plasma layer is at the 100% mark. The hematocrit value is where the top of the red blood cell layer falls on the scale (see Figure 13-24). The two values of the microhematocrits (one from each tube) should match within 2%.

Strep Screening

Someone with a sore throat that presents suddenly, accompanied by fever but no cold symptoms (such as coughing or sneezing), may have strep throat. **Strep screening** is used to determine if the bacteria Group A *Streptococcus* is present in the throat, causing strep throat. This bacterium can also cause rheumatic fever and autoimmune disease if left undetected and untreated. Many manufacturers produce kits for Group A strep testing, which are immunoassay tests (using antibodies to bacterial antigens to create a reaction, such as a color change). Some strep screening test procedures have several reagents that must be applied in a particular sequence and timing.

The strep test kits that are most appropriate for the waived testing laboratory require that the throat swab be placed in a testing vial that contains premeasured amounts of extraction reagent (which removes the bacteria from the swab). The vial is set onto a testing device that is treated with antibodies to the bacterial antigens and

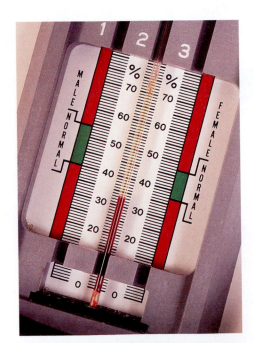

Figure 13-24 Compare the column of packed red blood cells in the capillary tube with the hematocrit scale and record the results. In this example, the hematocrit measures 33%.

color developers. Controls are built into the test device in order to verify that the test has been performed correctly. In Figure 13-25, the letter "T" on the test device indicates the location of the patient's specimen reaction. The two devices on the left of the image show positive reactions, whereas the one on the right is negative. The letter "C" indicates the location of the control reaction. The control reaction must be present or the test is invalid. Each manufacturer's strep screening kits have their own procedures and means of interpreting results. Be sure to follow the instructions specific for each kit.

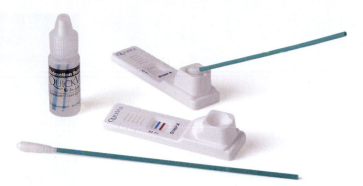

Figure 13-25 Testing devices used for rapid detection of Group A *Streptococcus* infections. Throat swab specimens are obtained and antigen is extracted; results can be reported in less than 10 minutes. (QuickVue In-Line Strep A, Quidel, San Diego, CA)

Urine Pregnancy Testing

Urine pregnancy tests are performed on women to confirm or rule out pregnancy when pregnancy is suspected, as well as on women of childbearing age prior to invasive surgical procedures, such as gallbladder removal, cardiac surgery, or neurosurgery. During pregnancy, the placenta produces **human chorionic gonadotropin (hCG).** This hormone is detectable in urine as early as 10 days after conception, rises during pregnancy, and usually returns to non-detectable levels in the third trimester.

Pregnancy test kits are available for home testing as well as for performance at waived testing laboratories. Procedures for pregnancy tests vary by manufacturer, so you must follow the instructions specific to the test kit used by your facility.

In general, the required number of drops of urine are deposited onto the testing device and allowed to react for the required amount of time. Some devices display a positive (+) or negative (−) symbol to indicate the presence or absence of detectable amounts of hCG. A built-in control indicator verifies that the test has been performed correctly (see Figure 13-26).

Urine Chemical Screening

Urine chemical screening is part of a **urinalysis,** which is a tool used to evaluate substances found in urine. Urine tests can help determine the state of the human body if collected and analyzed properly. A complete urinalysis consists of three parts: a physical component, a chemical component, and a microscopic component. The physical component is the evaluation of color and clarity of the urine. The chemical component consists of measuring pH (acidity or alkalinity) and specific gravity (level of concentration) as well as detecting blood, bilirubin, glucose, ketones, leukocytes, protein, nitrites, and urobilinogen that may be abnormally present in urine. The microscopic component consists of pouring a well-mixed urine sample into a centrifuge tube, then spinning it down to obtain the sediment. The sediment is used to make a slide to view under a microscope to check for various cells, crystals, microorganisms, and urine casts (which are formed inside the kidney and shaped like tiny tubes). Urine microscopic examination is NOT a waived procedure, and therefore is not performed by phlebotomists.

A phlebotomist who is properly trained may be asked to perform a urine chemical screening using a **dipstick** test (a plastic strip with reagent pads) (see Figure 13-27). These pads contain chemicals that react with a particular substance in urine and change color in precise ways. These changes indicate the presence of that substance and the amount or concentration of the substance in the urine specimen.

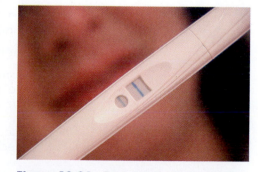

Figure 13-26 Test results from ready-purchased kits are easy to read. This pregnancy test gives a color reaction in the shape of a plus or minus sign. The test shown here is negative.

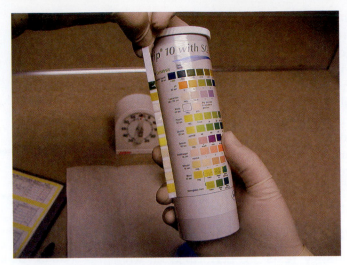

Figure 13-27 Reagent strips are dipped into the urine and then compared to colors on the reagent bottle to determine the results.

For example, when a reagent strip is used to test for blood, the color on the strip, after it is allowed to react with the urine for the proper amount of time, will correspond to a specific concentration of blood or show that no blood is present in the urine. A small amount of blood may produce a green-blue color, whereas a large amount of blood will produce a dark blue color.

Urine Chemical Screening Procedure

To perform a urine chemical screening test, first verify the patient and collection information on the label to ensure that the correct specimen is being tested. Use all appropriate PPE (lab coat, gloves, and face shield) as required by your facility.

Competency Check 13-8

Urine Chemical Screening

1. Double check that the specimen is correctly identified and matches the chart where you will record the results.

2. Allow the urine to come to room temperature; then mix the urine thoroughly.

3. Remove the reagent strip from the bottle and replace the cap.

4. Remove the cap from the urine container and dip the reagent strip into the urine, making sure that all the reagent pads come into contact with the urine.

5. Remove the reagent strip immediately (drag strip across the top of the container to prevent dripping). Some facilities suggest removing excess urine by touching the side edge of the reagent strip to an absorbent material. Never blot the tops of the pads on the strip and do not allow urine from one pad to run over onto another.

6. Begin timing immediately.

7. Compare the colors of the reagent pads to those of the color chart on the reagent strip bottle at the time designated by the manufacturer, to avoid erroneous results.

8. Record the test result for each chemical component in the patient's medical record.

Although the process is essentially the same for all reagent strip tests, there are variations in time intervals before reading results. Test reactions must be read at the designated time to avoid inaccurate results. Figure 13-28 shows the urine chemical screening procedure.

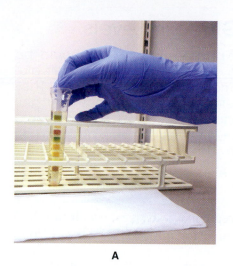 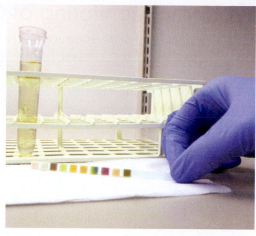 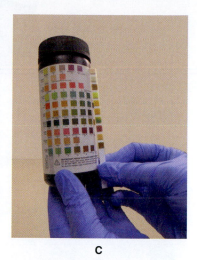

A   B   C

Figure 13-28 (A) Dip the urinalysis strip into the patient's urine. Be sure that all the reagent pads come in contact with the urine specimen. Promptly remove the reagent strip. (B) Remove any excess urine from the strip, but do not blot the strip. (C) Using the chart provided by the manufacturer and following the timing requirements, compare the color of each reagent pad located on the urinalysis strip to the chart. Record all results.

Several manufacturers produce urine reagent strips. Some of these strips are more sensitive to certain chemicals than others. You must choose the appropriate strip according to the chemical test requested. All reagent strips are used once and then discarded.

Follow the directions that come with the reagent strips used by your facility to ensure accurate results. For quality assurance, take these basic precautions:

- Keep strips in tightly closed containers in a cool, dry area.
- Never remove strips from the container until immediately before testing.
- Never touch the pads on the strip with your fingers or gloved hands.
- Examine strips for discoloration before use; discard discolored strips.
- Check the expiration date on the bottle; do not use strips that have expired.
- Use strips within 6 months of opening the container.
- Every time you open a new supply of reagents, run control samples to check for proper operation. Write the date opened on the bottle.

Use the competency checklist *Urine Chemical Screening* at the end of this chapter to review and practice the procedure.

Point-of-Care Testing (POCT)

Point-of-care testing (POCT), or near-patient testing, is designed to reduce healthcare costs while enhancing patient care by making results available quickly. These tests involve collecting a sample and immediately testing it on an instrument typically at the patient's side. The purpose of POCT is to reduce the turnaround time for test results. POCT instruments are typically portable, internally calibrated, easy-to-use, self-contained devices that can be operated with minimal training. The instruments are designed to make tests less dependent on the technical skill of the operator. Depending on the health-care environment, these tests are usually performed by a phlebotomist, nurse, patient care technician, or medical assistant.

Some POCT blood tests are glucose, hemoglobin, sodium, potassium, chloride, bicarbonate, ionized calcium, cholesterol, blood ketones, blood gases, and coagulation studies, such as prothrombin time (PT). Other waived tests, mentioned earlier, may also be performed as POCT tests, including urine

Home Monitoring of Glucose Levels

Patients who are monitoring their glucose at home should be instructed in the proper handling and maintenance of their glucose meter, as well as the correct method for glucose testing. They should also be informed of factors besides diet that affect their glucose level, such as physical and emotional stress. Patients should keep a detailed log of all the glucose testing they perform at home and provide this information to their primary care provider.

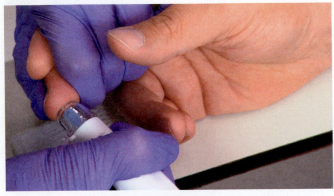

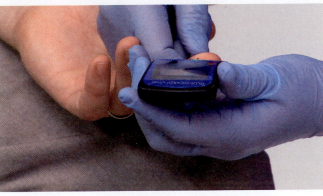

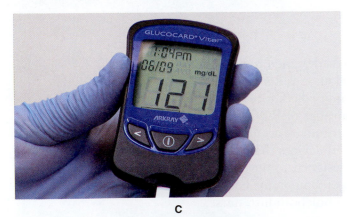

Figure 13-29 For POCT glucose monitoring, (A) a fingerstick puncture is performed, (B) a drop of blood is applied directly to the test strip while in the glucometer, and (C) after testing is complete, the results are read and documented in the appropriate records.

dipstick, urine pregnancy tests, fecal occult (hidden) blood, and screening for infections, such as Group A *Streptococcus.*

POCT tests typically require a small amount of blood from a dermal puncture. However, each instrument is specific to the type of test, so the type and collection requirements of the specimen depend on the manufacturer's recommendations. All POCT instruments should be calibrated on a regular basis. Calibration and testing procedures are found in the manufacturer's directions. Regular calibration and instrument checking must be documented in a logbook at the facility where you are employed.

Glucose Testing

Glucose testing is used to screen for abnormal glucose levels and to monitor glucose levels in patients with diabetes mellitus (high blood glucose levels). Glucose testing is a critical part of diabetes management. Patients can even perform these tests at home. A POCT glucose determination allows frequent monitoring of a patient's blood at any time in any location. Changes in blood sugar can be handled immediately, and patients tend to be more compliant when they obtain immediate results. Testing provides the opportunity for better regulation of the patient's medication and condition.

Several brands of glucose meters are available for POCT glucose. Methods vary by manufacturer. Phlebotomists and other meter operators should refer to the specific operator's manual for their meters for proper instrument maintenance, storage, and handling of reagent strips, test performance, and interpretation. Control substances should always be run and levels verified to be within acceptable limits prior to running any patient samples.

Glucose POCT Procedure

In general, most POCT procedures for glucose testing follow a procedure similar to the one outlined in Competency Check 13-9 and shown in Figure 13-29.

Glucose Point-of-Care Testing

1. Properly identify the patient.
2. Use PPE appropriate to the procedure and as required by your facility.
3. Assemble the dermal/capillary puncture equipment.
4. Verify that controls have been run on the glucose instrument and are in range.
5. Prepare the glucose instrument for testing (insert test strip).
6. Perform a routine dermal/capillary puncture.
7. Wipe away the first drop (the first drop may contain fluid from the tissue and give elevated results).
8. Apply a drop of blood to the test strip (following the manufacturer's requirements).
9. Testing should begin automatically.
10. Provide post-puncture patient care.
11. Properly dispose of biohazards.
12. After the test is complete, read and record the results.

Use the competency checklist *Point-of-Care Glucose Testing* at the end of this chapter to review and practice the procedure.

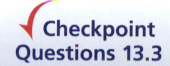

Checkpoint Questions 13.3

1. What substances may cause a false positive result when testing occult blood by the guaiac method?
2. Briefly describe the proper way to obtain a microhematocrit specimen using dermal puncture.
3. What is the purpose of POCT?
4. When performing urine chemistry tests using a reagent strip, why can't all the test results be read at the same time?
5. Why should the first drop of blood be wiped away after dermal puncture before testing the blood glucose level by POCT methods?

Chapter Summary

Learning Outcome	Key Concepts/Examples	Related NAACLS Competency
13.1 Explain how to collect various non-blood specimens. Pages 355–367.	Phlebotomists may need to collect, or instruct patients about how to collect, non-blood specimens. Each non-blood specimen has a unique method of collection and unique specimen containers.	4.00, 4.2, 4.3, 5.4, 7.00, 7.2, 7.6
13.2 Differentiate among waived tests, moderately complex tests, and high complexity testing. Pages 367–370.	• The Clinical Laboratory Improvement Amendments of 1988 (CLIA '88) identified the following levels of complexity for medical laboratory tests: waived tests, moderately complex tests, provider-performed microscopy, and high complexity tests. • A Certificate of Waiver is needed for facilities wishing to perform waived testing.	N/A
13.3 Describe procedures for various waived and point-of-care tests that a phlebotomist may be asked to perform, including quality controls. Pages 370–381.	• Phlebotomists and other healthcare workers may perform waived tests, including point-of-care testing (POCT), where licensure regulations allow. • Some waived or POCT tests include erythrocyte sedimentation rates, fecal occult blood testing, microhematocrit, strep screening, urine pregnancy testing, urine chemical screening, and bedside glucose testing. Each procedure must be performed according to standard operating procedures, which include the performance of quality control checks prior to patient testing.	4.3, 4.5, 5.00, 5.1, 5.2

Chapter Review

A: Labeling

Label the areas on the hematocrit test shown in this image.

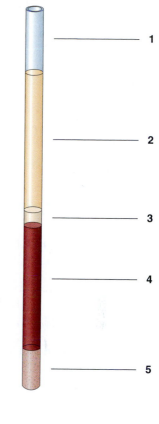

1. [LO 13.3] _____

2. [LO 13.3] _____

3. [LO 13.3] _____

4. [LO 13.3] _____

5. [LO 13.3] _____

B: Matching

Match each specimen with its use in laboratory testing.

____**6.** [LO 13.1] semen specimen

____**7.** [LO 13.1] sputum expectorant

____**8.** [LO 13.1] stool specimen

____**9.** [LO 13.1] throat swab

____**10.** [LO 13.1] urine specimen

a. fertility status of the male reproductive system

b. microorganisms of the lower respiratory system

c. status of the digestive system

d. status of the renal system and overall metabolism

e. strep infection of the upper respiratory system

C: Fill in the Blanks

Write in the word(s) to complete the statement or answer the question.

11. [LO 13.3] A strep test is used to screen for Group _____ *Streptococcus.*

12. [LO 13.3] A(n) _____ is a plastic strip containing pads that are impregnated with reagents.

13. [LO 13.3] Methods for performing erythrocyte sedimentation rates include _____, _____, and _____.

14. [LO 13.3] If occult blood is present in a stool specimen, the guaiac card will turn _____ when the sample is added and _____ is applied.

D: Sequencing

Place each step of the throat swab collection procedure in order.

15. [LO 13.1] _____ Discard tongue depressor.

16. [LO 13.1] _____ Explain the procedure.

17. [LO 13.1] _____ Hold the tongue down with the tongue depressor.

18. [LO 13.1] _____ Identify the patient.

19. [LO 13.1] _____ Label the specimen while the patient is still present.

20. [LO 13.1] _____ Obtain a tongue depressor.

21. [LO 13.1] _____ Place the swab back into its sterile container.

22. [LO 13.1] _____ Put on PPE.

23. [LO 13.1] _____ Remove the sterile swab from the container (do not set it down).

24. [LO 13.1] _____ Rub the back of the throat and each tonsil with the swab.

25. [LO 13.1] _____ Withdraw the swab, then the tongue depressor.

26. [LO 13.1] _____ Remove PPE and wash hands.

E: Case Study/Critical Thinking

27. [LO 13.1] When collecting a throat swab, you find that the patient has a difficult time suppressing the gag reflex. What can you do and have the patient do to help with this collection process?

28. [LO 13.1] A patient must collect a sputum specimen. You have explained the procedure and asked the patient to repeat it back to you. The patient says, "Okay, I spit in the tube." What further instructions should you give the patient?

29. [LO 13.1] A patient must have a urinalysis and urine culture performed. How should the patient be instructed in the collection of this specimen? What must you do with the specimen to prepare it for transport to the laboratory?

30. [LO 13.3] A specimen is tested for occult blood and found to be positive. A brief history on the patient revealed that he had recently eaten a meal that included steak with horseradish dressing. What is the most appropriate course of action?

31. [LO 13.3] When performing urine chemistry screening using reagent strips, you notice that the urobilinogen pad is already brown when you remove the strip from the container. What is your course of action? How might this strip have become discolored?

F: Exam Prep

Choose the best answer for each question.

32. [LO 13.1] Swabs used in the collection of specimens from the back of the throat should be (*Choose all that apply*)
   a. calcium alginate.
   b. cotton.
   c. Dacron.
   d. sterile.

33. [LO 13.1] When collecting a throat swab, rub the following areas. (*Choose all that apply.*)
   a. Back of throat
   b. Both tonsils
   c. Sides of mouth
   d. Uvula

34. [LO 13.1] The mouth and teeth should be avoided when collecting throat cultures because
   a. touching these areas causes a gag reflex.
   b. these areas contain normal bacteria.
   c. these areas do not contain bacteria.
   d. these areas contain too much saliva.

35. [LO 13.1] A sputum specimen is collected when
   a. saliva is spit out of the mouth into a sterile cup.
   b. the mouth is rinsed with water and spit into a sterile cup.
   c. coughing onto a microbiology culture media plate.
   d. mucus that is coughed up from deep within the lungs is spit into a sterile cup.

36. [LO 13.1] A stool specimen is used to test for (*Choose all that apply*)

    a. digestive problems.
    b. pathogenic bacteria.
    c. ova and parasites.
    d. gastrointestinal bleeding.

37. [LO 13.1] Errors in test results on stool specimens can be caused by which of the following factors? (*Choose all that apply.*)

    a. The presence of urine in the specimen
    b. The patient's following a prescribed diet prior to specimen collection
    c. The patient's having had an enema before the specimen was collected
    d. Specimen collection before the patient has taken barium sulfate

38. [LO 13.1] The best urine specimen to use for general health assessment is the

    a. 24-hour collection.
    b. clean-catch specimen.
    c. first morning void.
    d. random void.

39. [LO 13.1] During collection of a clean-catch urine specimen, which portion is collected into the sterile container?

    a. Beginning of the stream
    b. Middle of the stream
    c. End of the stream
    d. All of the urine

40. [LO 13.1] The gray-topped urine collection tube contains (*Choose all that apply*)

    a. sodium borate.
    b. sodium fluoride.
    c. sodium formate.
    d. sodium propionate.

41. [LO 13.1] When adding preservatives to 24-hour urine collection containers, you should (*Choose all that apply*)

    a. wear goggles, gloves, and a chemical apron.
    b. add preservatives in a fume hood.
    c. label the container with an appropriate caution label.
    d. add water to acid, if required to dilute the acid.

42. [LO 13.2] Levels of laboratory testing complexity were established by

    a. CAP.
    b. CLIA.
    c. CLSI.
    d. COLA.

43. [LO 13.3] An erythrocyte sedimentation rate is

    a. the distance RBCs settle in a calibrated tube after 1 hour.
    b. the speed at which RBCs move through an automated analyzer.
    c. how far red blood cells settle in the EDTA tube.
    d. the percentage of red blood cells in a centrifuged capillary tube.

44. [LO 13.3] A microhematocrit is

    a. the percentage of red blood cells in a centrifuged capillary tube.
    b. the amount of hemoglobin in the average red blood cell.
    c. the number of red blood cells seen using a microscope.
    d. none of these.

45. [LO 13.3] The guaiac card occult blood test is commonly performed on what type of specimen?

    a. Sputum
    b. Stool
    c. Throat swab
    d. Urine

46. [LO 13.3] False-positive results may occur in a fecal occult blood test if patients have ingested (*Choose all that apply*)

    a. alcohol.
    b. bananas.
    c. milk.
    d. horseradish.

47. [LO 13.3] A microhematocrit test is used to screen for

    a. anemia.
    b. diabetes mellitus.
    c. occult blood.
    d. strep infection.

48. [LO 13.3] Testing for human chorionic gonadotropin assesses the status of

   a. pregnancy in women.

   b. male fertility.

   c. *Streptococcus* infection.

   d. none of these.

49. [LO 13.3] Points of concern when using reagent strips for urine chemical testing include *(Choose all that apply)*

   a. the time urine is in contact with reagent pads.

   b. the removal of excess urine off the reagent pads.

   c. correct comparison of the color changes of the reagent pads.

   d. the time of day the specimen was collected.

50. [LO 13.3] What is POCT?

   a. Physician-ordered chemistry test

   b. Patient-operated cholesterol test

   c. Point-of-care testing

   d. Personnel occupational care training

51. [LO 13.3] The blood glucose test is performed by

   a. applying blood to a strip inserted into a specially designed electronic meter.

   b. using a urine reagent strip to test for glucose.

   c. allowing blood to settle in a calibrated tube and measuring the distance.

   d. applying blood to a guaiac card and adding hydrogen peroxide.

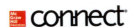

Enhance your learning by completing these exercises and more at connect.mheducation.com

References

Cox, P., & Wilken, D. (2011). *Palko's medical laboratory procedures* (3rd ed.). New York: McGraw-Hill.

Department of Health and Human Services, Centers for Medicare & Medicaid Services. (2013). *Clinical Laboratory Improvement Amendments (CLIA)*. Retrieved July 30, 2013, from www.cms.gov/Outreach-and-Education/Medicare-Learning-Network-MLN/MLNProducts/downloads/CLIABrochure.pdf

Department of Health and Human Services, Centers for Medicare & Medicaid Services. (2006). *How to obtain a CLIA Certificate of Waiver*, Brochure #6. Retrieved September 10, 2013, from www.cms.gov/Regulations-and-Guidance/Legislation/CLIA/Downloads/HowObtainCertificateofWaiver.pdf

Harmening, D. (2007). *Laboratory management principles and processes* (2nd ed.). St. Petersburg, FL: D. H. Publishing & Consulting.

Mundt, L., & Shanahan, K. (2011). *Graff's textbook of urinalysis and body fluids* (2nd ed.). Philadelphia: Lippincott.

National Accrediting Agency for Clinical Laboratory Sciences. (2010). *NAACLS entry-level phlebotomist competencies*. Rosemont, IL. NAACLS.

Sinatra, M. A., St. John, D. J. B., & Young, G. P. (1999). Interference of plant peroxidases with guaiac-based fecal occult blood tests is avoidable. *Clinical Chemistry, 45,* 123–126.

COMPETENCY CHECKLIST: THROAT SWAB COLLECTION

Procedure Steps	Practice			Performed		
	1	2	3	Yes	No	Master
Preprocedure						
1. Examines the requisition.						
2. Greets the patient; introduces self.						
3. Properly identifies the patient.						
4. Explains the procedure to the patient.						
5. Puts on gloves, mask, and eye protection.						
6. Obtains equipment (sterile tongue depressor and culture swab).						
Procedure						
7. Carefully removes the swab from its container; does not set it down (maintains sterility of the swab).						
8. Asks the patient to tilt his or her head back and stick out the tongue.						
9. Correctly uses the tongue depressor to hold down the tongue.						
10. Rubs the correct areas with the sterile swab (back of throat and each tonsil).						
11. Avoids other oral structures during swab collection.						
12. Withdraws the swab, then the tongue depressor.						
13. Places the swab back into its sterile container and crushes the media ampule when required.						
Postprocedure						
14. Discards the tongue depressor.						
15. Correctly labels the specimen.						
16. Properly removes and discards PPE and washes hands.						
17. Thanks the patient.						

COMMENTS: _____
_____
_____
_____

SIGNED

EVALUATOR: _____

STUDENT: _____

NAME: _____ DATE: _____

COMPETENCY CHECKLIST: NASAL SWAB COLLECTION

Procedure Steps	Practice			Performed		
	1	2	3	Yes	No	Master
Preprocedure						
1. Examines the requisition.						
2. Greets the patient; introduces self.						
3. Properly identifies the patient.						
4. Explains the procedure to the patient.						
5. Puts on gloves, mask, and eye protection.						
6. Obtains equipment (culture swab).						
Procedure						
7. Carefully removes the swab from its container; does not set it down (maintains sterility of the swab).						
8. Asks the patient to tilt his or her head back and supports the back of head with a hand.						
9. Correctly swabs the inside of both nares.						
10. Withdraws the swab.						
11. Slowly releases head-supporting hand.						
12. Places the swab back into its sterile container and crushes the media ampule when required.						
Postprocedure						
13. Properly removes and discards PPE and washes hands.						
14. Correctly labels the specimen.						
15. Thanks the patient.						

COMMENTS: _____
_____
_____
_____

SIGNED

EVALUATOR: _____
STUDENT: _____

COMPETENCY CHECKLIST: NASOPHARYNGEAL SWAB COLLECTION

Procedure Steps	Practice			Performed		
	1	2	3	Yes	No	Master
Preprocedure						
1. Examines the requisition.						
2. Greets the patient; introduces self.						
3. Properly identifies the patient.						
4. Explains the procedure to the patient.						
5. Puts on gloves, mask, and eye protection.						
6. Has the patient clear nasal drainage if present (provides tissue).						
7. Obtains equipment (culture swab, viral transport medium, and scissors).						
Procedure						
8. Loosens cap on viral transport medium container (but does not remove cap).						
9. Carefully removes the swab from its container; does not set it down (maintains sterility of the swab).						
10. Asks the patient to tilt his or her head back and supports the back of the head with a hand.						
11. Inserts the swab through the nasal passage and to the nasopharynx (stops if resistance is met and tries the other nasal passage).						
12. Withdraws the swab.						
13. Slowly releases the head-supporting hand.						
14. Removes the cap from the viral transport medium container (maintains sterility of the cap) and inserts the swab into the medium.						
15. Cuts off the swab handle with scissors and replaces the cap.						
Postprocedure						
16. Properly removes and discards PPE and washes hands.						
17. Correctly labels the specimen.						
18. Thanks the patient.						

COMMENTS: _____

_____

_____

_____

SIGNED

EVALUATOR: _____

STUDENT: _____

COMPETENCY CHECKLIST: URINE CHEMICAL SCREENING

Procedure Steps	Practice			Performed		
	1	2	3	Yes	No	Master
Preprocedure						
1. Examines the requisition.						
2. Matches requisition identification with the specimen identification.						
3. Labels a report form correctly with the patient's identification or opens the correct patient's electronic laboratory test reporting form.						
4. Dons appropriate PPEs (lab coat, gloves, eye protection or face shield).						
5. Assembles appropriate equipment (reagent strips, absorbent material, biohazard waste container).						
Procedure						
6. Ensures that the specimen is at room temperature.						
7. Thoroughly mixes the specimen before removing the cap.						
8. Correctly removes a reagent strip from its bottle (does not contaminate other strips; replaces cap on the bottle).						
9. Correctly dips the reagent strip into the urine (submerges all reagent pads).						
10. Immediately removes strip, dragging it across the top of the container to eliminate dripping.						
11. Begins timing immediately.						
12. Compares reagent strip pad colors to the chart on the bottle at the correct time.						
13. Selects the correct reaction reading for each test pad on the reagent strip.						
14. Correctly records results onto the result form or patient chart (or electronic record).						
Postprocedure						
15. Properly disposes of reagent strip, specimen, and PPEs.						

COMMENTS: _____

_____

_____

_____

SIGNED

EVALUATOR: _____

STUDENT: _____

COMPETENCY CHECKLIST: POINT-OF-CARE GLUCOSE TESTING

Procedure Steps	Practice			Performed		Master
	1	2	3	Yes	No	
Preprocedure						
1. Performs quality control on the glucose meter.						
2. Records quality control and verifies the meter is in control.						
3. Examines the requisition.						
4. Greets the patient; introduces self.						
5. Identifies the patient verbally using two identifiers, including comparing the identification band with the requisition.						
6. Explains the procedure to the patient.						
7. Verifies diet restrictions or instructions.						
8. Puts on gloves.						
9. Selects the correct equipment and supplies.						
10. Assembles the equipment and supplies properly.						
11. Conveniently places the equipment.						
12. Reassures the patient.						
13. Selects the appropriate finger.						
14. Warms the finger, if necessary.						
15. Selects the dermal puncture site.						
16. Cleanses the puncture site.						
17. Allows the site to air dry.						
Procedure						
18. Applies the lancet across the fingerprints.						
19. Uses adequate pressure when activating the lancet.						
20. Wipes away the first drop of blood.						
21. Follows the manufacturer's procedure for performing glucose analysis.						
22. Places gauze over the puncture site.						
23. Records the glucose level correctly.						

(continued)

Procedure Steps	Practice			Performed			Master
	1	2	3	Yes	No		
Postprocedure							
24. Thanks the patient.							
25. Disposes of used supplies appropriately.							
26. Removes gloves and washes hands.							
27. Documents the results in the computer system (if required).							

COMMENTS: _____

_____

_____

_____

SIGNED

EVALUATOR: _____

STUDENT: _____

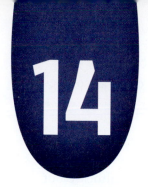

14

Practicing Professional Behavior

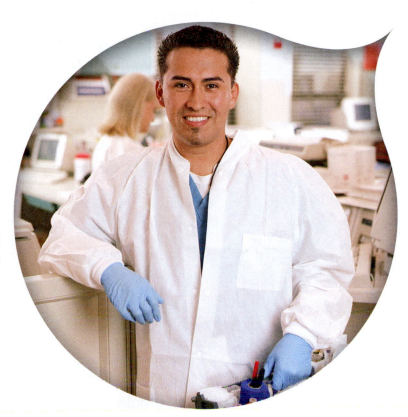

Learning Outcomes

14.1 Model professional behavior and appearance.

14.2 Summarize healthcare diversity and competent professional communications.

14.3 Discuss risk management and policies and protocol designed to avoid medicolegal problems.

14.4 List the causes of stress in the workplace and discuss the coping skills used to deal with workplace stress.

14.5 Recognize the different elements of the professional community of the phlebotomist.

Related NAACLS Competencies

9.00 Communicate (verbally and nonverbally) effectively and appropriately in the workplace.

9.1 Maintain confidentiality of privileged information on individuals, according to federal regulations (e.g., HIPAA).

9.2 Demonstrate respect for diversity in the workplace.

9.3 Interact appropriately and professionally.

9.6 Model professional appearance and appropriate behavior.

9.8 Define and use medicolegal terms and discuss policies and protocol designed to avoid medicolegal problems.

9.9 List the causes of stress in the workplace and discuss the coping skills used to deal with workplace stress.

Introduction

This chapter provides insights into professional behaviors, cultural competence, and professional life after phlebotomy training.

14.1 Professional Behavior

The concept of professional behavior is important not only in healthcare but also in nearly any field in which a person works, whether this person is an auto mechanic, a butcher, a fashion retailer, or an investment banker. Consider what the phrase "professional behavior" means to you and the images that you might associate with such behavior. A **professional** is an individual who performs a vocation or job requiring specialized educational training. **Professionalism** is behavior that exhibits the traits or features that correspond to the models and standards of that profession, which, in this case, is phlebotomy. Models and standards are developed by professional organizations, such as the American Society for Clinical Laboratory Science, the National Phlebotomy Association, and some state and other governmental entities. In addition, some organizations have developed a list of professional standards, called a code of ethics. A code of ethics is a statement adopted by a profession that states the expected professional and personal conduct of its members. It is a moral framework that is used to assist professionals in understanding and applying professional behavior in everyday practice and especially in challenging situations. Phlebotomy Code of Ethics statements and Pledges to the Profession can be found on the professional society websites listed in Table 14-2 near the end of this chapter. Community needs and cultures also play roles in developing standards of professionalism.

Two types of skills are needed in any profession:

1. **Hard skills**—technical skills that require specific training as well as operational proficiencies within a professional's scope of practice.

   Hard skills usually require training and represent the minimum proficiencies necessary to do the job. Examples of hard skills for phlebotomists are

   - dermal and venipuncture techniques
   - specimen handling and processing
   - computer data entry

   The ability to perform hard skills is readily observable by trainers and supervisors who can help students or employees correct any deficiencies. The hard skill set is the first screen employers use to determine if applicants are qualified for the position.

2. **Soft skills**—personal **attributes** (defining qualities) or behaviors that enhance an individual's interactions, job performance, and career prospects

   Soft skills are more elusive and less concrete. These are the characteristics, attributes, or attitudes—such as respect, dependability, and integrity—that people develop throughout their lives and bring with them to their educational programs and jobs. Although these are generally personal attributes, when they are sought after and significant for specific jobs, they are also professional attributes or behaviors. Keep in mind that technical (hard) skills associated with phlebotomy are the reasons most graduates are hired. However, the lack of a specific soft skill or professional behavior is the reason for most terminations. Weakness in the soft skills is also a major reason that students do not successfully complete their phlebotomy education. Therefore, knowing how to do something is important, but behaving professionally while practicing is essential. The practical application of soft skills in the workplace is treated throughout this book. The chapter *Phlebotomy and Healthcare* discusses professional dress and patient communications. Patient communications and the application of healthcare ethics are examined in the chapter *Patient and Specimen Requirements*.

1. Define *professionalism*.
2. What is the difference between a hard skill and a soft skill?

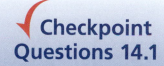 **Checkpoint Questions 14.1**

14.2 Diversity in Healthcare

Have you heard the expression "It takes all kinds"? Professionalism involves understanding people who are different from you and respecting their right to be different. After all, from their point of view, you are the one who is different! **Diversity** is a term used to encompass variations of a category, such as the various types of life found on earth, the various ways one can invest money, and the various cultures displayed by human beings. **Culture** is usually understood to mean a specific ethnic, religious, or social-economic background (see Figure 14-1).

Culturally Aware Communication

Every person has a basic worldview that shapes his/her beliefs about health and disease, the methods for treating disease, and the role of healthcare providers. These belief systems can create challenges for the healthcare worker because individual preferences affect how patients respond to healthcare. National standards have been developed by the Office of Minority Health, within the U.S. Department of Health and Human Services, to serve as a guide for the delivery of quality healthcare to diverse populations. These standards are called the *National Standards for Culturally and Linguistically Appropriate Services in Health Care* (**CLAS Standards**). The intent of these standards is to help eliminate misunderstandings in healthcare interactions, improve patient compliance, and eliminate healthcare disparities. See Table 14-1 to read the CLAS Standards in full.

Communicating with people of diverse backgrounds can be difficult because of barriers that may naturally result from diversity. For example, **stereotypes** are one type of barrier to communicating with people from different cultures. Stereotypes are beliefs and concepts about a specific cultural group of people that are often based on assumptions about that cultural group. Phlebotomists and other healthcare workers should avoid stereotyping individuals and realize that everyone is different, even if they come from the same culture or a different one. Although people of the same culture or background

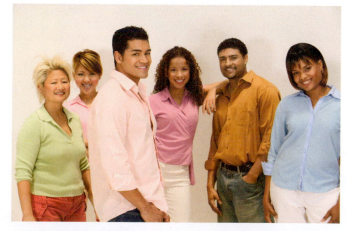

Figure 14-1 Healthcare workers and patients come from a variety of backgrounds.

TABLE 14-1 National Standards for Culturally and Linguistically Appropriate Services in Health Care

Principal Standard:

1. Provide effective, equitable, understandable, and respectful quality care and services that are responsive to diverse cultural health beliefs and practices, preferred languages, health literacy, and other communication needs.

Governance, Leadership, and Workforce:

2. Advance and sustain organizational governance and leadership that promotes CLAS and health equity through policy, practices, and allocated resources.
3. Recruit, promote, and support a culturally and linguistically diverse governance, leadership, and workforce that are responsive to the population in the service area.
4. Educate and train governance, leadership, and workforce in culturally and linguistically appropriate policies and practices on an ongoing basis.

Communication and Language Assistance:

5. Offer language assistance to individuals who have limited English proficiency and/or other communication needs, at no cost to them, to facilitate timely access to all health care and services.
6. Inform all individuals of the availability of language assistance services clearly and in their preferred language, verbally and in writing.
7. Ensure the competence of individuals providing language assistance, recognizing that the use of untrained individuals and/or minors as interpreters should be avoided.
8. Provide easy-to-understand print and multimedia materials and signage in the languages commonly used by the populations in the service area.

Engagement, Continuous Improvement, and Accountability:

9. Establish culturally and linguistically appropriate goals, policies, and management accountability, and infuse them throughout the organization's planning and operations.
10. Conduct ongoing assessments of the organization's CLAS-related activities and integrate CLAS-related measures into measurement and continuous quality improvement activities.
11. Collect and maintain accurate and reliable demographic data to monitor and evaluate the impact of CLAS on health equity and outcomes and to inform service delivery.
12. Conduct regular assessments of community health assets and needs and use the results to plan and implement services that respond to the cultural and linguistic diversity of populations in the service area.
13. Partner with the community to design, implement, and evaluate policies, practices, and services to ensure cultural and linguistic appropriateness.
14. Create conflict and grievance resolution processes that are culturally and linguistically appropriate to identify, prevent, and resolve conflicts or complaints.
15. Communicate the organization's progress in implementing and sustaining CLAS to all stakeholders, constituents, and the general public.

can share the same beliefs, many factors affect the way an individual reflects and acts on these beliefs. The following are a few of these factors:

- Place of birth
- Place of upbringing (urban, suburban, rural)
- Current place of residence
- Family history
- Social status
- Economic status
- Education
- Spiritual beliefs
- Superstitions and folklore
- Length of time in the United States
- Level of **acculturation** (changes made by minorities in response to the dominant culture) to mainstream American culture

Avoiding Culture Clashes

When two or more groups from different backgrounds have a long historical relationship with one another, it is often perceived that the only differences among them are physical characteristics. When this assumption is made, communications may fail, causing frustration and even anger in both parties. For example, a healthcare worker may be caring for a patient from a different culture. Her assumption is that the only difference between them is their ethnicity and this may cause her to ignore requests that seem silly to the healthcare worker but that are rooted in the patient's cultural beliefs and important for that patient's perception of quality care.

These factors influence the way patients view healthcare and their expectations for quality. A general rule of practice is to treat others like we would like to be treated. However, treating every patient the same as you want to be treated is not always appropriate because differences in culture and background may cause differences in expectations of treatment.

During your interactions with patients, they may express their cultural beliefs. If this occurs, refrain from judgment. Some patients may, for example, take offense at being greeted by a person of the opposite gender or by being touched, such as with a handshake. The following practices will help make communications more pleasant for both the phlebotomist and the patient:

- Determine the appropriateness of your communication style. You may need to modify your approach depending on the patient's age, capacity to communicate, or ability to understand your instructions.

- Adapt to patient needs, expectations, and perceptions of various healthcare functions. Do not assume that the patient is familiar with blood or other specimen collection procedures.

- Honor the patient's decisions and decision-making process. A patient may wish to refuse a procedure once it is explained.

- Do not dictate to patients about specimen collection procedures but provide them with opportunities to feel in control by asking them their preferences.

- Do not make assumptions about similarities or differences between your background and the patient's.

Culture Perspectives

Healthcare employees who deliver care must be aware of the **multicultural** backgrounds of their patients. However, they should avoid stereotyping on the basis of cultural beliefs. Beliefs and customs that are common among people of a specific culture may or may not be held by all individuals of that culture.

In general, when interacting with patients, be sure to introduce yourself using your title and address the patient by title (Mr., Mrs., etc.) and family name rather than using the patient's first name. Make an attempt to assess the basic communication needs of your patients and speak on a level they can understand, without being condescending. Do not be judgmental when they express cultural beliefs that vary from your own. Each patient is an individual and should not be judged or treated differently because of his or her beliefs.

The following is a list of beliefs you may encounter and some additional practices you should understand while working as a phlebotomist.

- Some people believe in the harmonious relationship of body, mind, and soul with nature. This may cause patients to deny terminal diagnoses and seek treatments that will restore harmony to the body rather than conventional approaches to healing.

- Some people believe that blood is a person's essence and to have some taken for tests may upset the body's natural balance and cause weakness. This belief can cause patients to feel extreme anxiety over phlebotomy procedures.
- Some people view health not simply as the absence of illness, but rather as a state of physical and emotional well-being.
- Some people view suffering as a blessing from God, whereas others see illness as a punishment from God.
- Certain people prefer to use home remedies, and others wear religious symbols to ward off illness.
- Some people rely more on physician's skills in diagnosis and view blood collection procedures as unnecessary or perceived as indicating a very serious illness.
- Be aware that some individuals may feel that making eye contact with persons in authority, such as a healthcare worker, is being disrespectful. However, some people feel that not making eye contact, or looking down when speaking indicates that something is being held back.
- In some cases individuals may expect medical decisions to be made for them rather than by them and can seem to be uncooperative because they are waiting for someone to tell them what to do.
- Communications with individuals of certain cultures may be successful if the healthcare worker is of the same gender as the patient.
- Individuals of some cultures may have a very strong sense of family and a high appreciation for family support. Patients may desire to have family present during their time in a healthcare facility even though you may feel that this violates HIPAA requirements. The husband may be the one who communicates for his wife, as this is thought to be a sign of caring for her.
- Patients may not ask questions because they highly desire privacy and independence, not wanting to "bother" anyone or have family members worried.
- Some people have a different perspective on the concept of time, which may make scheduling appointments, especially for timed tests, difficult.
- In certain cultures older persons hold higher status and young healthcare practitioners may be viewed as untrustworthy and as having inadequate skills. These patients may ask for an older phlebotomist whom they perceive as being more experienced.
- Being warm and friendly, but not informal, can ease communications with patients who are from cultures where formality is not the norm. However, smiling while they are speaking may be viewed as an expression of disagreement with their opinions. Exercising common social politeness, such as shaking hands and addressing patients by title and family name (Mr. A, Mrs. B, etc.) shows respect and is generally expected.

Patient Education & Communication

Directing Communication

When communicating with people who have immigrated to the United States, a trained interpreter may need to be provided for interpretation. Phlebotomists and other healthcare workers should direct their questions, instructions, and communications to the patient, even though someone else is communicating the responses.

A Family Decision

In some cultures, major decisions, including an individual's healthcare, are often handled as a family decision. Other cultures defer to the eldest son for major decisions. In addition, older immigrants sometimes rely on family members belonging to a younger generation to understand the English language and American culture. These situations may pose concerns regarding HIPAA compliance. You must ensure that if anyone other than the patient is involved in decisions concerning medical procedures or test results, they are informed of HIPAA regulations and have signed the required documentation.

Interprofessional Communications

Cultural diversity also applies to **interprofessional** (people from different professions) communications in an industry. Differences exist among professions within healthcare, and stereotyping of professions can make communications difficult, as it does with multicultural interactions. Misperceptions about each other's scope of practice or approach to patient care may create barriers to effective communication between healthcare workers from different professions. Although healthcare professionals share a medical language, their views about various activities and functions in the delivery of healthcare may vary based on their professional discipline. A few of the healthcare professionals with whom phlebotomists interact are physicians, nurses, and laboratory, respiratory, and X-ray technicians. A phlebotomist may also serve on multidisciplinary or interprofessional healthcare teams and committees. Phlebotomists must always remember to adjust their communication to each interaction, whether multicultural, interdisciplinary, or both. When encountering an interprofessional situation that you are not sure how to handle, it is best to seek the advice of your supervisor/manager. Use the competency checklist *Patient Communication* at the end of this chapter to review and practice the procedure.

A Question of Practice

Sometimes you may encounter a situation where you are being asked for information or to perform tasks that are not part of your job description. The healthcare professional making this request may not be aware of your scope of practice. A graceful response or, if needed, a referral to your supervisor/manager will help to minimize misunderstandings.

Social Media

Social media have become popular outlets for frustrations encountered on the job. Be careful how you use this technology when discussing your employer or co-workers. Disparaging comments may lead to disastrous results including a lawsuit and job loss if the entity who is the target of your comments perceives harm in any way.

✓ Checkpoint Questions 14.2

1. What is a stereotype?
2. Name at least three practices that can help improve your communication with patients.
3. What should you do if you feel communications between yourself and another healthcare professional did not go well?

14.3 Risk Management

An enormous amount of potential for injury exists in healthcare facilities. **Risk management** departments generate policies and procedures to protect patients, employees, and employers from loss and injury. Hospital risk management departments may also develop policies and procedures that protect the institution from **liability** (legal obligation to compensate for loss or damages) and **litigation** (legal action).

Patient Issues

Patients are susceptible to numerous risks when they enter a healthcare facility, from minor falls to the unjustifiable loss of a limb. Venipuncture procedures, if improperly performed, can cause temporary or permanent injury to an extremity.

The Clinical and Laboratory Standards Institute (CLSI) has specific standards that apply to everyone who performs venipuncture. These standards provide guidelines for the accurate and safe performance of phlebotomy procedures. Most injuries resulting from phlebotomy procedures fall under **malpractice** (incorrect treatment of a patient by a healthcare worker) or **negligence** (failure to perform reasonably expected duties to patients). For example, as discussed in the chapter *Patient and Specimen Requirements*, failure to secure the patient's consent for a procedure can result in charges of assault or battery.

Law & Ethics

Patient-Disclosed Information

Communication with patients must be handled with tact and professionalism. In the event a patient discloses to you any dissatisfaction with a practitioner or another team member, discuss this with the appropriate person so that the problem can be resolved. Do not lead the patient to believe that this disclosed information will be kept confidential because addressing customer concerns is important in limiting litigations.

Litigation related to healthcare issues appears to be commonplace. Patients are considered healthcare consumers. They have a certain level of knowledge and expect a certain level of service to be provided. In the event a patient thinks negligence or malpractice has occurred, the patient is required to prove that such events have taken place. The healthcare facility is not required to prove that malpractice or negligence did not occur. The burden of proof is always the responsibility of the patient or the person filing the complaint.

Preventing Liability Suits

All healthcare personnel must understand and exercise their legal duty to the patient. Phlebotomists must be aware of the standards of care, as well as their boundaries and limitations of practice. Attempting procedures that you are not fully trained to perform can lead to poor-quality care and perceived negligence. Other health team members may attempt to delegate tasks, such as arterial puncture, that go beyond the phlebotomist's level of training and expertise. Never perform any procedures you are not fully trained to perform. Many healthcare facilities train employees to perform skills they were not formally trained to do in their educational programs. This allows the employee to use these skills within the healthcare facility where they were trained. All persons performing phlebotomy must do so according to the established standard of care to prevent potential litigation.

In addition to performing procedures according to established care standards, phlebotomists must avoid destructive and unethical criticism of other team members. Patients hearing negative comments about other team members may develop negative perceptions about them and the facility before they ever interact with them. Never discuss a former practitioner or another team member involving a negative experience. Allow patients to discuss their concerns, but do not add comments to the discussion that might be construed as an admission of fault.

Proper documentation is another vital link in preventing liability. Remember to properly record results or variances immediately to prevent errors and liability. Documentation serves as a blueprint of the healthcare facility's account of the patient's care and treatment. Good record keeping is often the only account of an event that healthcare facilities can rely on when faced with potential liability. The patient record is also a communication medium used by the health team members when planning and evaluating care. Each member is responsible for properly documenting essential information.

Healthcare personnel take several measures to prevent patient injuries and thus reduce liability. The same determination must be exercised to prevent employee injuries and exposure to bloodborne pathogens.

Healthcare Personnel Issues

Exposure to bloodborne pathogens presents a great risk to healthcare employees. Phlebotomists must adhere to CDC and OSHA guidelines. As discussed in the chapter *Infection Control and Safety*, the CDC established standard precautions while OSHA requires use of personal protective equipment (PPE) in potential exposure situations. In addition, OSHA mandates that all healthcare institutions maintain individualized exposure plans. These plans serve not only as a step-by-step guide to be followed in the event of exposure but also as documentation of the event and a recommendation for the course of treatment. All employees at risk of exposure to bloodborne pathogens are to be given, free of charge, the hepatitis B vaccination, according to OSHA guidelines.

Phlebotomists are at risk with every venipuncture procedure; therefore, safety measures must be taken at all times. The phlebotomist must properly apply PPE and dispose of all sharps (such as needles) correctly in the designated biohazard containers.

Another safety issue in the laboratory is the presence of chemicals and substances that are potentially hazardous. A branch of OSHA called the OSHA Hazardous Communication Standard (OSHA HazCom) governs the identification of chemicals and substances that are potentially hazardous. Remember that phlebotomists may need to handle chemicals, especially when preparing preservative containers for use by patients collecting urine specimens at home. Phlebotomists must be familiar with all potential hazards to ensure their safety, as well as that of co-workers and patients.

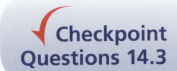

Checkpoint Questions 14.3

1. What is the purpose of a risk management department?
2. List three components that can help prevent liability lawsuits.

14.4 Coping with Stress

Healthcare professionals, including phlebotomists, may experience high levels of **stress** (the body's nonspecific response to change or demands) in their work environment. Stress can result from a feeling of being under pressure, or it can be a reaction to anger, frustration, or a change in your routine. Stress can increase your blood pressure, speed up your breathing and heart rate, and cause muscle tension. Stress can also be a barrier to communication when working. For example, if you are feeling very pressured at work, you might snap at a co-worker or patient, or you might forget to properly label a specimen. To minimize stress—for the sake of your health as well as to prevent errors—it is helpful to understand some basic information about stress.

Preventing Burnout

Burnout is an energy-depleting condition that can affect your health and career. It is the result of prolonged periods of stress without relief. Certain personality types are more prone to burnout. If you are highly driven and perfectionistic, you are more susceptible to burnout. Experts often refer to such a person as having a characteristic type A personality. A more relaxed, calm individual is considered a type B person. Type B personalities are less prone to burnout but have the potential to suffer from it, especially if they work in healthcare.

The burnout process has five phases. These five phases, according to Lyle Miller and Alma Dell Smith in the book *The Stress Solution*, are summarized here:

1. *The Honeymoon Phase.* During the honeymoon phase, your job is wonderful. You have boundless energy and enthusiasm, and all things seem possible. You love the job and the job loves you. You believe it will satisfy all your needs and desires and solve all your problems. You are delighted with your job, your co-workers, and the organization.

2. *The Awakening Phase.* The honeymoon wanes and the awakening stage starts with the realization that your initial expectations were unrealistic. The job isn't working out the way you thought it would. It doesn't satisfy all your needs, your co-workers and the organization are less than perfect, and rewards and recognition are scarce. As disillusionment and disappointment grow, you become confused. Something is wrong, but you can't quite put your finger on it. Typically, you work harder to make your dreams come true. But working harder doesn't change anything and you become increasingly tired, bored, and frustrated. You question your competence and ability and start losing your self-confidence.

3. *The Brownout Phase.* As brownout begins, your early enthusiasm and energy give way to chronic fatigue and irritability. Your eating and sleeping patterns change, and you indulge in escapist behaviors, such as partying, overeating, recreational drugs, alcoholism, and binge

shopping. You become indecisive and your productivity drops. Your work deteriorates. Co-workers and managers may comment on it. Unless interrupted, brownout slides into later stages. You become increasingly frustrated and angry and project the blame for your difficulties onto others. You are cynical, detached, and openly critical of the organization, superiors, and co-workers. You are beset with depression, anxiety, and physical illness.

4. *The Full-Scale Burnout Phase.* Unless you wake up and interrupt the process or someone intervenes, brownout drifts remorselessly into full-scale burnout. Despair is the dominant feature of this final stage. It may take several months to get to this phase, but in most cases it takes 3 to 4 years. You experience an overwhelming sense of failure and a devastating loss of self-esteem and self-confidence. You become depressed and feel lonely and empty. Life seems pointless, and there is a paralyzing "what's the use" pessimism about the future. You talk about "just quitting and getting away." You are exhausted physically and mentally. Physical and mental breakdowns are likely. Suicide, stroke, or heart attack is not unusual as you complete the final stage of what all started with such high hopes, energy, optimism, and enthusiasm.

5. *The Phoenix Phenomenon.* You can arise from the ashes of burnout (like a phoenix), but it takes time. First, you need to rest and relax. Don't take work home. If you're like many people, the work won't get done and you'll only feel guilty for being "lazy." Second, be realistic in your job expectations as well as your aspirations and goals. Whomever you're talking to about your feelings can help you, but be careful. Your readjusted aspirations and goals must be yours, not those of someone else. Trying to be and do what someone else wants you to be or do is a surefire recipe for continued frustration and burnout. Third, create balance in your life. Invest more of yourself in family and other personal relationships, social activities, and hobbies. Spread yourself out so that your job doesn't have such an overpowering influence on your self-esteem and self-confidence.

Types and Causes of Stress

A certain amount of stress is normal. A little bit of stress—the kind that makes you feel excited or challenged by the task at hand—can motivate you to get things done and push you toward a higher level of productivity. For example, your manager may ask you to learn a new procedure. Learning something new, although in itself stressful, can be an exciting challenge and a welcome change of pace. This is considered "good" stress. Ongoing stress, however, can be overwhelming and affect you physically. This is considered "bad" stress.

Bad stress can lower your resistance to colds and other infections and increase your risk of developing heart disease, diabetes, high blood pressure, ulcers, allergies, asthma, colitis, and cancer. It can also increase your risk for certain autoimmune diseases, which cause the body's immune system to attack normal tissue. Some people develop anxiety disorders or have panic attacks when repeatedly under stress (see Figure 14-2).

Stress is not the same for everyone. What is perceived as bad stress by one person may be normal for another. It is important to

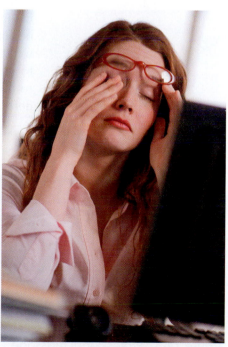

Figure 14-2 Stress is expressed differently by each person.

understand what causes you stress. The following are some potential causes of stress:

- Children leaving or returning home
- Death of a spouse or family member
- Divorce or separation
- Having a new baby
- Hospitalization (yours or a family member's)
- Marriage or reconciliation from a separation
- Moving or remodeling your home
- Sexual problems
- Significant change in your financial status (for better or worse)
- Significant personal success (public recognition)
- Substantial debt, such as a mortgage or overspending on credit cards due to injury or illness
- Trips or vacations (planning as well as taking)

Work-related causes of stress include the following:

- Job change
- Learning new job tasks
- Loss of a job or retirement
- Observation for evaluation by a supervisor or inspector
- Restructuring of the organization, such as your boss's retiring, that may put your job at risk
- Success at work, such as a promotion

Once you recognize the cause of your stress, it is easier for you to manage it.

Managing Stress

Some stress at work is inevitable, so an important goal is to learn how to manage or reduce it. Take into account your strengths and limitations, and be realistic about how much you can handle at work and in your life outside work. Pushing yourself a certain amount can be motivating. Pushing yourself too much is dangerous. Consider using the following tips for reducing stress to improve your health and work performance. Remember, you will need to determine what works for you.

- Allow time for yourself and plan time to relax.
  - Avoid foods high in caffeine, salt, sugar, and fat.
  - Be organized. Good planning can help you manage your workload.
  - Change some of the things you have control over.
  - Do something for fun, such as seeing a funny movie.
  - Eat balanced, nutritious meals and healthful snacks.
  - Exercise regularly.
  - Get enough sleep.
  - Get professional massages to help relieve mental stress as well as physical tension (see Figure 14-3).
  - Identify sources of conflict and try to resolve them.
  - Keep yourself focused. Focus your full energy on one thing at a time and finish one project before starting another.

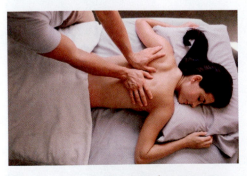

Figure 14-3 Professional massage therapy can help reduce the effects of stress.

- Learn and use relaxation techniques, such as deep breathing, meditation, or imagining yourself in a quiet, peaceful place.
- Maintain a healthy balance in your life among work, family, and leisure activities.
- Maintain a healthy sense of humor. Laughter can help relieve stress. Joke with friends after work.
- Redirect excess energy constructively—clean your closet, work in the garden, do volunteer work, have friends over for dinner, and exercise.
- Rely on the support that family, friends, and co-workers have to offer. Don't be afraid to share your feelings.
- Seek help from social or professional support groups, if necessary.
- Try not to overreact. Ask yourself if a situation is really worth getting upset or worried about.
- Try to be realistic about what you can and cannot do. Do not be afraid to admit that you cannot take on another responsibility.
- Try to set realistic goals for yourself. Remember that there are always choices, even when there appear to be none.

1. What are the five phases of the burnout process?
2. What are the differences between good stress and bad stress?

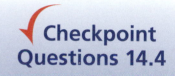
Checkpoint Questions 14.4

14.5 Professional Community

Work Experience Requirements

As of this text's publication in early 2015, phlebotomy positions are plentiful in many areas of the United States. According to the Bureau of Labor and Statistics, phlebotomists are in great need, with a 27% job growth rate. Of course, the more on-the-job experience you acquire, the more marketable you will be as a phlebotomist. In addition, experiences such as being active within your professional community will help you advance in your phlebotomy career. Professional communities are comprised of new and seasoned members of a given discipline—in this case, phlebotomists. The professional community also includes professional organizations or societies. Professional societies, such as the American Society for Clinical Laboratory Science (ASCLS), offer support to their members in the form of opportunities for professional development, outlets for leadership advancement, continuing education, networking, and benefits such as personal and professional insurance policies. Professional development (growing into a profession) includes training and education that helps you enter your chosen profession, maintain your credential, and/or advance to another career (such as the phlebotomist to MLT to MLS career track). Obtaining and maintaining a credential, such as a certification, registration, or licensure, is usually expected of professional community members.

Certification, Registration, and Licensure

Certification, in general, consists of a two-part process: the successful completion of defined academic and training requirements as well as the validation of these studies through a national examination. In any profession, mastering certification requirements ensures an individual's ability to perform the program's competencies. Passing a national examination affords the right to a title and professional credentials.

Although not all employers make certification mandatory for employment as a phlebotomist, it is often required for career advancement. Holding certification in phlebotomy shows patients as well as other healthcare professionals that you possess a certain level of competence and understand the standards of your profession. Certification is granted by a nongovernmental agency and usually requires examination by a testing board. Agencies responsible for providing phlebotomy certification are listed in Table 14-2. Each agency sets standards for the number and type of actual "sticks" a candidate must perform before he or she can become certified. For example, for the National Healthcareer Association's certification, a student must have a minimum of 30 successful venipunctures and 10 successful capillary sticks. These venipunctures and capillary sticks must be performed on live individuals.

Although some phlebotomy certification agencies also accredit phlebotomy programs, many of these agencies follow the requirements of the National Accrediting Agency for Clinical Laboratory Sciences (NAACLS). The required training that NAACLS-approved phlebotomy programs must provide includes at least 40 hours of classroom exposure and a minimum of 100 hours of applied experience, with no less than 100 blood collections. It is the educational institution's duty to ensure that phlebotomy technician students learn all competencies set forth by the certifying agency. In addition,

TABLE 14-2 Phlebotomy Certification Agencies

Agency	Address	Phone	Fax	Website
American Academy of Phlebotomy Technicians (AAPT)	6609 Reisterstown Rd., Suite 208 Baltimore, MD 21215	410-347-1433		www.aaopt.net
American Certification Agency (ACA)	P.O. Box 58 Osceola, IN 46561	574-277-4538	574-277-4624	www.acacert.com
American Medical Technologists (AMT)	10700 W. Higgins Rd., Suite 150 Rosemont, IL 60018	847-823-5169	847-823-0458	www.americanmedtech.org
American Society for Clinical Pathology (ASCP)	33 W. Monroe St., Suite 1600 Chicago, IL 60603	312-541-4999	312-541-4998	www.ascp.org
American Society of Phlebotomy Technicians (ASPT)	P.O. Box 1831 Hickory, NC 28603	828-294-0078	828-327-2969	www.aspt.org
National Center for Competency Testing (NCCT)	7007 College Blvd., Suite 385 Overland Park, KS 66211	800-875-4404	913-498-1243	www.ncctinc.com
National Healthcareer Association (NHA)	11161 Overbrook Rd. Leawood, KS 66211	800-499-9092	913-661-6291	www.nhanow.com
National Phlebotomy Association (NPA)	1901 Brightseat Rd. Landover, MD 20785	301-386-4200	301-386-4203	www.nationalphlebotomy.org

program officials must prove that the training they provide meets the requirements of their state's regulatory body. For instance, the State of California has particular requirements, as outlined in Table 14-3. Evidence of practice and completion must be clearly documented for each student. Students must practice and complete all required skills and then be evaluated by an instructor who is proficient at these skills. A passing grade must be accomplished on each competency. Procedure or competency sheets are used to document that the student has demonstrated competence in each skill.

Registration is different from certification. Registration means that you are on a list maintained by a nongovernmental agency or association. For example, the ASCP keeps a registry of all the individuals who have been certified by the BOR. A professional group may choose to identify themselves as

TABLE 14-3 Phlebotomy Certification Agencies' Requirements

Agency	Didactic Training Requirement	Clinical Training Requirement
American Academy of Phlebotomy Technicians (AAPT) (certifying agency)	AAPT Path 1: high school graduate (or equivalent) AND graduate of AAPT-approved program	AAPT Path 2: high school graduate (or equivalent) AND one year of full-time employment (2080 hours) or equivalent part-time employment as a phlebotomy technician
American Certification Agency (ACA) (certifying agency)	ACA: completion of a formal program that includes phlebotomy	ACA: 100 clinical hours with at least 100 successful venipunctures and 10 skin punctures
American Medical Technologists (AMT) (certifying agency)	AMT: minimum of 120 hours of didactic instruction	AMT: minimum of 120 hours of clinical practicum
American Society for Clinical Pathology (ASCP) (most common and well-recognized certifying agency)	ASCP Route 1: high school graduation (or equivalent) AND completion of a NAACLS-approved phlebotomy program with at least 40 hours of classroom or a phlebotomy program approved by the California Department of Public Health	Completion of a NAACLS-approved phlebotomy program with a minimum of 100 hours of applied experiences to include no less than 100 blood collections
American Society of Phlebotomy Technicians (ASPT) (certifying agency)	ASPT: successful completion of an accredited phlebotomy training program; current ASPT membership	100 documented successful venipunctures and 5 documented skin punctures
National Center for Competency Testing (NCCT) (certifying agency)		NCCT: requires documentation of experience
National Healthcareer Association (NHA) (certifying agency)	NHA: high school diploma and successful completion of an NHA-approved training program	
National Phlebotomy Association (NPA) (accrediting body and certifying agency)	NPA: at least 160 contact hours of lecture	NPA: minimum of 220 hours of practical experience with either mannequins or clinical practicum or a combination
Laboratory Field Services branch of the California Department of Public Health (approves programs and recognizes these phlebotomy exams: ACA, AMT, ASCP, NCCT, NCA, and NHA)		California requires 50 venipunctures and 10 capillary draws; 40 hours of practicum

either certified or registered. For example, nurses who hold a certification at a particular level of practice identify themselves as registered nurses (RN). Facilities may check a prospective employee's credentials by calling the agency that provides the credential.

Critical Thinking

Certification with a Small *C*

When attending a seminar or a course, participants are often awarded a certificate to document their attendance at the event. This type of certification is not the same as having a credential that states you are "certified" in a particular profession. Someone attending a one-day course in phlebotomy who receives a certificate of completion or attendance is not as qualified as a phlebotomist who has completed an accredited course of study and passed a national certification examination.

Law & Ethics

Certification Required

Employers of healthcare professionals, such as phlebotomists, must demonstrate employee competence to their accrediting agencies. An employer who hires uncertified workers is at risk for a lawsuit if these workers make errors. Hiring a phlebotomist without certification may become a liability to the employer.

Licensure is a process similar to certification, but it is enforced by a governmental agency that grants permission to people meeting predetermined qualifications that are set in place by state or local laws. Certification is voluntary, whereas licensure is mandatory. A license to practice a specific trade is attained after a person who completes the requirements for education and experience in that trade successfully meets the qualifications of the governmental agency. Sometimes licensing agencies use licensing examinations, or passing a national certification examination, as the basis for awarding a licensure. Currently, phlebotomists are not licensed in the United States, but California does require specific California certification. State public health departments may be contacted for specific licensure information.

Continuing Education

In addition to certification, participation in **continuing education** (education after professional training) assists in establishing a professional public image. Most certifying agencies have specific guidelines regarding how much and what kind of continuing education are required to maintain certification. Some employers also require documentation of continuing education in order to remain employed or to receive pay increases. A number of employers also keep records, such as the one shown in Figure 14-4, for each employee and these help demonstrate continuing educational and professional involvement. You may want to keep a similar document for your own records or portfolio. However, more importantly, as a professional phlebotomist, continuing education is a lifelong process necessary to stay current in your field. The desire to learn more about the work of a phlebotomist and how it impacts patients is part of the nature of a dedicated, caring, and competent healthcare professional.

Continuing Education Record

A Name _____ Position _____ Time Period _____
Facility _____ Dept/Unit _____

Professional Organization Memberships (List Expiration Date)

	Attended	Expiration
B CPR.................		
Yearly Safety Review...		
OSHA...............		
Competency Validation		
Age Related Competency		
Other................		
....		

_____ **E**
_____
_____

Hospital Committee Memberships

_____ **F**
_____
_____
_____

C

Dept/Unit Meeting Attendance			
Jan	Apr	July	Oct
Feb	May	Aug	Nov
Mar	June	Sept	Dec

Inservices Presented/Dept/Unit Projects

_____
_____ **G**
_____

Inservices / Seminars Attended

D

Date	Program Title	CEUs	Sponsor	Location

Figure 14-4 An employee's continuing education record may display (A) employee information, (B) required annual competency assessment, (C) attendance at department meetings, (D) a record of internally and externally obtained continuing education, (E) membership in professional organizations, (F) participation on various facility committees, and (G) inservices or training presented by the employee.

Continuing education can be obtained in a variety of ways. Certifying agencies (such as ASCP and NPA) and professional societies (such as ASCLS and NPA) provide opportunities to attend workshops and seminars (see Figure 14-5). In addition, manufacturers of phlebotomy and medical laboratory equipment often hold seminars, webinars, and workshops. Phlebotomists can also use the Internet to subscribe to learning modules or online tutorials provided by other continuing education providers (such as MediaLab and the Colorado Association for Continuing Medical Laboratory Education, Inc.). Online modules can be completed, scored, and sent to your certifying agency directly from your computer. Staff development programs are available at many healthcare facilities that provide additional continuing education opportunities. Staying current through education and membership in professional organizations is one way to strive for professional development.

Professional Development

Professional development refers to skills and knowledge attained for both personal development and career advancement. During training, students should strive to improve their knowledge and skills.

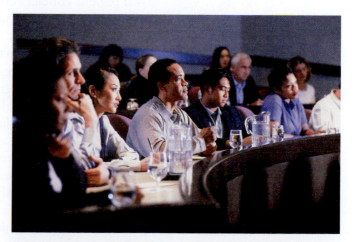

Figure 14-5 Participation in continuing education events provides healthcare workers the opportunity to stay current in their areas of specialty.

Appropriate training helps with transitioning into a job situation. Valuable knowledge and skills can be gained through volunteering prior to or in addition to clinical training, also called an **externship**, internship, or rotations.

During training and practice, phlebotomists must understand and work within their **scope of practice** (permitted procedures and processes).

Volunteer Programs

Volunteering (working without payment on behalf of others or a particular cause) is a rewarding experience. Even before beginning phlebotomy training, students can gain experience in a healthcare profession through volunteer work. Volunteers experience hands-on training and learn what it is like to assist patients who are ill, disabled, or frightened. Students may volunteer as an aide in a hospital, clinic, nursing home, or doctor's office or as a typist or filing clerk in a medical office or medical record room. These experiences may help students decide on a career as a phlebotomist or other healthcare professional. The American Red Cross also offers volunteer opportunities with its disaster relief programs locally, statewide, nationally, and abroad. As part of a disaster relief team at the site of a hurricane, tornado, storm, flood, earthquake, or fire, volunteers learn first-aid and emergency triage skills.

Red Cross volunteers gain valuable work experience that may help them obtain a job. Because volunteers are not paid, it is usually easy to find work opportunities. Just because you are not paid for volunteer work, however, does not mean the experience is not useful or meaningful for meeting your career goals. So be sure to include information about any volunteer work on your **résumé** (a document that summarizes your employment and educational history). Also, make sure to note specific duties, responsibilities, and skills you developed during the volunteer experience.

Continued Training

After becoming a phlebotomist, opportunities to advance your career are vast and include becoming a donor phlebotomist (a phlebotomist who can collect units of blood from donors for the blood bank), for which certification is also available. Phlebotomy is a good foundational skill for many healthcare professions. Some phlebotomists may want to become **multiskilled** or **cross-trained** (trained in more than one job function). Many hospitals and healthcare practices are embracing the idea of a multiskilled healthcare professional. There are two basic pathways for advancement: patient care or medical laboratory.

If patient contact is preferred, a phlebotomist may train to become a medical assistant, either certified (CMA) or registered (RMA). Advancement along this path can proceed from medical assisting to the nursing field, or phlebotomists may go directly into nursing and travel up the nursing ladder from licensed practical nurse (LPN) to registered nurse (RN) with either an associate's or a bachelor's degree.

Phlebotomists who decide to further their careers within the medical laboratory can follow the ladder of career progression from phlebotomy (PBT), to medical laboratory assistant (MLA), medical laboratory technician (MLT) with an associate's degree, and medical laboratory scientist (MLS) with a bachelor's degree or higher. Higher aspirations include laboratory management or pathologist's assistant (PA), and even specializing in pathology after completing medical school.

Phlebotomists may also advance into education. Teaching students who want to become phlebotomists can be very rewarding as you see them acquire skills and gain confidence. Some certifying agencies offer certification as a phlebotomy instructor. Table 14-4 lists agencies that offer phlebotomy instructor

TABLE 14-4 Advanced Certification for Phlebotomists

Agency	Advanced Certification Offered
American Academy of Phlebotomy Technicians (AAPT)	Phlebotomy Instructor
American Certification Agency (ACA)	Phlebotomy Instructor
	EKG Technician
	Patient Care Technician
American Medical Technologists (AMT)	Phlebotomy Instructor
American Society for Clinical Pathology (ASCP)	Donor Phlebotomy
	Point of Care Testing
American Society of Phlebotomy Technicians (ASPT)	Donor Phlebotomy
	Point of Care Testing
	Arterial Blood Gasses
	Drugs
National Center for Competency Testing (NCCT)	Post-Secondary Instructor
	Donor Phlebotomy
	ECG Technician
National Healthcareer Association (NHA)	Phlebotomy Instructor
National Phlebotomy Association (NPA)	Phlebotomy Instructor

certification as well as those agencies offering other types of advanced certification for which phlebotomists may be qualified after additional training.

Networking

Networking is building alliances, socially and professionally. It starts long before your job search. Networking is making contacts with relatives, friends, and acquaintances that may have information about how to find a job in your field. People in your network may be able to give you job leads or tell you about openings. By attending professional association meetings, conferences, or continuing education conferences, phlebotomists generate opportunities for employment as well as personal and professional growth.

Word-of-mouth referrals (finding job information by talking with other people) can be very helpful. Other people may be able to introduce you to or know people who work in your field. Networking is a valuable tool for advancing your career. Joining and being an active member of a professional society, such as the National Phlebotomy Association or American Society for Clinical Laboratory Science, is the easiest way to network. Attend local chapter meetings and talk with as many people as possible. Classmates are often also a good source of networking. It is important to build lasting friendships with classmates and keep in touch after graduation. Often, classmates will know of positions as they gain employment. Networking begins in the classroom and with friends and family.

1. Briefly describe the differences between certification, registration, and licensure.
2. Why is it important to participate in continuing education?

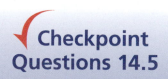

Checkpoint Questions 14.5

Chapter Summary

Learning Outcome	Key Concepts/Examples	Related NAACLS Competency
14.1 Model professional behavior and appearance. Pages 394–395.	Professionalism is demonstrated by the use of hard skills (job proficiency) and soft skills (personal characteristics and behavior).	9.6
14.2 Summarize healthcare diversity and professional communications. Pages 395–400.	• Respect for diversity in the workplace includes interacting appropriately and professionally in multicultural as well as interdisciplinary situations. • Phlebotomists must be aware of the potential for violation of patients' rights under HIPAA when involving family members in the patient's decision-making process.	9.00, 9.1, 9.2, 9.3
14.3 Discuss risk management and policies and protocol designed to avoid medicolegal problems. Pages 400–402.	Risk management policies and protocols are designed to avoid medicolegal complications and protect the employer, employee, patients, and visitors.	9.8
14.4 List the causes of stress in the workplace and discuss the coping skills used to deal with workplace stress. Pages 402–405.	Stress in the work environment is experienced and managed differently by each person. If stress is not kept under control, employees may experience burnout.	9.9
14.5 Recognize the different elements of the professional community of the phlebotomist. Pages 405–411.	• The professional community provides a means of support and professional growth for the phlebotomist. • Opportunities exist for networking, continuing education, and career advancement.	9.3

Chapter Review

A: Labeling

Explain what is recorded in each numbered area of this continuing education document.

Continuing Education Record

1 Name _____ 　 Position _____ Time Period _____
Facility _____ 　 Dept/Unit _____
Professional Organization Memberships (List Expiration Date)

	Attended	Expiration
2 CPR.................		
Yearly Safety Review...		
OSHA...............		
Competency Validation		
Age Related Competency		
Other.................		
....		

_____ **5**
_____
_____

Hospital Committee Memberships

_____
_____ **6**
_____
_____

3 Dept/Unit Meeting Attendance

Jan	Apr	July	Oct
Feb	May	Aug	Nov
Mar	June	Sept	Dec

Inservices Presented/Dept/Unit Projects

_____
_____
_____ **7**

Inservices / Seminars Attended

4

Date	Program Title	CEUs	Sponsor	Location

1. [LO 14.5] _____

2. [LO 14.5] _____

3. [LO 14.5] _____

4. [LO 14.5] _____

5. [LO 14.5] _____

6. [LO 14.5] _____

7. [LO 14.5] _____

B: Matching

Match these terms with their meanings.

_____ **8.** [LO 14.1] attributes

_____ **9.** [LO 14.4] burnout

_____ **10.** [LO 14.5] continuing education

_____ **11.** [LO 14.2] culture

_____ **12.** [LO 14.2] diversity

_____ **13.** [LO 14.2] interprofessional

_____ **14.** [LO 14.5] licensure

_____ **15.** [LO 14.3] malpractice

_____ **16.** [LO 14.2] multicultural

_____ **17.** [LO 14.5] multiskilled

_____ **18.** [LO 14.3] negligence

_____ **19.** [LO 14.1] professional

_____ **20.** [LO 14.5] registration

_____ **21.** [LO 14.3] risk management

_____ **22.** [LO 14.4] stress

a. depletion of energy after prolonged stress
b. enforced by a governmental agency
c. ethnic, religious, or social-economic background
d. failure to perform reasonably expected duties to patients
e. incorrect treatment of a patient by a healthcare worker
f. many different cultures
g. member of a vocation requiring specialized education
h. nonspecific response to change
i. placement on a list of a professional organization
j. post-professional training
k. protecting patients and employees from loss or injury
l. qualities that define a person
m. several different types of occupations
n. trained in more than one job function
o. variations of a category

C: Fill in the Blank

Write in the word(s) to complete the statement or answer the question.

23. [LO 14.2] The process of making changes to the beliefs and behavior of a minority group in response to the dominant culture is _____.

24. [LO 14.5] _____ is a process that ensures successful completion of defined academic and training requirements.

25. [LO 14.5] Training that phlebotomists receive in a clinical setting to become proficient is the _____.

26. [LO 14.1] Specific technical and operational proficiencies are part of a person's _____ skills.

27. [LO 14.1] _____ skills are a person's attributes or behaviors that enhance his or her interactions with others.

28. [LO 14.2] A(n) _____ is a commonly held belief about a specific group of people.

29. [LO 14.5] Building social and professional alliances is the purpose of _____.

30. [LO 14.5] A(n) _____ is a document that summarizes your employment and educational history.

D: Sequencing

Place the phases of burnout in the order in which they typically happen.

31. [LO 14.4] _____ Awakening Phase

32. [LO 14.4] _____ Brownout Phase

33. [LO 14.4] _____ Full-Scale Burnout Phase

34. [LO 14.4] _____ Honeymoon Phase

35. [LO 14.4] _____ Phoenix Phenomenon

E: Case Study/Critical Thinking

36. [LO 14.1] A phlebotomy supervisor received a complaint from a patient that the phlebotomist who collected her specimen never said a word after the initial identification process. Though the procedure went smoothly, the patient felt ignored. Explain what type of skills would be helpful while communicating with patients and how to use these skills.

37. [LO 14.2] While collecting specimens from a female patient, the phlebotomist realizes that the patient's husband insists on doing all the communicating. What may be the reason for this behavior, and how should the phlebotomist proceed?

38. [LO 14.3] A phlebotomist is asked to collect a venipuncture specimen from a patient whose specimen could not be obtained by another phlebotomist. What are the possible consequences for the employer if the phlebotomist performing the re-collection shares negative opinions about her co-worker with the patient?

39. [LO 14.4] During an exceptionally busy time at work, a co-worker begins to show signs of burnout. What self-care activities might you suggest to your co-worker to help her cope?

40. [LO 14.5] A student is interested in a career in healthcare but realizes that he does not know much about professions other than doctors and nurses. How might working as a volunteer at a local hospital assist this student with a career path choice?

F: Exam Prep

Choose the best answer for each question.

41. [LO 14.1] Professionalism (*Choose all that apply*)

a. is the same for every profession.

b. is model behavior for a specific line of work.

c. is a trait everyone is born with.

d. consists of hard and soft skills.

42. [LO 14.1] Hard skills (*Choose all that apply*)

a. require special training.

b. are specific job skills.

c. are behavior-based.

d. reflect attitudes.

43. [LO 14.2] *Diversity* refers to (*Choose all that apply*)

a. human cultural characteristics.

b. various types of plants and animals.

c. differences among industries.

d. the variety of healthcare jobs.

44. [LO 14.2] The term *culture* refers to (*Choose all that apply*)

a. ethnicity.

b. religious belief systems.

c. differences in hair color.

d. social-economic background.

45. [LO 14.2] Factors that influence individual beliefs include (*Choose all that apply*)

    a. family history.

    b. level of acculturation.

    c. place of upbringing.

    d. physical traits (such as eye and hair color).

46. [LO 14.2] Communication among people from different cultures is best when

    a. assumptions are made that the only differences are physical characteristics.

    b. people treat each other as they want to be treated.

    c. people understand that expectations might vary due to cultural differences.

    d. people base their communication style on perceived stereotypes.

47. [LO 14.2] When communicating with patients from cultures other than their own, phlebotomists should (*Choose all that apply*)

    a. treat everyone the same.

    b. adapt to each patient's needs.

    c. base their approach on stereotypes.

    d. not dictate; rather, they should provide choices.

48. [LO 14.2] Some people feel that they are being disrespectful if they

    a. answer questions using an interpreter.

    b. ask for clarification of a procedure.

    c. make direct eye contact with healthcare personnel.

    d. provide healthcare personnel with name and identification when asked.

49. [LO 14.2] Social customs that may not be observed by all cultures include (*Choose all that apply*)

    a. making eye contact while speaking.

    b. being on time for scheduled appointments.

    c. using titles and family names.

    d. being physically close when speaking.

50. [LO 14.3] In a malpractice lawsuit, the burden of proof is on the

    a. employee.

    b. employer.

    c. lawyer.

    d. patient.

51. [LO 14.3] Actions that will help prevent liability include (*Choose all that apply*)

    a. making negative comments about the phlebotomist who left a bruise on a patient's arm.

    b. agreeing with the patient that a procedure seems unnecessary.

    c. holding all patient complaints in confidence and not disclosing this information to supervisors.

    d. documenting any variances in the delivery of quality healthcare.

52. [LO 14.4] Stress is caused by (*Choose all that apply*)

    a. a feeling of being under pressure.

    b. a reaction to anger expressed by a patient.

    c. frustration at work or at home.

    d. a change from the daily routine.

53. [LO 14.4] The Awakening Phase of burnout produces (*Choose all that apply*)

    a. feelings of enthusiasm.

    b. realization of unrealistic expectations.

    c. satisfaction with a job.

    d. confusion and boredom.

54. [LO 14.4] When feeling stressed at work, the best thing to do is grab a snack that is (*Choose all that apply*)

    a. high in caffeine, such as a cup of coffee.

    b. high in salt, such as potato chips.

    c. high in sugar and fat, such as a candy bar.

    d. healthful, such as fresh fruit or yogurt.

55. [LO 14.5] Certification usually indicates that a phlebotomist has (*Choose all that apply*)

    a. successfully completed a weekend short course.

    b. passed a nationally recognized examination.

    c. paid the fees required by the state in which he or she lives.

    d. fulfilled the requirements of a structured program.

56. [LO 14.5] Education that occurs after a healthcare professional's initial certification training is called

    a. career education.

    b. continuing education.

    c. degreed education.

    d. supplemental education.

57. [LO 14.5] The career path a phlebotomist may take in the area of nursing includes all of these EXCEPT

   a. MA.

   b. CNA.

   c. RN.

   d. MLS.

58. [LO 14.5] Networking involves making contacts with *(Choose all that apply)*

   a. relatives and friends.

   b. classmates and co-workers.

   c. acquaintances within professional organizations.

   d. acquaintances at other healthcare institutions.

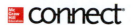

Enhance your learning by completing these exercises and more at connect.mheducation.com

References

American Academy of Phlebotomy Technicians. (2013). *Phlebotomy technician (CPT)*. Retrieved September 19, 2013, from www.aaopt.net/certification/phlebotomy-technician-cpt/

American Certification Agency. (n.d.). *Application for certification*. Retrieved June 28, 2011, from www.acacert.com/applications.htm

American Medical Technologists. (2011). *Phlebotomist certification*. Retrieved June 28, 2011, from www.americanmedtech.org/Certification/Phlebotomist.aspx

American Society of Clinical Pathologists. (2011). *Certification*. Retrieved June 28, 2011, from www.ascp.org/FunctionalNavigation/certification.aspx

American Society of Phlebotomy Technicians. (2009). *Phlebotomy certification*. Retrieved June 28, 2011, from www.aspt.org/phlebotomy.html

Bureau of Labor and Statistics. (2014). *Occupational outlook handbook: Phlebotomists*. Retrieved April 7, 2014, from www.bls.gov/ooh/healthcare/phlebotomists.htm

Cultural Diversity in Nursing. (2012). *Cultural competence*. Retrieved February 15, 2014, from www.culturediversity.org/cultcomp.htm

Larson, B. (2002). *Good stress, bad stress: An indispensable guide to identifying and managing your stress*. Jackson, TN. Da Capo Press.

Miller, L, & Dell Smith, A. (1993). *The stress solution: An action plan to manage the stress in your life*. New York, NY. Pocket Books.

National Accrediting Agency for Clinical Laboratory Sciences. (2010). NAACLS *entry-level phlebotomist competencies*. Rosemont, IL. NAACLS.

National Center for Competency Testing. (2011). *Certification information*. Retrieved June 28, 2011, from www.ncctinc.com/Certifications/

National Healthcareer Association. (n.d.). *Phlebotomy technician certification*. Retrieved June 28, 2011, from www.nhanow.com/phlebotomy-technician.aspx

National Phlebotomy Association. (2011). *Who we are*. Retrieved June 28, 2011, from www.nationalphlebotomy.org

Office of Minority Health. (n.d.). *National CLAS standards*. Accessed February 15, 2014, from http://minorityhealth.hhs.gov

Salimbene, S. (2005). *What language does your patient hurt in?* (2nd ed.). St. Paul, MN. EMC Paradigm.

Spector, R. E. (2009). *Cultural diversity in health and illness* (7th ed.). Upper Saddle River, NJ. Pearson Prentice Hall.

UNAIDS. (2009). *Preventing career burnout: Inter-mission care and rehabilitation society*. New York. WHO.

COMPETENCY CHECKLIST: PATIENT COMMUNICATION

Procedure Steps	Practice			Performed		Master
	1	2	3	Yes	No	Master
Preprocedure						
1. Identifies the patient with a smile.						
2. Introduces self and explains procedure.						
Procedure						
3. Identifies sources of anxiety, anger, or lack of understanding.						
4. Remains calm and demonstrates respect to patient throughout interaction.						
5. Listens attentively and with an open mind.						
6. Obtains assistance through interpreter if needed.						
7. Leaves room if feels threatened or patient becomes violent.						
8. Notifies supervisor or other staff if assistance is needed.						
Postprocedure						
9. Completes the specimen collection or notifies supervisor of patient refusal.						

COMMENTS: _____
_____
_____
_____

SIGNED

EVALUATOR: _____
STUDENT: _____

Appendix A

Standard Precautions*

Standard Precautions are the minimum infection prevention practices that apply to all patient care, regardless of the suspected or confirmed infection status of the patient, in any setting where healthcare is delivered. These practices are designed to both protect healthcare personnel (HCP) and prevent HCP from spreading infections among patients.

Standard Precautions apply to (1) blood; (2) all body fluids, secretions, and excretions, except sweat, regardless of whether or not it contains visible blood; (3) nonintact skin; and (4) mucous membranes. OSHA defines other potentially infectious materials (OPIM) as

- human body fluids: semen, vaginal secretions, cerebrospinal fluid, synovial fluid, pleural fluid, pericardial fluid, peritoneal fluid, amniotic fluid, saliva in dental procedures, any body fluid that is visibly contaminated with blood, and all body fluids in situations where it is difficult or impossible to differentiate between body fluids
- any unfixed tissue or organ (other than intact skin) from a human (living or dead)
- HIV-containing cell or tissue cultures, organ cultures, and HIV- or HBV-containing culture medium or other solutions; and blood, organs, or other tissues from experimental animals infected with HIV or HBV

Standard precautions are designed to reduce the risk of transmission of microorganisms from both recognized and unrecognized sources of infection in healthcare facilities. Standard Precautions are used for the care of all patients, regardless of their diagnosis or presumed infection status.

Standard Precautions include (1) hand hygiene, (2) use of personal protective equipment (e.g., gloves, gowns, masks), (3) safe injection practices, (4) safe handling of potentially contaminated equipment or surfaces in the patient environment, and (5) respiratory hygiene/cough etiquette.

Hand Hygiene

Key situations where hand hygiene should be performed include

- before touching a patient, even if gloves will be worn
- before exiting the patient's care area after touching the patient or the patient's immediate environment
- after contact with blood, body fluids or excretions, or wound dressings
- prior to performing an aseptic task (e.g., placing an IV, preparing an injection)
- if hands will be moving from a contaminated-body site to a clean-body site during patient care
- after glove removal

Use soap and water when hands are visibly soiled (e.g., blood, body fluids) or after caring for patients with known or suspected infectious diarrhea (e.g., *Clostridium difficile*, norovirus). Otherwise, the preferred method of hand decontamination is with an alcohol-based hand rub.

Personal Protective Equipment (PPE)

Personal protective equipment (PPE) refers to a variety of barriers and respirators used alone or in combination to protect mucous membranes, airways, skin, and clothing from contact with infectious agents. Gloves, gowns, and face protection are the most common forms of PPE. The selection of PPE is based on the nature of the patient interaction and/or the likely mode(s) of transmission.

Gloves

Wear gloves (clean, nonsterile gloves are adequate) when touching blood, body fluids, secretions, excretions, and contaminated items. Put on clean gloves just before touching mucous membranes and nonintact skin. Change gloves between tasks and procedures

---

*Information adapted from the following: *Guide to Infection Prevention for Outpatient Settings: Minimum Expectations for Safe Care* (www.cdc.gov); *Occupational Safety and Health Administration Bloodborne Pathogens—1910.1030* (www.osha.gov); *2007 Guidelines for Isolation Precautions: Preventing Transmission of Infectious Agents in Healthcare Settings* (www.cdc.gov).

on the same patient after contact with material that may contain a high concentration of microorganisms. Do not wear the same pair of gloves for the care of more than one patient. Do not wash gloves for the purpose of reuse. Remove gloves promptly after use, before touching noncontaminated items and environmental surfaces, and before going to another patient. Wash hands immediately to avoid transfer of microorganisms to other patients or environments.

Gowns

Wear a gown (a clean, nonsterile gown is adequate) to protect skin and to prevent soiling of clothing during procedures and patient-care activities that are likely to generate splashes or sprays of blood, body fluids, secretions, or excretions. Select a gown that is appropriate for the activity and the amount of fluid likely to be encountered. Remove a soiled gown as promptly as possible and wash hands to avoid transfer of microorganisms to other patients or environments. Do not wear the same gown for the care of more than one patient.

Face Protection

Wear a mask and eye protection or a face shield to protect the mucous membranes of the eyes, nose, and mouth during procedures and patient-care activities that are likely to generate splashes or sprays of blood, body fluids, secretions, and excretions.

Remove and discard all PPE before leaving the patient's room or area.

Safe Injection Practices

Injection safety includes practices intended to prevent transmission of infectious diseases between one patient and another, or between a patient and a healthcare provider during preparation and administration of parenteral medications. Although phlebotomists do not administer medications, they do use sharps. Two key recommendations of this standard are appropriate to a phlebotomist:

- Dispose of used syringes and needles at the point of use in a sharps container that is closable, puncture-resistant, and leak-proof.
- Adhere to federal and state requirements for protection of HCP from exposure to bloodborne pathogens.

OSHA defines work practice controls related to the use of sharps and the prevention of transmission of bloodborne pathogens that are federal requirements.

These controls require HCP to take care to prevent injuries when using needles, scalpels, and other sharp instruments or devices; when handling sharp instruments after procedures; when cleaning used instruments; and when disposing of used needles. The guidelines state the following:

- Never recap used needles, or otherwise manipulate them using both hands, or use any other technique that involves directing the point of a needle toward any part of the body.
- Use either a one-handed "scoop" technique or a mechanical device designed for holding the needle sheath.
- Do not remove used needles from disposable syringes by hand and do not bend, break, or otherwise manipulate used needles by hand.
- Place used disposable syringes and needles, scalpel blades, and other sharp items in appropriate puncture-resistant containers, which are located as close as practical to the area in which the items were used.
- Place reusable syringes and needles in a puncture-resistant container for transport to the reprocessing area.

Patient Environment

Handle used patient-care equipment soiled with blood, body fluids, secretions, and excretions in a manner that prevents skin and mucous membrane exposures, contamination of clothing, and transfer of microorganisms to other patients and environments. Ensure that reusable equipment is not used for the care of another patient until it has been cleaned and reprocessed appropriately. See that single-use items are discarded properly.

Verify that the healthcare facility has adequate procedures for the routine care, cleaning, and disinfection of environmental surfaces, beds, bedrails, bedside equipment, and other frequently touched surfaces and ensure that these procedures are being followed.

Use mouthpieces, resuscitation bags, or other ventilation devices as an alternative to mouth-to-mouth resuscitation methods in areas where the need for resuscitation is predictable.

Place a patient who contaminates the environment or who does not (or cannot be expected to) assist in maintaining appropriate hygiene or environmental control in a private room. If a private room is not available, consult with infection control professionals regarding patient placement or other alternatives.

Respiratory Hygiene/Cough Etiquette

Implement measures to contain respiratory secretions in patients and accompanying individuals who have signs and symptoms of a respiratory infection, beginning at point of entry to the facility and continuing throughout the duration of the visit.

- Post signs at entrances with instructions to patients with symptoms of respiratory infection to
  - cover their mouths/noses when coughing or sneezing
  - use and dispose of tissues
  - perform hand hygiene after hands have been in contact with respiratory secretion

- Provide tissues and no-touch receptacles for disposal of tissues.
- Provide resources for performing hand hygiene in or near waiting areas.
- Offer masks to coughing patients and other symptomatic persons upon entry to the facility.
- Provide space and encourage persons with symptoms of respiratory infections to sit as far away from others as possible. If available, facilities may wish to place these patients in a separate area while waiting for care.

Educate all health care personnel on the importance of infection prevention measures to contain respiratory secretions to prevent the spread of respiratory pathogens when examining and caring for patients with signs and symptoms of a respiratory infection.

Appendix B

Transmission-Based Precautions*

Transmission-Based Precautions (i.e., Airborne Precautions, Droplet Precautions, and Contact Precautions) are recommended to provide additional precautions beyond Standard Precautions to interrupt the transmission of pathogens in hospitals.

Transmission-Based Precautions can be used for patients who are known or suspected to be infected or colonized with epidemiologically important pathogens that can be transmitted by airborne or droplet transmission or by contact with dry skin or contaminated surfaces. These precautions should be used in addition to Standard Precautions:

- Airborne Precautions are used for infections spread in small particles in the air such as chicken pox.
- Droplet Precautions are used for infections spread in large droplets by coughing, talking, or sneezing such as influenza.
- Contact Precautions are used for infections spread by skin-to-skin contact or contact with other surfaces such as herpes simplex virus.

Airborne Precautions, Droplet Precautions, and Contact Precautions may be combined for diseases that have multiple routes of transmission. Whether used singularly or in combination, they are always implemented in addition to Standard Precautions.

Contact Precautions

Contact Precautions are intended to prevent transmission of infectious agents, including important microorganisms, that are spread by direct or indirect contact with the patient or the patient's environment. Contact Precautions are required for patients infected or colonized with multidrug-resistant organisms. Contact Precautions also apply where the presence of excessive wound drainage, fecal incontinence, or other discharges from the body suggest an increased potential for extensive environmental contamination and risk of transmission. A single-patient room is preferred for patients who require Contact Precautions. When a single-patient room is not available, consultation with infection control personnel is recommended to assess the various risks

associated with other patient placement options (e.g., cohorting, keeping the patient with an existing roommate). In multipatient rooms, at least 3 feet of spatial separation between beds is advised to reduce the opportunities for inadvertent sharing of items between the infected/colonized patient and other patients. Healthcare personnel caring for patients on Contact Precautions wear a gown and gloves for all interactions that may involve contact with the patient or potentially contaminated areas in the patient's environment. Healthcare personnel don PPE before entering the patient's room and discard it before exiting the room. This is done to contain pathogens, especially those that are transmitted through environmental contamination, such as vancomycin-resistant enterococci, *C. difficile*, noroviruses, and other intestinal tract pathogens.

Droplet Precautions

Droplet Precautions are intended to prevent transmission of pathogens spread through respiratory or mucous membrane contact with the respiratory secretions of an infected person. Because these pathogens do not remain infectious over long distances in a healthcare facility, special air handling and ventilation are not required to prevent droplet transmission. Infectious agents for which Droplet Precautions are indicated include *pertussis*, influenza virus, adenovirus, rhinovirus, *N. meningitides*, and group A *Streptococcus* (for the first 24 hours of antimicrobial therapy). A single-patient room is preferred for patients who require Droplet Precautions. When a single-patient room is not available, consultation with infection control personnel is recommended to assess the various risks associated with other patient placement options (e.g., cohorting, keeping the patient with an existing roommate). Spatial separation of at least 3 feet and drawing the curtain between patient beds are especially important for patients in multibed rooms with infections transmitted by the droplet route. Healthcare personnel wear a mask (a respirator is not necessary) for close contact with infectious patients; the mask is generally donned upon room entry. Patients on Droplet

*Adapted from Centers for Disease Control Guidelines for Isolation Precautions 2007 (www.cdc.gov).

Precautions who must be transported outside the room should wear a mask, if tolerated, and follow Respiratory Hygiene/Cough Etiquette.

Airborne Precautions

Airborne Precautions prevent transmission of infectious agents that remain infectious over long distances when suspended in the air (e.g., rubeola virus [measles], varicella virus [chickenpox], *M. tuberculosis*, and possibly SARS-CoV). The preferred placement for patients who require Airborne Precautions is in an airborne infection isolation room (AIIR). An AIIR is a single-patient room that is equipped with special air handling and ventilation capacity that meet the American Institute of Architects/Facility Guidelines Institute (AIA/FGI) standards for AIIRs. Some states require the availability of such rooms in hospitals, emergency departments, and nursing homes that care for patients with M. tuberculosis. A respiratory protection program that includes education about use of respirators, fit-testing, and user seal checks is required in any facility with AIIRs. In settings where Airborne Precautions cannot be implemented due to limited engineering resources (e.g., physician offices), masking the patient, placing the patient in a private room (e.g., office examination room) with the door closed, and providing N95 or higher-level respirators or masks if respirators are not available for healthcare personnel will reduce the likelihood of airborne transmission until the patient is either transferred to a facility with an AIIR or returned to the home environment, as deemed medically appropriate. Healthcare personnel caring for patients on Airborne Precautions wear a mask or respirator mask that is donned prior to room entry. Whenever possible, non-immune healthcare workers should not care for patients with vaccine-preventable airborne diseases (e.g., measles, chickenpox, and smallpox).

Applications of Transmission-Based Precautions

Diagnosis of many infections requires laboratory confirmation. Since laboratory tests, especially those that depend on culture techniques, often require 2 or more days for completion, Transmission-Based Precautions must be implemented while test results are pending based on the clinical presentation and likely pathogens. Use of appropriate Transmission-Based Precautions at the time a patient develops symptoms or signs of transmissible infection, or arrives at a healthcare facility for care, reduces transmission opportunities.

Discontinuation of Transmission-Based Precautions

Transmission-Based Precautions remain in effect for limited periods of time (i.e., while the risk for transmission of the infectious agent persists or for the duration of the illness). For some diseases (e.g., pharyngeal or cutaneous diphtheria, RSV), Transmission-Based Precautions remain in effect until culture or antigen-detection test results document eradication of the pathogen and, for RSV, symptomatic disease is resolved. For other diseases (e.g., *M. tuberculosis*), state laws and regulations, and healthcare facility policies, may dictate the duration of precautions. In immunocompromised patients, viral shedding can persist for prolonged periods of time (many weeks to months) and transmission to others may occur during that time; therefore, the duration of contact and/or droplet precautions may be prolonged for many weeks.

Application of Transmission-Based Precautions in Ambulatory and Home Care Settings

Transmission-Based Precautions apply in all healthcare settings; however, the environment dictates changes. For example, in home care, AIIRs are not available. Typically family members already exposed to diseases such as varicella and tuberculosis would not use masks or respiratory protection, but visiting phlebotomists or other healthcare workers would need to use such protection. Similarly, management of patients colonized or infected with multidrug-resistant organisms may necessitate Contact Precautions in acute-care hospitals and in some long-term care facilities when there is continued transmission, but the risk of transmission in ambulatory care and home care has not been well defined. Consistent use of Standard Precautions is essential. In ambulatory care centers, screening for potentially infectious symptomatic and asymptomatic individuals is necessary at the start of the initial patient encounter.

Appendix C

Prefixes, Suffixes, and Word Roots in Commonly Used Medical Terms

Prefixes

a-, an- without, not

ab- from, away

ad- `to, toward

ambi-, amph-, amphi- both, on both sides, around

ante- before

antero- in front of

anti- against, opposing

auto- self

bi- twice, double

brachy- short

brady- slow

cata- down, lower, under

centi- hundred

cephal- head

chol-, chole-, cholo- gall, bile

chromo- color

circum- around

co-, com-, con- together, with

contra- against

cryo- cold

de- down, from

deca- ten

deci- tenth

demi- half

dextro- to the right

di- double, twice

dia- through, apart, between

dipla-, diplo- double, twin

dis- apart, away from

dys- difficult, painful, bad, abnormal

e-, ec-, ecto- away, from, without, outside

em-, en- in, into, inside

endo- within, inside

ento- within, inner

epi- on, above

erythro- red

eu- good

ex-, exo- outside of, beyond, without

extra- outside of, beyond, in addition

fore- before, in front of

gyn-, gyno-, gyne-, gyneco- woman, female

hemi- half

hetero- other, unlike

homeo-, homo- same, like

hyper- above, over, increased, excessive

hypo- below, under, decreased

idio- personal, self-produced

im-, in-, ir- not

in- in, into

infra- beneath

inter- between, among

intra-, intro- into, within, during

juxta- near, nearby

kata-, kath- down, lower, under

kineto- motion

leuco-, leuko- white

levo- to the left

macro- large, long

mal- bad

mega-, megalo- large, great

meio- contraction

melan-, melano- black

mes-, meso- middle

meta- beyond

micro- small

mio- smaller, less

mono- single, one

multi- many

neo- new

non-, not- no

nulli- none

ob- against

olig-, oligo- few, less than normal

ortho- straight

oxy- sharp, acid

pachy- thick

pan- all, every

par-, para- alongside of, with; woman who has given birth

per- through, excessive

peri- around

pes- foot

pluri- more, several

pneo- breathing

poly- many, much

post- after, behind

pre-, pro- before, in front of

presby-, presbyo- old age

primi- first

pseudo- false

quadri- four

re- back, again

retro- backward, behind

semi- half

steno- contracted, narrow

stereo- firm, solid, three-dimensional

sub- under

super-, supra- above, upon, excess

sym-, syn-   with, together
tachy-   fast
tele-   distant, far
tetra-   four
tomo-   incision, section
trans-   across
tri-   three
tropho-   nutrition, growth
ultra-   beyond, excess
uni-   one
veni-   vein
xanth-, xantho-   yellow

Suffixes

-ad   to, toward
-aesthesia, -esthesia   sensation
-al   characterized by
-algia   pain
-ase   enzyme
-asthenia   weakness
-cele   swelling, tumor
-centesis   puncture, tapping
-cidal   killing
-cide   causing death
-cise   cut
-coele   cavity
-cyst   bladder, bag
-cyte   cell, cellular
-dynia   pain
-ectomy   cutting out, surgical removal
-emesis   vomiting
-emia   blood
-esthesia   sensation
-form   shape
-fuge   driving away
-gene, -genic, -genetic, -genesis, -genous   arising from, origin, formation
-gram   recorded information
-graph   instrument for recording
-graphy   the process of recording

-ia   condition
-iasis   condition of
-ic, -ical   pertaining to
-ism   condition, process, theory
-itis   inflammation of
-ium   membrane
-ize   to cause to be, to become, to treat by special method
-kinesis, -kinetic   motion
-lepsis, -lepsy   seizure, convulsion
-lith   stone
-logy   science of, study of
-lysis   setting free, disintegration, decomposition
-malacia   abnormal softening
-mania   insanity, abnormal desire
-meter   measure
-metry   process of measuring
-odynia   pain
-oid   resembling
-ole   small, little
-oma   tumor
-opia   vision
-opsy   to view
-osis   disease, condition of
-ostomy   to make a mouth, opening
-otomy   incision, surgical cutting
-ous   having
-pathy   disease, suffering
-penia   too few, lack, decreased
-pexy   surgical fixation
-phagia, -phage   eating, consuming, swallowing
-phobia   fear, abnormal fear
-phylaxis   protection
-plasia   formation or development
-plastic   molded
-plasty   operation to reconstruct, surgical repair

-plegia   paralysis
-pnea   breathing
-rrhage, -rrhagia   abnormal or excessive discharge, hemorrhage, flow
-rrhaphy   suture of
-rrhea   flow, discharge
-sclerosis   hardening
-scope   instrument used to examine
-scopy   examining
-sepsis   poisoning, infection
-spasm   cramp or twitching
-stasis   stoppage
-stomy   opening
-therapy   treatment
-thermy   heat
-tome   cutting instrument
-tomy   incision, section
-tripsy   surgical crushing
-trophy   nutrition, growth
-tropy   turning, tendency
-uria   urine

Word Roots

adeno-   gland, glandular
adipo-   fat
aero-   air
andr-, andro-   man, male
angio-   blood vessel
ano-   anus
arterio-   artery
arthro-   joint
bili-   bile
bio-   life
blasto-, blast-   developing stage, bud
bracheo-   arm
broncho-   bronchial (windpipe)
carcino-   cancer
cardio-   heart
cerebr-, cerebro-   brain
cephalo-   head
cervico-   neck

chondro- cartilage

chromo- color

colo- colon

colp-, colpo- vagina

coro- body

cost-, costo- rib

crani-, cranio- skull

cysto- bladder, bag

cyto- cell, cellular

dacry-, dacryo- tears, lacrimal apparatus

dactyl-, dactylo- finger, toe

dent-, denti-, dento- teeth

derma-, dermat-, dermato- skin

dorsi-, dorso- back

encephalo- brain

entero- intestine

esthesio- sensation

fibro- connective tissue

galact-, galacto- milk

gastr-, gastro- stomach

gingiv- gums

glosso- tongue

gluco-, glyco- sugar, sweet

gravid-, gravida- pregnant female

haemo-, hemato-, hem-, hemo- blood

hepa-, hepar-, hepato- liver

herni- rupture

hidro- sweat (perspiration)

histo- tissue

hydra-, hydro- water

hyster-, hystero- uterus

ictero- jaundice

ileo- ileum

karyo- nucleus, nut

kera-, kerato- horn, hardness, cornea

lact- milk

laparo- abdomen

latero- side

linguo- tongue

lipo- fat

lith- stone

lobo- lobe

mast-, masto- breast

med-, medi- middle

mening- meninges (covers the brain)

metro-, metra- uterus

my-, myo- muscle

myel-, myelo- marrow

narco- sleep

nas-, naso- nose

necro- dead

nephr-, nephro- kidney

neu-, neuro- nerve

niter-, nitro- nitrogen

nucleo- nucleus

oculo- eye

odont- tooth

omphalo- navel, umbilicus

onco- tumor

oo- ovum, egg

oophor- ovary

ophthalmo- eye

orchid- testicle

os- mouth, opening

oste-, osteo- bone

oto- ear

palpebro- eyelid

path-, patho- disease, suffering

pedo- child

pepso- digestion

phag-, phago- eating, consuming, swallowing

pharyng-, pharyngo- throat, pharynx

phlebo- vein

pleuro- side, rib

pneumo- air, lungs

pod- foot

procto- rectum

psych- the mind

pulmon-, pulmono- lung

pyelo- pelvis (renal)

pyo- pus

pyro- fever, heat

reni-, reno- kidney

rhino- nose

sacchar- sugar

sacro- sacrum

salpingo- tube, fallopian tube

sarco- flesh

sclero- hard, sclera

septi-, septic-, septico- poison, infection

stomato- mouth

teno-, tenoto- tendon

thermo- heat

thio- sulfa

thoraco- chest

thrombo- blood clot

thyro- thyroid gland

tricho- hair

urino-, uro- urine, urinary organs

utero- uterus, uterine

uvulo- uvula

vagin- vagina

vaso- vessel

ventri-, ventro- abdomen

vesico- blister

Appendix D

Abbreviations and Symbols Commonly Used in Medical Notations

Abbreviations

a before

$\overline{\text{aa}}$, $\overline{\text{AA}}$ of each

ABGs arterial blood gases

a.c. before meals

ADD attention deficit disorder

ADL activities of daily living

ad lib as desired

ADT admission, discharge, transfer

AIDS acquired immunodeficiency syndrome

AKA above knee amputation

a.m.a. against medical advice

AMA American Medical Association

amp. ampule

amt amount

aq., AQ water; aqueous

ASHD atherosclerotic heart disease

ausc. auscultation

ax axis

Bib, bib drink

b.i.d., bid, BID twice a day

BKA below knee amputation

BM bowel movement

BP, B/P blood pressure

BPC blood pressure check

BPH benign prostatic hypertrophy

bpm beats per minute

BSA body surface area

$\overline{\text{c}}$ with

Ca, CA calcium; cancer

CABG coronary artery bypass graft

cap, caps capsules

CBC complete blood (cell) count

C.C., CC chief complaint

CDC Centers for Disease Control and Prevention

CHF congestive heart failure

chr chronic

cm centimeter

CNS central nervous system

Comp, comp compound

COPD chronic obstructive pulmonary disease

CP chest pain

CPE complete physical examination

CPR cardiopulmonary resuscitation

CSF cerebrospinal fluid

CT computed tomography

CV cardiovascular

CVA cerebrovascular accident

CXR chest X-ray

d day

D&C dilation and curettage

DEA Drug Enforcement Administration

Dil, dil dilute

DM diabetes mellitus

DNR do not resuscitate

DOB date of birth

Dr. doctor

DTaP diphtheria-tetanus-acellular pertussis vaccine

DTs delirium tremens

DVT deep venous thrombosis

D/W dextrose in water

Dx, dx diagnosis

ECG, EKG electrocardiogram

ED emergency department

EEG electroencephalogram

EENT eyes, ears, nose, and throat

EP established patient

ER emergency room

ESR erythrocyte sedimentation rate

FBS fasting blood sugar

FDA Food and Drug Administration

FH family history

Fl, fl , fld fluid

fl oz fluid ounce

F/u follow-up

FUO fever of unknown origin

Fx fracture

g gram

GBS gallbladder series

GI gastrointestinal

Gm, gm gram

gr grain

gt, gtt drop, drops

GTT glucose tolerance test

GU genitourinary

GYN gynecology

HA headache

HB, Hgb hemoglobin

hct hematocrit

HEENT head, ears, eyes, nose, throat

HIV human immunodeficiency virus

HO   history of
HPI   history of present illness
HPV   human papillomavirus
Hx   history
ICU   intensive care unit
I&D   incision and drainage
IDDM   insulin-dependent diabetes mellitus
IM   intramuscular
inf.   infusion; inferior
inj   injection
I&O   intake and output
IT   inhalation therapy
IUD   intrauterine device
IV   intravenous
KUB   kidneys, ureters, bladder
L   liter
L1, L2, etc.   lumbar vertebrae
lab   laboratory
lb   pound
liq   liquid
LLE   left lower extremity (left leg)
LLL   left lower lobe
LLQ   left lower quadrant
LMP   last menstrual period
LUE   left upper extremity (left arm)
LUQ   left upper quadrant
m   meter
M   mix (Latin *misce*)
mcg   microgram
mg   milligram
MI   myocardial infarction
mL   milliliter
mm   millimeter
MM   mucous membrane
mmHg   millimeters of mercury
MRI   magnetic resonance imaging
MS   multiple sclerosis
NB   newborn
NED   no evidence of disease

NIDDM   noninsulin-dependent diabetes mellitus
NKA   no known allergies
no, #   number
noc, noct   night
npo, NPO   nothing by mouth
NPT   new patient
NS   normal saline
NSAID   nonsteroidal anti-inflammatory drug
NTP   normal temperature and pressure
N&V, N/V   nausea and vomiting
NYD   not yet diagnosed
OB   obstetrics
OC   oral contraceptive
oint   ointment
OOB   out of bed
OPD   outpatient department
OPS   outpatient services
OR   operating room
OT   occupational therapy
OTC   over-the-counter
oz   ounce
p̄   after
PA   posteroanterior
Pap   Pap smear
Path   pathology
p.c., pc   after meals
PE   physical examination
per   by, with
PH   past history
PID   pelvic inflammatory disease
PMFSH   past medical, family, social history
PMS   premenstrual syndrome
po   by mouth
p/o   postoperative
POMR   problem-oriented medical record
P&P   Pap smear (Papanicolaou smear) and pelvic examination

p.r.n., prn, PRN   whenever necessary
pt   pint
Pt   patient
PT   physical therapy
PTA   prior to admission
pulv   powder
PVC   premature ventricular contraction
q.   every
q2, q2h   every 2 hours
q.a.m., qam   every morning
q.h., qh   every hour
qns, QNS   quantity not sufficient
qs, QS   quantity sufficient
qt   quart
RA   rheumatoid arthritis; right atrium
RBC   red blood cells; red blood (cell) count
RDA   recommended dietary allowance, recommended daily allowance
REM   rapid eye movement
RF   rheumatoid factor
RLE   right lower extremity (right leg)
RLL   right lower lobe
RLQ   right lower quadrant
R/O   rule out
ROM   range of motion
ROS/SR   review of systems/ systems review
RUE   right upper extremity (right arm)
RUQ   right upper quadrant
RV   right ventricle
Rx   prescription, take
s̄   without
SAD   seasonal affective disorder
SIDS   sudden infant death syndrome
sig   sigmoidoscopy
Sig   directions

SL   sublingual

SOAP   subjective, objective, assessment, plan

SOB   shortness of breath

sol   solution

S/R   suture removal

Staph   staphylococcus

stat, STAT   immediately

STI   sexually transmitted infection

Strep   streptococcus

subcu, subcut   subcutaneous

subling   sublingual

surg   surgery

S/W   saline in water

SX   symptoms

T1, T2, etc.   thoracic vertebrae

T&A   tonsillectomy and adenoidectomy

tab   tablet

TB   tuberculosis

tbs., tbsp   tablespoon

TIA   transient ischemic attack

t.i.d., tid, TID   three times a day

tinc, tinct, tr   tincture

TMJ   temporomandibular joint

top   topically

TPR   temperature, pulse, and respiration

TSH   thyroid stimulating hormone

tsp   teaspoon

Tx   treatment

U   unit

UA   urinalysis

UCHD   usual childhood diseases

UGI   upper gastrointestinal

ung, ungt   ointment

URI   upper respiratory infection

US   ultrasound

UTI   urinary tract infection

VA   visual acuity

VD   venereal disease

VF   visual field

VS   vital signs

WBC   white blood cells; white blood (cell) count

WNL   within normal limits

wt   weight

y/o   year old

Symbols

Weights and Measures

\#   pounds

°   degrees

′   foot; minute

″   inch; second

mEq   milliequivalent

mL   milliliter

dL   deciliter

mg%   milligrams percent; milligrams per 100 mL

Mathematical Functions and Terms

\#   number

+   plus; positive; acid reaction

−   minus; negative; alkaline reaction

±   plus or minus; either positive or negative; indefinite

×   multiply; magnification; crossed with, hybrid

÷, /   divided by

=   equal to

≈   approximately equal to

>   greater than; from which is derived

<   less than; derived from

$\nleq$ not less than

$\ngeq$ not greater than

≤   equal to or less than

≥   equal to or greater than

≠   not equal to

√   square root

$\sqrt[3]{\ }$ cube root

∞   infinity

:   ratio; "is to"

∴   therefore

%   percent

π   pi (3.14159)—the ratio of circumference of a circle to its diameter

Chemical Notations

Δ   change; heat

⇌   reversible reaction

↑   increase

↓   decrease

Warnings

Ⓒ   Schedule I controlled substance

Ⓒ   Schedule II controlled substance

Ⓒ   Schedule III controlled substance

Ⓒ   Schedule IV controlled substance

Ⓒ   Schedule V controlled substance

☠   poison

☢   radiation

☣   biohazard

Others

℞   prescription; take

□, ♂   male

○, ♀   female

†   one

††   two

†††   three

Appendix E

Medical Laboratory Tests

TABLE E-1 Alphabetical Listing of Blood Tests (partial list)

Lab Test	Abbreviation (may vary by laboratory)	Specimen Requirement (specimen requirements vary by laboratory method)	Tube Cap Colors (BD product)	Laboratory Section
ABO group & Rh type	ABO&Rh	EDTA; special patient identification and banding	pink, lavender	Blood Bank
Acetone		SST, keep on ice	gold	Chemistry
Acid-fast bacillus (in blood culture)	AFB	Blood culture bottles, or yellow-SPS tubes	yellow	Microbiology
Acid phosphatase (prostatic form)	ACP	SST or nonadditive; centrifuge, separate, and freeze	gold, red	Chemistry
Adrenocorticotropic hormone	ACTH	EDTA; centrifuge, separate, and freeze	purple	Chemistry
Alanine transferase	ALT	SST or PST; centrifuge, separate, and refrigerate	gold, green	Chemistry
Albumin	Alb	SST or PST; centrifuge, separate, and refrigerate	gold, green	Chemistry
Alcohol	ETOH	Oxalate, heparin, SST, EDTA, or nonadditive; no alcohol prep, keep on ice	gray, green, gold, lavender, red	Chemistry or Toxicology
Aldolase		SST; centrifuge, separate, and refrigerate	gold	Chemistry
Aldosterone	Aldo	Nonadditive; centrifuge, separate, and refrigerate. Patient must be "up-right" for at least ½ hour prior to collection	red	Chemistry
Alkaline phosphatase	ALP	PST or SST; centrifuge, separate; fasting specimen	green, gold	Chemistry
Alpha-fetoprotein	AFP	SST; centrifuge, separate	gold	Chemistry
Aluminum	Al	Trace-element-free (nonadditive or EDTA)	navy blue	Chemistry
Ammonia	NH3	PST; transport on ice; separate and refrigerate	green	Chemistry
Amylase	Amy	PST or SST; centrifuge, separate, and refrigerate	green, gold	Chemistry
Antidiuretic hormone	ADH	EDTA; centrifuge, separate, and freeze	lavender	Chemistry

Lab Test	Abbreviation (may vary by laboratory)	Specimen Requirement (specimen requirements vary by laboratory method)	Tube Cap Colors (BD product)	Laboratory Section
Antinuclear antibodies	ANA	SST; centrifuge, separate, and refrigerate	(gold)	Immunology
Antistreptolysin	ASO	PST or SST; centrifuge, separate, and refrigerate	(green) (gold)	Immunology
Antithrombin	AT-III	Citrate; centrifuge, separate, and freeze	(light blue)	Coagulation
Apolipoprotein		PST or SST; centrifuge, separate, and freeze; fasting specimen	(green) (gold)	Chemistry
Arterial blood gasses	ABGs	Heparin or heparinized syringe; transport on ice	(green)	Chemistry
Aspartate aminotransferase	AST	PST or SST; centrifuge, separate, and refrigerate	(green) (gold)	Chemistry
Basic metabolic profile	BMP	PST or SST; centrifuge, separate; fasting specimen	(green) (gold)	Chemistry
Beta human chorionic gonadotropin	Beta hCG	PST or SST; centrifuge, separate	(green) (gold)	Chemistry
Beta-type natriuretic protein	BNP	EDTA; separate and freeze	(lavender)	Chemistry
Bilirubin, – direct Bili – total Bili	Bili	PST or SST; centrifuge, separate, and refrigerate; protect from light	(green) (gold)	Chemistry
Blood culture – aerobic – anaerobic	BC	Blood culture bottles, or yellow-SPS tubes	(yellow)	Microbiology
Blood urea nitrogen	BUN	PST or SST; centrifuge, separate, and refrigerate	(green) (gold)	Chemistry
Cadmium		Trace-element-free EDTA	(navy)	Chemistry
Calcitonin		Nonadditive; centrifuge, separate, freeze; fasting specimen	(red)	Chemistry
Calcium	Ca	PST or SST; centrifuge, refrigerate	(green) (gold)	Chemistry
Carbon monoxide	CO	EDTA; refrigerate; tube must be full	(lavender)	Chemistry
Carcinoembryonic antigens	CEA	SST; centrifuge, separate, and refrigerate	(gold)	Chemistry
Carcinogenic antigen	Ca 125	PST or SST; centrifuge, separate, and refrigerate; freeze if testing is delayed	(green) (gold)	Chemistry
Carotene, beta		SST; centrifuge, separate, and freeze; protect from light	(gold)	Chemistry

(continued)

TABLE E-1 Alphabetical Listing of Blood Tests (partial list) *(continued)*

Lab Test	Abbreviation (may vary by laboratory)	Specimen Requirement (specimen requirements vary by laboratory method)	Tube Cap Colors (BD product)	Laboratory Section
Ceruloplasmin		PST or SST; centrifuge, separate, and freeze; fasting specimen	light green, gold	Chemistry
Chlamydia antibodies		SST; centrifuge, separate, and refrigerate	gold	Immunology
Cholesterol, total – HDL – LDL – VLDL	Chol	PST or SST; centrifuge, separate, and refrigerate; fasting specimen	light green, gold	Chemistry
Chromium	Cr	Trace element-free (nonadditive); centrifuge, separate, and refrigerate	dark blue	Chemistry
Cluster of differentiation (Flow cytometry)	CD markers (Flow)	Heparin or EDTA; transport immediately	green, lavender	Special Hematology
Cold agglutinins		EDTA; keep warm and place in laboratory water bath 37°C	lavender, pink	Immunology or Blood Bank
Complement	C1-C8	PST; centrifuge, separate, and refrigerate	light green	Immunology
Complete blood count – WBC – RBC – Hgb – Hct – MCV – MCH – MCHC – Platelets	CBC	EDTA; Hgb and Hct may be ordered separately; platelet count may be ordered separately; CBC may include differential	lavender, pink	Hematology
Copper	Cu	Trace-element-free (nonadditive or EDTA); centrifuge, separate into copper-free transfer tube, and refrigerate	dark blue	Chemistry or Toxicology
Cortisol		PST or SST; centrifuge, separate, and refrigerate	light green, gold	Chemistry
C-reactive protein	CRP	PST or SST; centrifuge, separate, and refrigerate	light green, gold	Immunology
Creatine kinase, total – CK-BB – CK-MB – CK-MM	CK	PST or SST; centrifuge, separate, and refrigerate	light green, gold	Chemistry
Creatinine	Creat	PST or SST; centrifuge, separate, and refrigerate	light green, gold	Chemistry
Cryoglobulin		Clot activator or SST; centrifuge, separate; keep warm	red, gold	Chemistry
Cystic fibrosis gene mutation		EDTA; refrigerate, DO NOT separate	lavender, pink	Molecular

TABLE E-1 Alphabetical Listing of Blood Tests (partial list) (continued)

Lab Test	Abbreviation (may vary by laboratory)	Specimen Requirement (specimen requirements vary by laboratory method)	Tube Cap Colors (BD product)	Laboratory Section
Cyclosporine		EDTA; centrifuge, separate, and refrigerate	(purple) (pink)	Chemistry
Cytomegalovirus	CMV	EDTA; centrifuge, separate, and freeze	(purple) (pink)	Microbiology
D-Dimer	D-Di	Citrate; centrifuge, separate, and freeze	(blue)	Coagulation
Dehydroepiandrosterone	DHEA	SST; centrifuge, separate, refrigerate; 6:00–10:00 a.m. draw	(yellow)	Chemistry
Differential – % WBC types – RBC morphology – Platelet estimate	Diff	EDTA or blood smears	(purple)	Hematology
Direct antiglobulin test	DAT, Coombs	EDTA; special patient identification and banding	(pink) (purple)	Blood Bank
Disseminated intravascular coagulation panel	DIC	Citrate; centrifuge, separate, and freeze	(blue)	Coagulation
Drug monitoring – Amikacin – Barbiturates – Carbamazepine – Digoxin – Gentamicin – Lithium – Phenytoin – Salicylates – Theophylline – Tobramycin – Vancomycin		SST; centrifuge, separate; indicate peak or trough level if appropriate	(yellow)	Chemistry
Electrolytes – sodium – potassium – chloride – carbon dioxide	Lytes – Na – K – Cl – CO_2	PST or SST; centrifuge, separate, and refrigerate. Each test may be ordered separately.	(green) (yellow)	Chemistry
Eosinophil count	Eos	EDTA; included in CBC with differential	(purple)	Hematology
Epstein-Barr	EBV	SST; centrifuge, separate, and refrigerate	(yellow)	Immunology
Erythrocyte sedimentation rate	ESR	EDTA, citrate, or special black dependent on method	(purple) (blue)	Hematology
Estradiol		PST; centrifuge, separate, and refrigerate	(green)	Chemistry
Estrogen		EDTA; centrifuge, separate, and refrigerate	(purple)	Chemistry

(continued)

TABLE E-1 Alphabetical Listing of Blood Tests (partial list) (continued)

Lab Test	Abbreviation (may vary by laboratory)	Specimen Requirement (specimen requirements vary by laboratory method)	Tube Cap Colors (BD product)	Laboratory Section
Factor assays		Citrate; centrifuge, separate, and freeze	(light blue)	Coagulation
Factor V Leiden	FVL	EDTA or citrate	(lavender) (light blue)	Molecular or Coagulation
Febrile agglutinin		SST; centrifuge, separate, and refrigerate	(gold)	Immunology
Ferritin		PST or SST; centrifuge, separate, and refrigerate	(green) (gold)	Chemistry
Fibrin degradation/split products FDP/FSP		Special light blue or black dependent on kit; contains thrombin and trypsin		Coagulation
Fibrinogen	Fibr	Citrate	(light blue)	Coagulation
Fluorescent treponemal antibody	FTA-ABS	Clot activator or SST; centrifuge, separate, and refrigerate	(red) (gold)	Immunology
Folate (RBC)		EDTA; refrigerate	(lavender)	Chemistry
Folate (serum)		PST or SST; centrifuge, separate, and refrigerate	(green) (gold)	Chemistry
Follicle stimulating hormone	FSH	PST or SST; centrifuge, separate, and refrigerate	(green) (gold)	Chemistry
Gamma-glutamyl transferase	GGT	PST or SST; centrifuge, separate, and refrigerate	(green) (gold)	Chemistry
Gastrin		SST; centrifuge, separate, and freeze; fasting specimen	(gold)	Chemistry
Glucose (fasting)	Glu, FBS	Fluoride, PST or SST; centrifuge, separate, and refrigerate	(gray) (green) (gold)	Chemistry
Glucose-6-phosphate dehydrogenase	G-6-PD	EDTA, heparin or ACD; refrigerate	(lavender) (pink) (green) (yellow)	Chemistry
Glucose tolerance test	GTT	Fluoride; centrifuge, separate, and refrigerate	(gray)	Chemistry
Glycosylated hemoglobin	Hgb A1c	EDTA; refrigerate	(lavender)	Chemistry
Growth hormone	GH	PST or SST; centrifuge, separate, and refrigerate	(green) (gold)	Chemistry
Haptoglobin	Hapt	Mint or gold; centrifuge, separate, and refrigerate	(green) (gold)	Chemistry
Hemoglobin electrophoresis	HBEP	EDTA; refrigerate	(lavender) (pink)	Hematology

Lab Test	Abbreviation (may vary by laboratory)	Specimen Requirement (specimen requirements vary by laboratory method)	Tube Cap Colors (BD product)			Laboratory Section
Hepatitis A virus	HAV	PST or SST; centrifuge, separate, and refrigerate	🟢	🟡		Immunology
Hepatitis B surface antibody	HBsAb	PST or SST; centrifuge, separate, and refrigerate	🟢	🟡		Immunology
Histamine	Hist	Heparin or EDTA; centrifuge, separate, and freeze	🟢	🟣		Chemistry
Homocystine		EDTA; centrifuge, separate, and refrigerate	🟣			Chemistry
Human chorionic gonadotropin	HCG	Heparin; centrifuge, separate, and refrigerate	🟢			Chemistry
Human immunodeficiency virus	HIV	EDTA; centrifuge, separate, and refrigerate	🟣			Immunology
Human leukocyte	HLA	ACD	🟡			Blood Bank
Helicobacter pylori antibodies	Hpylor-ABS	SST, EDTA, or heparin; centrifuge, separate, and refrigerate	🟡	🟣	🟢	Immunology
Immunoglobulins – IgA – IgD – IgE – IgG – IgM	Ig	SST; centrifuge, separate, and refrigerate	🟡			Chemistry
Insulin		SST or EDTA; centrifuge, separate, and refrigerate	🟡	🔴		Chemistry
Iron and total iron binding capacity	Fe & TIBC	PST or SST; centrifuge, separate, and refrigerate; fasting specimen preferred	🟢	🟡		Chemistry
Kleihauer-Betke		EDTA; refrigerate	🔴			Blood Bank or Hematology
Lactate dehydrogenase	LD	SST; centrifuge, separate, and refrigerate	🟡			Chemistry
Lactic acid	LA	Fluoride; transport on ice; no tourniquet draw	🟤			Chemistry
Lead	Pb	Lead-free or trace-element-free (EDTA)	🟠	🟣		Chemistry or Toxicology
Leukocyte alkaline phosphatase/neutrophil alkaline phosphatase	LAP or NAP	Heparin	🟢			Hematology
Lipase	Lip	SST; centrifuge, separate, and refrigerate	🟡			Chemistry
Magnesium	Mg	SST; centrifuge, separate, and refrigerate	🟡			Chemistry

(continued)

Lab Test	Abbreviation (may vary by laboratory)	Specimen Requirement (specimen requirements vary by laboratory method)	Tube Cap Colors (BD product)	Laboratory Section
Malaria		EDTA or thick and thin blood smears	(lavender)	Microbiology
Methylenetetrahydrofolate reductase gene mutation	MTHFR	EDTA or citrate	(lavender) (light blue)	Molecular or Coagulation
Mononucleosis screen	Mono or Monospot	SST; centrifuge, separate, and refrigerate	(gold)	Immunology
Myoglobin	Myo	PST or SST; centrifuge, separate, and refrigerate	(green) (gold)	Chemistry
Partial thromboplastin time (activated)	PTT/APTT	Citrate; centrifuge, separate, and freeze	(light blue)	Coagulation
Phenylketonuria	PKU	Collect on special test paper		Chemistry
Phosphorus	P, PO4	SST; centrifuge, separate, room temperature	(gold)	Chemistry
Plasminogen		Citrate; centrifuge, separate, and freeze	(light blue)	Coagulation
Platelet aggregation	Plat Agg	Citrate; **do not** centrifuge or freeze	(light blue)	Coagulation
Platelet function assay	PFA	Citrate (must collect discard tube first)	(light blue)	Coagulation
Platelet response (aspirin or Plavix)		Citrate (must collect discard tube first)	(light blue)	Coagulation
Prostatic specific antigen	PSA	SST; centrifuge, separate, and freeze	(gold)	Chemistry
Prothrombin gene mutation	PGM	EDTA or citrate	(lavender) (light blue)	Molecular or Coagulation
Prothrombin time	PT	Citrate; centrifuge, separate, and freeze	(light blue)	Coagulation
Rapid plasmin reagin	RPR	SST; centrifuge, separate, and refrigerate	(gold)	Immunology
Renin		EDTA; centrifuge, separate, and freeze; collect between 8 and 10 a.m. after 2 hours of upright position	(lavender) (pink)	Chemistry
Reticulocyte count	Retic	EDTA	(lavender)	Hematology
Rheumatoid factor	RF	SST; centrifuge, separate, and refrigerate	(gold)	Immunology
Rh immune globulin	Rhogam	EDTA; special patient identification and banding	(pink) (lavender)	Blood Bank
Rubella		SST; centrifuge, separate, and refrigerate	(gold)	Chemistry

Lab Test	Abbreviation (may vary by laboratory)	Specimen Requirement (specimen requirements vary by laboratory method)	Tube Cap Colors (BD product)	Laboratory Section
Rubeola		SST; centrifuge, separate, and refrigerate	(gold)	Chemistry
Salicylate		Nonadditive; centrifuge, separate, and refrigerate	(red)	Chemistry or Toxicology
Serotonin		SST; centrifuge, separate, and freeze within 1 hour	(gold)	Chemistry
Serum protein electrophoresis	SPE	SST; centrifuge, separate, and refrigerate	(gold)	Chemistry
Sickle cell screen	Sickle	EDTA	(lavender)	Hematology
Testosterone	Test	PST or SST; centrifuge, separate, and refrigerate	(green) (gold)	Chemistry
Thyroid profile – Triiodothyronine – Thyroxine – Thyroid stimulating hormone	T3 T4 TSH	SST; centrifuge, separate, and refrigerate	(gold)	Chemistry
Transferrin		SST; centrifuge, separate, and refrigerate	(gold)	Chemistry
Triglycerides	Trig	SST; centrifuge, separate, and refrigerate; fasting specimen	(gold)	Chemistry
Troponin	Tn	PST; centrifuge, separate, and refrigerate	(green)	Chemistry
Uric acid	Uric	SST; centrifuge, separate, and refrigerate	(gold)	Chemistry
Vitamins – Vitamin A – Vitamin B_{12} – Vitamin D – Vitamin K	Vit A Vit B_{12} Vit D Vit K	SST; centrifuge, separate, and refrigerate	(gold)	Chemistry
Von Willebrand factor – activity – antigen – multimers		Citrate; centrifuge, separate, and freeze	(blue)	Coagulation
West Nile virus	WNV	SST; centrifuge, separate, and refrigerate	(gold)	Chemistry
White blood cell count	WBC	EDTA	(lavender)	Hematology
Zinc (RBC)	ZNRBC	Trace-element-free (EDTA); centrifuge, separate, and refrigerate	(dark blue)	Chemistry
Zinc (serum)	Zn	Trace-element-free (nonadditive); centrifuge, separate, and refrigerate	(dark blue)	Chemistry

TABLE E-2 Alphabetical Listing of Non-Blood Tests (partial list)

Lab Test	Abbreviation (may vary by laboratory)	Specimen Requirement (specimen requirements vary by laboratory method)	Laboratory Section
Body fluid cell counts	BF Cell Cnt	Body fluid (CSF, serous, synovial, etc.) in appropriate container; transport STAT	Hematology
Body fluid chemistry	BF Chem	Body fluid (CSF, serous, synovial, etc.) in appropriate container; transport STAT	Chemistry
Body fluid cultures	BF Cult	Body fluid (CSF, serous, synovial, etc.) in sterile container; transport immediately	Microbiology
Culture and sensitivity	C&S	Culture swab appropriate for tissue being cultured; transport STAT	Microbiology
DNA test for chlamydia and gonorrhea	CT/GC	Culture swab appropriate for tissue being cultured; transport STAT	Molecular or Microbiology
Human papiloma virus	HPV	Cervix sample or other tissue	Molecular, Immunology, or Microbiology
Occult blood		Stool specimen	Hematology or Microbiology
Ova, cysts and/or parasites	O&P or OCP	Stool specimen	Microbiology
Sputum for tuberculosis		Early morning sample	Microbiology
Streptococcus screen	Strep Screen	Throat culture swab; transport STAT	Immunology or Microbiology
Urinalysis	UA	Urine in appropriate container	Urinalysis

Glossary

A

abdominopelvic cavity   Body cavity containing the abdominal organs: stomach, small and large intestines, gallbladder, liver, spleen, kidneys, and pancreas, and the pelvic organs: bladder and internal reproductive organs.

ABO antigens   Blood type proteins.

accession number   Sequential number assigned in the order received.

accreditation   Process by which a governmental agency evaluates a program or an institution according to established guidelines or standards.

acculturation   Changes made by minorities in response to the dominant culture.

accuracy   Achieving complete correctness or acceptable measures as close as possible to the true value.

acid citrate dextrose (ACD)   Additive that maintains red cell viability.

additive   Substance, such as an anticoagulant, an antiglycolytic agent, a separator gel, a cell preservative, or a clot activator, added to a blood collection tube.

additive-to-blood ratio   Balance between the amount of additive or anticoagulant and the amount of blood.

aerobic   Microorganism that can live and grow in the presence of oxygen or air.

aerosol   Fine mist of substances or particles suspended in a gas or the air.

agglutination   Clumping of red blood cells that occurs from the binding of antibodies and antigens.

airborne transmission   Spread of disease by small particles carried through the air.

aliquoting   Dividing or separating samples into separate containers.

ambulatory   Walking about.

American Certification Agency (ACA)   National certification agency for healthcare professionals, including phlebotomists and phlebotomy instructors.

American Medical Technologists (AMT)   Organization that provides certification to phlebotomy personnel and approves phlebotomy programs.

American Society of Clinical Pathologists (ASCP)   Agency responsible for providing clinical laboratory personnel certification, including phlebotomists.

American Society of Phlebotomy Technicians (ASPT)   Professional organization for phlebotomists that also provides certification.

anaerobic   Microorganism that can live and grow in the absence of oxygen or air.

analyte   Substance undergoing analysis, such as glucose or cholesterol.

anatomical position   Body facing forward with the arms at the sides and the palms of the hands facing forward.

anatomy   Study of the structure of the body.

anesthesiology   Management of pain before, during, and after surgery.

antecubital fossa   Area in the middle of the arm, in front of the elbow, that houses the veins most commonly used for venipuncture.

anterior   Toward the front of the body.

antibody   Complex protein substance produced in the presence of foreign substances, such as bacteria, viruses, lipids, or carbohydrates, in order to protect the body.

antibiotic removal device (ARD)   A special resin designed to remove antibiotics from a patient's blood stream in order to increase the chances of recovering microorganisms in the blood culture.

anticoagulant   Agent that prevents blood from clotting.

antigen   Substance that causes the formation of an antibody when introduced into blood or tissue.

antiglycolytic   Glucose preservative found in some blood collection tubes.

antiseptic   Germicidal solution used to clean the skin prior to venipuncture or dermal puncture.

aorta   Largest artery in the body.

arterial puncture   The procedure used to obtain blood samples from the artery.

arteriole   Smaller branch of an artery; a miniature artery.

artery   Blood vessel that carries blood from the heart to the tissues.

ASAP   Abbreviation for "as soon as possible."

aseptic   Pertaining to a condition that is free of disease-producing microorganisms (germs).

assault   Unlawful act of threatening or causing a person to experience fear.

assay   Test, examination, or laboratory analysis of a substance.

atoms   Simplest units of matter.

atrium (atria)   One of two top chambers of the heart, known as the holding chambers.

attribute   Defining quality or personal characteristic.

audit   Review of records and documents.

autoantibody   Immunoglobulin created in response to damaged antigens on the surface of one's own blood or body cells.

autoimmune disease   A disease in which the body fights against itself.

autologous   Pertaining to oneself, as in donating blood for self-use.

B

bacteremia   Presence of bacteria in the blood.

bacteriostatic   Substance that is capable of inhibiting the growth of bacteria.

basal state   Metabolic condition after 12 hours of fasting and lack of exercise.

basilic vein   Vein, used for venipuncture, that is not well anchored and tends to roll.

basophil   Least numerous type of leukocytes; the granules are large and stain dark blue from basic dyes and often obscure the nucleus.

battery   Unlawful use of physical force or contact toward another individual.

B-cell lymphocyte   Type of lymphocyte that produces antibodies upon stimulation.

bedside manner   Behavior that puts a patient at ease while healthcare personnel perform a procedure.

bevel   Point of the needle that has been cut on a slant for ease of entry.

biconcave   Having two concave sides.

biohazard   Risk associated with exposure to biological substances that can threaten human health.

biotinidase   Enzyme that breaks down the vitamin biotin.

bloodborne pathogens   Disease-causing organisms that are carried in the blood.

Bloodborne Pathogens Standard   Federal guidelines developed by OSHA, specifying practices that ensure safe handling of specimens that may contain pathogens.

blood type   Description, based on the ABO classification system, of the presence of specific antigens on the surface of red blood cells.

brachium   Arm.

burnout   Result of prolonged periods of stress without relief.

butterfly needle set   Winged infusion set; used mostly for small veins or difficult venipuncture.

C

calcaneus   Heel bone in the foot.

calibration   Comparison of a known constant to the test equipment reading or measurement.

cannula   Hollow tube used for temporary access to a vein or an artery to administer medication or draw blood.

capillary   Smallest of all blood vessels, which allow the exchange of nutrients and oxygen between the cells and blood; capillaries connect arteries to veins.

capillary action   Process in which blood automatically flows into a thin tube.

capillary puncture   Use of a sharp device to make an incision into the skin for the collection of small amounts of blood.

capillary tube   Disposable, small-diameter tube that fills by capillary action.

cardiovascular system   Body system of organs that work to circulate blood throughout the body.

catheter   Medically approved tube that can be inserted in the body to treat diseases, perform a surgical procedure, or collect specimens.

catheterization   Insertion of a hollow tube into the bladder, used for urine collection.

caudal plane   Toward the feet.

cells   Smallest living units in the body.

Centers for Disease Control and Prevention (CDC)   Federal agency responsible for identifying, monitoring, and reporting diseases, especially infectious diseases capable of becoming widespread or epidemic.

Centers for Medicare & Medicaid Services (CMS)   Federal agency that established regulations to implement CLIA'88 and COLA.

centrifugation   Process of separating components of a specimen using a centrifuge.

centrifuge   Instrument that spins contents at high speeds, used to separate cells from plasma or serum.

centrifuging   The act of using the centrifuge.

cephalic vein   Vein, used for venipuncture, that may be difficult to palpate.

Certificate of Waiver   Certification that allows laboratories to perform waived testing.

certification   Process that ensures successful completion of defined academic and training requirements.

chain of custody   Protocol that must be strictly followed and documented for specimen accountability.

chain of infection   Six steps (links) that must take place for infection to occur (reservoir, infectious agent, portal of exit, mode of transmission, portal of entry, and susceptible host).

chemical hazard   Contamination of an area with harmful or potentially harmful chemicals.

chemical hygiene plan   A plan that specifies practices to ensure safe handling of chemicals.

citrate   Additive, usually sodium citrate, that prevents coagulation by binding calcium.

CLAS Standards   A set of standards that attempt to help eliminate misunderstandings in healthcare interactions, improve patient compliance, and eliminate healthcare disparities. Also known as National Standards for Culturally and Linguistically Appropriate Services in Health Care.

clean-catch midstream specimen   Urine collection procedure for culture, which requires skin cleansing and collection of the mid-portion of the urine stream.

Clinical and Laboratory Standards Institute (CLSI)   Nonprofit organization that sets recommendations, guidelines, or standards for all areas of the laboratory to improve the quality of medical care.

clinical chemistry   Evaluation of chemical constituents that normally occur in the human body, such as glucose, sodium, and potassium.

Clinical Laboratory Improvement Advisory Committee (CLIAC)   A committee that provides scientific and technical advice and guidance to the Department of Health and Human Services (HHS) that pertain to issues related to improvement in clinical laboratory quality and laboratory medicine practice as well as the specific questions related to CLIA standards.

Clinical Laboratory Improvement Amendments (CLIA '88)   Federal legislation that became effective in 1992; it mandates that all laboratories be regulated using the same standards, regardless of size, type, or location.

clot activator   An additive that speeds up the clotting of blood in a collection tube.

clotted specimen   Specimen in which plasma has changed to serum and now contains a solid mass of cells.

coagulation   Cessation of bleeding; clot formation.

code of ethics   Rules of behavior that govern the practices of a profession or person.

cold agglutinin   Antibody present in certain disease conditions, such as primary atypical pneumonia; located on the surface of the red blood cells, and at temperatures lower than normal body temperature they cause the blood cells to clump together.

collapsed vein   An abnormal retraction of the vessel walls, stopping blood flow.

College of American Pathologists (CAP)   Agency that accredits medical laboratories.

combining vowel   Vowel placed between a word root and a suffix to make pronunciation easier.

Commission on Office Laboratory Accreditation (COLA)   Agency that accredits physician office laboratories.

competency assessment   Method of documenting an employee's ability to perform assigned tasks correctly.

concentric circles   Circular motion starting from the center and moving outward in ever-widening, even circles.

confidentiality   Privacy regarding patient information.

congenital   A disorder or disease existing at birth.

consent   Permission to perform a procedure.

contact transmission   Spread of disease through physical transfer of pathogens from reservoir to susceptible host (person).

continence   Abstinence (used in reference to sexual activity).

continuing education   Education that occurs after professional training in order to enhance skills.

continuous quality improvement (CQM)   Another term for quality assessment and process improvement.

control material   A liquid or cellular material or substance with a known range of analyte values used for performing equipment system checks.

coronal   Toward the head.

corrective action   Steps to remedy a problem.

cranial   Pertaining to the brain.

cross-trained   Being trained to perform multiple tasks.

Culturally and Linguistically Appropriate Services (CLAS) Standards   A set of standards specified by the Department of Health and Human Services that attempt to help eliminate misunderstandings in healthcare interactions, improve patient compliance, and eliminate healthcare disparities.

culture   (1) Specific ethnic, religious, or socioeconomic background. (2) Growing microorganisms under controlled conditions (verb); groups of microorganisms that are grown under controlled conditions (noun).

culture media   Material added to blood collection tubes that enhances the growth of microorganisms.

cystic fibrosis   Systemic disorder that causes particular damage to the respiratory and digestive systems.

cytology   Study of human cells for the presence of cancer.

cytoplasm   Area of the cell outside the nucleus.

D

deep   Internally away from the surface of the body.

delta check   Amount of change in patient results from one time to the next.

deoxygenated   Presence of a larger quantity of carbon dioxide than oxygen.

deoxyribonucleic acid (DNA)   Genetic code that contains all the information needed for body processes.

Department of Health and Human Services (HHS)   Federal agency that oversees the Centers for Medicare & Medicaid Services (CMS).

dermal   Pertaining to the skin.

dermal puncture   Use of a sharp device to make an incision into the skin for the collection of small amounts of blood.

diabetes mellitus   Any of several related endocrine disorders characterized by an elevated level of glucose in the blood, caused by a deficiency of insulin or insulin resistance at the cellular level.

diapedesis   Process by which certain white blood cells can exit the capillaries and enter the tissues in response to pathogens.

diaphragm   Muscle that separates the thoracic and abdominopelvic cavities.

differential   Hematology test that is a microscopic examination of a monolayer stained blood smear; indicates the percentage of different types of white blood cells, the number of both platelets and white blood cells, red blood cell size and shape, and any other blood abnormalities, such as leukemia.

digestive system   Body system that takes in and digests food, absorbs nutrients, and removes solid waste.

dilate   To enlarge or increase the diameter.

dipstick   Plastic strip with reagent pads containing chemicals for urine or blood testing.

disinfectant   Solution that contains an agent intended to kill or irreversibly inactivate microorganisms.

distal   Away from the point of attachment or farther from the trunk of the body.

distal phalanx   Situated away from the center of the finger.

diurnal variation   Normal changes in laboratory values throughout the day.

diversity   Variation of a category.

dorsal   Pertaining to the backside.

dorsal cavity   Body cavity containing the cranial cavity and spinal cavity.

double-bagging   Enclosing contaminated equipment in a biohazard bag and placing that bag within a second biohazard bag.

droplet transmission   Spread of disease through droplets propelled short distances.

E

ecchymosis   Discoloration or bruising caused by the seeping of blood underneath the skin.

edema   Accumulation of fluid in the tissues, usually resulting in swelling.

edematous Marked by edema; the result of swelling due to fluid accumulation.

electrical hazard Contact with electrical equipment or the failure of equipment that creates a dangerous condition.

electronic health records (EHRs) Medical information stored in computerized formats.

electronic medical record (EMR) Another term used to describe computerized documents.

emergency preparedness Readiness for response during times of crisis.

endocrine system The body system that regulates body functions by releasing hormones into the bloodstream.

Environmental Protection Agency (EPA) Ensures that healthcare providers follow the Medical Waste Tracking Act.

eosinophil Leukocyte whose granules stain bright orange-red from eosin; aids the body in fighting parasites and numbers increase in allergies.

ergonomics The practice of adapting the job task or equipment so that you can perform the task safely and productively.

erythrocyte Red blood cell; an anuclear, biconcave disk-shaped blood cell that is responsible for transporting oxygen.

erythrocyte sedimentation rate (ESR) Rate at which red blood cells settle in whole blood (measured in millimeters) in 1 hour of falling.

ethics Area of philosophy that examines values, actions, and choices to determine right and wrong.

ethylenediaminetetraacetic acid (EDTA) Additive that prevents coagulation by binding calcium.

evacuated collection tube Stoppered glass or plastic tube used for collecting blood; contains a premeasured vacuum.

evacuated tube holder Specialized plastic adaptor that holds both a needle and a tube for blood collection; *adaptor* and *barrel* are also common names.

evaluation Examination of the evidence found when measuring the indicators.

examination Events during the analysis of blood and other specimens.

expectorate Generate a cough from deep within the lungs and bronchi.

exposure control plan A protocol to be followed in the event an employee is exposed to bloodborne pathogens.

external respiration The exchange of air between the lungs and the outside environment.

exsanguination Process of blood loss to a degree sufficient to cause death.

externship Training in a clinical setting.

F

false-negative Test result that does not indicate a condition or substance that is actually present.

false-positive Test result that indicates a positive result that is not true.

fasting Abstinence from food and liquids (except for water) for a specified period.

fecal occult blood Small amounts of blood found in the feces/stool.

female reproductive system The organs of a female that are involved in sexual reproduction.

femoral Pertaining to the thigh.

fibrin Filamentous protein formed by the action of thrombin on fibrinogen.

fibrinogen Protein found in plasma; essential for clotting blood.

fire and explosive hazard Situation in which the likelihood of fire or explosions exists.

first morning void Urine that is produced during the night and collected in the morning at the first void.

fistula Surgically inserted shunt (U-shaped tube) connecting an artery and a vein.

fomite Inanimate object capable of transmitting infectious organisms.

Food and Drug Administration (FDA) Federal agency that approves medical and diagnostic equipment, pharmaceuticals, reagents, diagnostic tests, and content labeling.

forensic specimens Specimens requiring special handling for criminal investigations.

frontal plane Plane dividing the body into front and back portions.

G

galactosemia Increased levels of galactose in the blood caused by the inability to break down the milk sugar galactose.

gauge Unit of measure assigned to the diameter of the lumen (hole) of a needle.

gestational diabetes Elevated blood sugar during pregnancy.

Globally Harmonized System (GHS) An internationally agreed-upon system for communicating chemical hazards.

glucose testing Measurement of blood glucose levels.

glycolysis Normal body reaction in which glucose is converted to lactic acid.

granulocytes White blood cells containing granuoles of various colors and chemical makeup: basophils, eosinophils, and neutrophils.

H

hand hygiene A general term that includes both handwashing and the use of alcohol-based hand rubs.

hard skills Specific technical and operational proficiencies.

hazardous materials (HAZMATS) Chemicals that pose a hazard when exposure occurs.

hazard statement Description of the nature and degree of a chemical's hazard(s).

healthcare-associated infections (HAIs) Infections acquired in healthcare settings.

Health Insurance Portability and Accountability Act (HIPAA) Federal law that establishes a national standard for electronic healthcare transactions and protects the privacy and confidentiality of patient information; among other provisions, HIPAA states that information about a patient must not be discussed with individuals other than the patient unless the patient has given written or verbal permission.

heel warmer   Chemically activated heating device.

hematocrit   Percentage of space taken up by red blood cells in a whole blood sample; also referred to as *packed cell volume and microhematocrit.*

hematology   Study of blood and blood-forming tissues.

hematoma   Collection of blood under the skin due to leakage of blood from a punctured vein or artery.

hematopoietic   Blood-forming tissues.

hemochromatosis   Disorder of iron metabolism in which too much iron is stored in the body, reaching toxic levels.

hemoconcentration   Rapid increase in the ratio of blood components (cells) to plasma (liquid).

hemodilution   Increase in plasma water.

hemoglobin   Iron-rich protein molecules found in red blood cells; transports oxygen and carbon dioxide.

hemolysis   Destruction of red blood cells that allows hemoglobin to be released from the red blood cells.

hemostasis   Coagulation, or clot formation, that repairs vessel damage and stops blood loss.

heparin   Additive that prevents coagulation by inactivating thrombin.

heparin lock   Winged needle set that remains in a patient's vein for a certain amount of time.

hepatitis   Inflammation of the liver from viral or toxic origin; can be caused by transmission through blood and body fluids.

high complexity   Classification of laboratory tests that require close attention to detail and specialized training.

histology   Study of human body tissues and cells.

hospital information system (HIS)   Computerized information system used by hospitals.

human chorionic gonadotropin (hCG)   Hormone produced by the placenta.

human immunodeficiency virus (HIV)   Virus that causes acquired immune deficiency syndrome (AIDS).

hypothyroidism   Decreased thyroid function.

I

iatrogenic anemia   Lowering of a patient's red blood cell count due to a medical treatment such as excessively repeated phlebotomy.

icteric   Greenish-yellow coloring indicating an elevated level of bilirubin.

immune system   The body system responsible for protecting the body against microorganisms, toxins, and cancer.

immunohematology (blood bank)   Collection and preparation of donor blood for transfusion.

immunology   Study of how the body resists allergies and other agents that affect the body's immune system; also called *serology.*

incident forms   Documents recording procedural or process errors.

indicators   Observable events used as evidence.

infection   Invasion of the body by pathogens and their multiplication.

infection control   Eliminating or minimizing the spread of infection.

inferior   Below or toward the feet.

informed consent   Permission granted by the patient to perform any treatment; obtained only after the patient has been told what to expect, the risks, and usually the consequences of the procedure.

integumentary system   Body system that provides protection, regulates temperature, prevents water loss, and synthesizes vitamin D.

interfering substance   Substance that produces incorrect laboratory test results.

internal respiration   The gas exchange between the blood and body cells.

interprofessional   Pertaining to people from different professions.

interstitial fluid   Fluid between cells and tissues.

Isolation Precautions   Practices to prevent the spread of infection based on how the infectious agent is transmitted.

J

jaundice   Yellow coloration to skin, eyes, and mucous membranes.

Joint Commission on the Accreditation of Healthcare Organizations (JCAHO)   Now called The Joint Commission.

K

keloid   Sharply elevated, irregularly shaped, progressively enlarging scar formed by excessive collagen in the skin during healing.

L

laboratory information system (LIS)   Computerized information system used by laboratories.

lancet   Small cutting instrument that controls the depth of the cutting blade.

lateral   Away from the middle of the body.

law   Rule of conduct or action prescribed or formally recognized as binding or enforced by a controlling authority.

legal specimens   Specimens requiring special handling for criminal investigation.

leukocyte   White blood cell; round cell with a nucleus whose main function is to combat infection and remove disintegrating tissues.

Levey-Jennings chart   Graph showing acceptable limits for results of control substance testing.

liability   Legal obligation to compensate another for loss or damages.

licensure   Process that is enforced by a governmental agency to ensure adequacy of training.

ligament   Fibrous tissue connecting bones to other bones.

light-sensitive   Type of substances for which specimens need to be covered.

lipemia/lipemic Cloudy serum or plasma following or caused by increased lipids (fats).

litigation Legal action or lawsuit.

lymphatic system Body system that removes foreign substances from the blood and lymph.

lymphocyte Leukocyte produced in the lymphoid tissue; a nongranular leukocyte that has a role in the body's immune system.

lymphoid Pertaining to the lymphatic system or resembling lymphocytes.

lymphostasis Lack of fluid drainage in the lymph system, usually caused by lymph node removal.

M

malaria Type of blood parasite.

male reproductive system The organs of a male that are involved in sexual reproduction.

malpractice Incorrect treatment of a patient by a healthcare worker.

medial Close to the middle of the body.

median cubital vein Most commonly used vein for venipuncture; located in the middle of the forearm.

medical microbiology Study of one-cell organisms (microorganisms) that are usually visible only under a microscope; the main focus is on bacteria.

microcollection Process of obtaining blood using a dermal (skin) puncture procedure; also known as *microtechnique*.

microhematocrit Manual procedure for determining hematocrit that requires only a small amount of blood.

microsample Sample of less than 1 milliliter.

microsurgery Surgery involving reconstruction of small tissue structures.

microtechnique Process of obtaining blood using a dermal (skin) puncture procedure; also known as *microcollection*.

midsagittal plane Plane dividing the body into equal left and right halves.

midstream specimen Urine collection procedure requiring the patient to collect only the mid-portion of a stream of urine.

mindset Group-held assumptions that cause the adoption of specific behaviors.

moderate complexity Classification of laboratory tests that fall between low (waived) and high complexity tests with respect to the complexity of the test and the training required.

molecular diagnostics Detection and classification of disease states using molecular and DNA-based testing.

molecules Atoms that have bonded together.

monocyte Large leukocyte formed in bone marrow, with abundant cytoplasm and a kidney-shaped nucleus; ingests bacteria, dying cells, and debris in tissues.

mononuclear Having a single-lobed nucleus.

multicultural Many different cultures.

multiskilled Trained in more than one job function.

muscular system Body system that produces movement, maintains posture, and produces body heat.

myeloid Developed from bone marrow.

N

nasal swab Used to collect a specimen from the cavities just inside the nose; also called the nares.

nasopharyngeal swab Used to collect a specimen from the area behind the nasal sinuses.

National Accrediting Agency for Clinical Laboratory Sciences (NAACLS) Organization that provides accreditation to phlebotomy training programs and offers certification for structured educational programs.

National Center for Competency Testing (NCCT) Independent third-party organization that provides certification testing for phlebotomy technicians.

National Credentialing Agency for Medical Laboratory Personnel (NCA) One of the agencies responsible for laboratory personnel certification.

National Healthcareer Association (NHA) Agency that provides certification and continuing education to healthcare professionals, including certified phlebotomy technicians.

needlestick injury Accidental puncture of skin with a needle.

Needlestick Safety and Prevention Act Legislation that mandates the use of safety devices that reduce needlestick injuries in the clinical setting.

natural killer (NK) cells Type of lymphocytes that can attack and destroy tumor cells or cells that have been infected by viruses.

negligence Intentional or unintentional error or wrongdoing; failure to perform reasonably expected duties to patients.

nervous system Body system that is responsible for conscious and unconscious actions.

networking Building social and professional alliances.

neutrophil Leukocyte that engulfs and digests pathogens found in tissues; its granules stain lavender.

normal flora Microorganisms that typically live on and in the body, normally causing no harm to the host.

nosocomial infections Infections acquired while in a hospital or other medical setting.

O

Occupational Safety and Health Administration (OSHA) Federal body responsible for preventing and minimizing employee injuries and exposure to harmful agents.

organelles Parts of a cell, such as nuclei, lysosomes, and mitochondria.

organism Living creature composed of organ systems.

organs Combination of two or more tissue types to form a system.

osteomyelitis Infection or inflammation of the bone or bone marrow.

other potentially infectious materials (OPIM) Body fluids, soiled laundry, or any item that may be contaminated with pathogens.

outcome Result of a test or procedure.

oxygenated Containing a higher concentration of oxygen than carbon dioxide.

P

packed cell volume (PCV) Hematocrit.

palmar Pertaining to the palm side of the hand.

palpable Detectable or noticeable by using touch; capable of being palpated.

palpate Examine by touching with the fingers, using pressure, then releasing.

parameters Limitations.

pathology Study and diagnosis of disease.

Patient Care Partnership Formerly called the Patient's Bill of Rights, a list of standards that patients can expect in healthcare.

peak level Specimen collected when a serum drug level is at its highest level, usually 15 to 30 minutes after administration.

performance improvement Effort of all team members to improve the quality of an entire healthcare facility, not just of services requiring clinical skills; involves employees learning from their mistakes and from the input of co-workers.

personal protective equipment (PPE) Protective coverings, such as gloves, goggles, gowns, and masks, that are worn to minimize exposure to blood and body fluids; required by OSHA to be worn when handling body fluids.

petechiae Small, nonraised, red spots appearing on the skin due to minor hemorrhage in underlying tissue.

phagocytosis Process by which bacteria and antigens are surrounded and engulfed by leukocytes.

phenylketonuria (PKU) Increased level of phenylketone in the blood.

phlebotomist Individual trained and skilled in obtaining blood samples for clinical testing.

phlebotomy Invasive procedure in which a sharp object is introduced into a vein to obtain blood.

phlebotomy cart/tray Storage and transport container for phlebotomy equipment.

physical hazards Nonbiological objects that may cause injury or illness.

physician office laboratory (POL) Small laboratory that is operated in a clinical practice office.

physiology Study of the function of the body.

pictogram A symbol that conveys specific information about the hazards of a chemical.

plantar Pertaining to the sole, or bottom, of the foot.

plasma Clear, pale yellow fluid component of blood that contains fibrinogen; obtained from a tube that has an anticoagulant and has been centrifuged.

platelet function assay (PFA) Blood test that determines platelet adhesion and aggregation.

pneumatic tube systems Transporting of tubes through pipes using vacuum forces.

point-of-care testing (POCT) Tests performed at the patient's bedside or work area, using a portable instrument.

polycythemia vera Condition in which there is an overproduction of red blood cells.

polymorphonuclear Having multiple-lobed nuclei.

posterior Toward the back of the body.

post-examination Events after the analysis of blood and other specimens, such as recording and reporting of test results.

postprandial After eating a meal.

precautionary statement Document that describes measures to minimize or prevent adverse effects resulting from exposure to a hazardous chemical.

precision Ability to give nearly the same result when performed repeatedly.

pre-examination Events before, during, or after the collection of blood and other specimens and before analysis.

prefix Placed at the beginning of a word to alter its meaning.

preventive action Activity that helps ensure that an error does not occur again.

process Procedure or duty that is to be done to a patient.

professional (1) A member of a vocation requiring specialized educational training; (2) A manner of behavior.

professional development Attaining skills and knowledge for both personal growth and career advancement.

professionalism Group of characteristics or qualities that display a positive image or code of ethics; behavior that exhibits the traits or features that correspond to the models and standards of a profession.

proficiency testing (PT) Means of evaluating the performance of a laboratory and its personnel in comparison with that of other similar laboratories.

prone Lying face down.

provider-performed microscopy procedures (PPMP) Subcategory of moderate complexity testing that allows healthcare providers to perform certain tests only for their own patients.

proximal Closer to the point of attachment or toward the trunk of the body.

pulmonary arteries Arteries that transport deoxygenated blood to the lungs.

pus Substance containing old leukocytes, pathogens, and other debris; created at the site of infection once the white blood cells undergo phagocytosis.

Q

quality assessment and process improvement (QAPI) The review of documentation to discover and eliminate weaknesses in a process and improve the quality of patient outcomes.

quality assurance (QA) System of planned activities that assess operational processes for the delivery of services or the quality of products provided to consumers, customers, or patients.

quality control (QC) Activities that ensure that specific steps in a process meet acceptable standards.

quality cost management (QCM) System to measure and manage the cost of quality.

quality management system (QMS) Establishment of quality objectives and the methods used to monitor the achievement of those objectives.

quantity not sufficient (QNS) Specimen amount is too small to perform the ordered test.

R

radioactive hazard A hazard that exists where ionizing radiation is present.

random Collected at any time of the day, usually requiring no special preparation.

random errors Errors that occur with no predictable pattern and may have several different causes.

rapport Behavior, courtesy, and respect given a patient.

reagents Chemicals used in performing laboratory tests.

real-time tracking Continuous monitoring of a specimen's status from the time of the test request to reporting of the results.

reference laboratory Offsite lab to which specimens are referred for testing; usually used for tests not routinely performed in physician offices.

reference values Expected values for a laboratory or population, usually established using patients in a basal state.

registration Placement on a membership list for a professional association (usually requiring certification).

reliable Believable and dependable.

reproductive system Body system that differs in males and females; produces male or female sex cells, provides a site for fertilization and fetal development, and produces milk for newborns.

requisition Documentation of a blood test order, usually generated by or at the request of a physician.

respiratory system Body system that provides oxygen to body cells and removes carbon dioxide.

respondeat superior The employer is responsible for the acts of his or her employees.

résumé Document summarizing employment and educational history.

Rh antigen Protein originally found on the red blood cells of Rhesus monkeys.

ribonucleic acid (RNA) Protein that assists in translating information from DNA.

risk management Policies and procedures to protect patients, employees, and the employer from loss or injury; generated and conducted by a department in healthcare facilities.

rouleaux formation The sticking of red bloods cells to one another in rows, usually caused by increased plasma proteins; these are not the same as clots.

S

safety data sheets (SDS) Documentation of specific chemical ingredients found in hazardous substances and emergency instructions to follow if abnormal contact occurs.

sagittal plane Plane dividing the body into left and right portions.

sclerosis Abnormal hardening of tissue.

scope of practice Procedures and processes permitted for a specific profession.

sedentary Not engaged in any physical activity.

semen Fluid produced by the male reproductive system, containing sperm and some substances necessary for fertilization.

septicemia Presence of pathogenic microorganisms in the blood, causing symptoms such as fever, chills, and changes in mental state.

septum Muscular wall between the left and right sides of the heart.

serology Identification of antibodies in the blood's serum.

serum Clear, pale yellow fluid that remains after blood clots and is separated; does not contain fibrinogen; plasma minus the clotting factors.

sharps container Clearly marked container that is rigid, leak-proof, and puncture resistant, for the disposal of needles, lancets, and other contaminated sharps.

shift Sudden jump in results that continues at a higher or lower level.

sickle cell disease Hemoglobin that causes red blood cells to have an abnormal structure due to a genetic mutation.

signal word A word or term (usually either "danger" or "warning") used on a label to indicate the relative level of severity of hazard.

skeletal system Body system that provides the body with protection and support.

sodium polyanethol sulfonate (SPS) Additive used in the collection of blood culture specimens.

soft skills Personal attributes or behaviors that enhance an individual's interactions on the job.

specimen transport bag Plastic zip-locked bags that displays a biohazard symbol; used for transporting laboratory specimens.

sputum Mucus that collects in the air passages of the respiratory system.

standard operating procedure (SOP) Purpose, specimen requirements, step-by-step procedure, limitations, normal and critical values, and interpretation for each procedure performed in the laboratory.

Standard Precautions Infection control guidelines issued by the CDC to decrease exposure to potentially infectious substances in acute care settings.

standards   Rules of practice.

STAT (ST)   Immediate need.

stereotype   Commonly held beliefs and concepts about a specific group of people.

sterile   Free of microorganisms.

stool specimens   Fecal matter that is waste discharged from the digestive system.

strep screening   Test used to determine if the bacteria Group A *Streptococcus* is present in the throat.

stress   The body's nonspecific response to change or demands.

suffix   Placed at the end of a word to alter its meaning.

superficial   Close to the surface of the body.

superior   Above or toward the head.

supine   Face upward, lying on the back.

suprapubic puncture   Urine collection procedure requiring the insertion of a needle through the area just above the pubic bone and directly into the bladder.

syncope   Fainting.

syringe   Device that consists of a plunger and a barrel graduated in milliliters or cubic centimeters.

systematic errors   Errors that occur due to differences in performance among staff.

T

T-cell lymphocyte   A type of lymphocyte that originates from the lymphoid tissue and assists the immune system through interactions with other leukocytes.

tendon   Fibrous tissue connecting bones to muscles.

The Joint Commission (formerly Joint Commission on the Accreditation of Healthcare Organizations)   Agency that accredits healthcare facilities to ensure high standards of patient care.

therapeutic drug monitoring (TDM)   Physician management of an effective drug dose.

therapeutic medication   Treatment, remedy, or cure of a disorder through the use of a medicinal substance.

therapeutic phlebotomy   Removal of large amounts of blood.

thick smear   Blood smear made by spreading a drop of blood on one slide with the corner of another placed in the center of the drop and moved in an outward, circular pattern.

thin smear   Blood smear made by spreading a drop of blood from one end of a slide with the edge of another slide placed across the drop at an angle and moved to the opposite end.

thixoptropic separator gel   Semisolid that forms a barrier between cells and plasma or serum upon centrifugation of blood specimens.

thoracic cavity   Body cavity that contains the lungs, heart, esophagus, and trachea.

throat swabs   Specimens taken from the back of the throat using a fabric-tipped applicator stick.

thrombin   Enzyme formed in response to an injury that converts fibrinogen to a fibrin clot.

thrombocyte   Smallest of the formed elements in the bloodstream; also called *platelet*.

tissue   A group of biological cells that perform a similar function.

total quality management (TQM)   identification of an organization's internal and external customers in an effort to design operations that produce the highest customer satisfaction.

tourniquet   Device that impedes or stops the flow of blood.

toxicology   Detection and study of agents that are harmful to the body.

training   Providing staff with the knowledge to perform their jobs correctly.

transmission-based precautions   Various levels of isolation and PPE uses that are based on how the infectious agent is transmitted.

transverse plane   Plane dividing the body into upper and lower portions.

trend   Results showing an upward or downward progression.

trough level   Specimen collected when a serum drug level is at its lowest level, usually immediately before the next scheduled dose is administered.

tunica adventitia   Outermost covering of arteries and veins.

tunica intima   Innermost layer of arteries and veins.

tunica media   Middle layer of arteries and veins.

twenty-four (24)-hour collection   Specimen collection procedure that requires patients to collect urine for a 24-hour period of time.

U

urinalysis   The testing of urine for physical, chemical, and microscopic characteristics.

urinary system   Body system that removes liquid waste from the blood and maintains the proper balance of water and salts in the body.

urine chemical screening   The testing of urine for various chemicals, most not normally present in the urine.

urine pregnancy tests   The testing of urine for the presence of human chorionic gonadotropin, indicating pregnancy.

V

validation   Ensuring accuracy and precision of laboratory test results.

valves   Flaps of tissue that open in one direction to let blood pass through.

variances   Deviations from the procedure.

vector-borne transmission   Spread of disease through insect or animal bites.

vehicle-borne transmission   Spread of disease through contact with contaminated items, such as food, linen, or equipment.

vein Blood vessel that transports blood from body tissues back to the heart.

vena cava Largest vein in the body.

venipuncture Procedure in which a sharp object is introduced into a vein for the purpose of withdrawing blood or instilling medications.

venous reflux Backward flow of blood into the patient's veins during venipuncture.

ventral Body cavity that contains the thoracic cavity and abdominopelvic cavity.

ventricle One of two bottom chambers of the heart, known as the pumping chambers.

venule Minute vein.

W

waived tests FDA-approved laboratory tests that are minimally complicated and pose little risk of harm to the patient.

winged infusion set Stainless steel collection needle connected to 5 to 12 inches of plastic tubing; also called a *butterfly needle set.*

word root Part of a medical term that contains the base meaning of the term.

Credits

Text/Line Art Credits

Chapter 2

Page 43, Figure 2.13: OSHA WEBSITE.

Page 44, Figure 2.14: OSHA WEBSITE.

Page 45, Figure 2.16: HMIS Color Bar Meanings. Copyright © by American Coating Association. The HMIS® trademark and related content are used under license of the American Coatings Association. All rights reserved. Used with permission.

Page 46, Figure 2.17: Hazardous Materials Identification System. Copyright © by American Coating Association. The HMIS® trademark and related content are used under license of the American Coatings Association. All rights reserved. Used with permission.

Page 50, Table 2.7: From Helen Houser and Terri Wyman, Administrative Medical Assisting 1e. New York, NY: McGraw-Hill Companies, 2011, p. 674. Copyright © 2011 by The McGraw-Hill Companies. All rights reserved. Used with permission.

Chapter 14

Page 395, Table 14.1: National Standards for Culturally and Linguistically Appropriate Services in Health Care. U.S. Department of Health and Human Services.

Appendix G

"Code of Ethics" and "Pledge to the Profession." http://www.ascls.org. Copyright © 2012-2014 by the American Society for Clinical Laboratory Science. All rights reserved. Used with permission.

Photo Credits

Design Elements

Patient Education & Communication: © Siri Stafford/Getty Images RF; Safety & Infection Control: © Walker and Walker/Getty Images RF; Law & Ethics: © Eyewire/Photodisc/PunchStock RF; Critical Thinking: © Brand New Images/Getty Images; Life Span Considerations: © Total Care Programming, Inc.

Chapter 1

Opener: © Keith Brofsky/Getty Images RF; Table 1.1(top): © Total Care Programming, Inc.; Table 1.1(bottom): © Lillian Mundt; 1.1: © Bettmann/Corbis; 1.2: © doc stock/Corbis; 1.3: © David Buffington/Getty Images RF; 1.4: © Total Care Programming, Inc.; 1.6: © Ingram Publishing RF; 1.7a-b: © Mitsu Yasukawa/Star Ledger/Corbis; 1.7c: © Mark Harmel/Getty Images; 1.8: © Adam Gault/age fotostock RF; 1.9, 1.10: © Blend Images RF; 1.11: © Getty Images RF; 1.12, 1.13: © Royalty-Free/Corbis; 1.14: © Photodisc Collection/Getty Images RF; 1.15: © Steve Allen/Getty Images RF.

Chapter 2

Opener: © studyoritim/Getty Images RF; 2.2: © McGraw-Hill Education/Sandra Mesrine, photographer; 2.3a: © McGraw-Hill Education/Jill Braaten, photographer; 2.3b: © Lillian Mundt; 2.5a-c: © McGraw-Hill Education/Jan L. Saeger, photographer; 2.6: © McGraw-Hill Education/Sandra Mesrine, photographer; 2.7: © Leesa Whicker; 2.8-2.10: © McGraw-Hill Education/Sandra Mesrine, photographer; 2.11(all): © David Kelly Crow; 2.12, 2.18a: © McGraw-Hill Education/Sandra Mesrine, photographer; 2.18b: © Phyllis; 2.19: © McGraw-Hill Education/Sandra Mesrine, photographer; 2.21: © Aaron Roeth RF; Table 2.7(Radiation Hazard): © Lillian Mundt.

Chapter 3

Opener: © Nancy Louie/Getty Images RF.

Chapter 4

Opener: © Stockbyte/Getty Images RF.

Chapter 5

Opener: Image © 2010 Nucleus Medical Media; 5.14b: © Bill Longcore/Science Source; Table 5.2(all): © Ed Reschke.

Chapter 6

Opener: © McGraw-Hill Education/Take One Digital Media, photographer; 6.1: © Creatas/PunchStock RF; 6.3: © Lillian Mundt; 6.4: © Plush Studios/Blend Images LLC RF; 6.5: © Purestock/Getty Images RF; 6.6: © Royalty-Free/Corbis; 6.8-6.11: © Lillian Mundt; 6.12: © GOODSHOOT/Alamy RF; 6.13: © Stockbyte/Getty Images RF; 6.14: © Brand X Pictures/PunchStock RF; 6.15: © JGI/Blend Images LLC RF; 6.16: © Chris Timken/Blend Images LLC RF; 6.17: © McGraw-Hill Education/Rick Brady, photographer; 6.19: © Keith Brofsky/Getty Images RF; 6.20: © Lillian Mundt; 6.21: © Don Farrall/Getty Images RF; 6.22: © Comstock Images/PictureQuest RF; p. 164: © Lillian Mundt.

Chapter 7

Opener: © Steve Allen/Getty Images RF; 7.1, 7.2a: © McGraw-Hill Education/Sandra Mesrine, photographer; 7.2b: © BSIP SA/Alamy; 7.2c: © Lillian Mundt; 7.3: © McGraw-Hill Education/Sandra Mesrine, photographer; 7.4: © Lillian Mundt; 7.5, 7.6: © McGraw-Hill Education/Sandra Mesrine, photographer; 7.7a-b: © Total Care Programming, Inc.; 7.8: © Lillian Mundt; 7.9a-b: © Total Care Programming, Inc.; 7.10-7.13a: © McGraw-Hill Education/Sandra Mesrine, photographer; 7.13b: © Total Care Programming, Inc.; 7.14: © Lillian Mundt; Table 7.2(3-5): Courtesy and © Becton, Dickinson and Company; 7.15, 7.16: © Lillian Mundt; 7.17a-b: © McGraw-Hill Education/Sandra Mesrine, photographer; 7.18, 7.19: © Lillian Mundt; 7.20a-c: Courtesy and © Becton, Dickinson and Company; 7.21, 7.22, 7.24: © Lillian Mundt; 7.25(left): © Total Care Programming, Inc.; 7.25(right): Courtesy and © Becton, Dickinson and Company; 7.26, 7.27: © Total Care Programming, Inc.; 7.28: © Lillian Mundt; Table 7.3, Table 7.4(all): Courtesy and © Becton, Dickinson and Company; Table 7.5(all), 7.29-7.31: © Lillian Mundt; 7.32, 7.33: © greiner bio-one. Photos provided by greiner bio-one; 7.34, 7.35(all): © greiner bio-one. Photos by Photo Affairs, Inc./Steve Rouben; 7.36-7.38: © Sarstedt, Inc.

Chapter 8

Opener: Jim Gathany/CDC; 8.1, 8.3, 8.4, 8.6: © Total Care Programming, Inc.; 8.7: © McGraw-Hill Education/Sandra Mesrine, photographer; 8.8, 8.9, 8.13, 8.14: © Total Care Programming, Inc.; 8.15: © Lillian Mundt; 8.16a: © Total Care Programming, Inc.; 8.16b: © Lillian Mundt; 8.17: © Total Care Programming, Inc.; 8.18: © McGraw-Hill Education/Sandra Mesrine, photographer; 8.20: © Total Care Programming, Inc.; 8.22, 8.25: © McGraw-Hill Education/Take One Digital Media, photographer; p. 227: © McGraw-Hill Education/Sandra Mesrine, photographer.

Chapter 9

Opener: © Ana Abejon/Getty Images RF; 9.1: © McGraw-Hill Education/Sandra Mesrine, photographer; 9.4: © Lillian Mundt; 9.5a-c: © McGraw-Hill Education/Take One Digital Media, photographer; 9.6: © Lillian Mundt; p. 251: © McGraw-Hill Education/Sandra Mesrine, photographer.

Chapter 10

Opener: © Lillian Mundt; 10.1-10.4: © McGraw-Hill Education/Sandra Mesrine, photographer; 10.6: © Getty Images RF; 10.7, 10.8: © McGraw-Hill Education/Sandra Mesrine, photographer; 10.9, 10.10: © Total Care Programming, Inc.; 10.11: © Lillian Mundt; 10.13: Courtesy of Tri-Tech Forensics, Inc.; 10.14: © Lillian Mundt; 10.15a: © Total Care Programming, Inc.; 10.16-10.18: © Lillian Mundt; 10.19: © McGraw-Hill Education/Sandra Mesrine, photographer; 10.20: © Lillian Mundt; 10.21, 10.22: © McGraw-Hill Education/Sandra Mesrine, photographer; 10.23: © Lillian Mundt.

Chapter 11

Opener: © Total Care Programming, Inc.; 11.1: © Lillian Mundt; 11.2: © Total Care Programming, Inc.; 11.3, 11.4: © Lillian Mundt; 11.5: Sickle Cell Foundation of Georgia/Jackie George, Beverly Sinclair/photo by Janice Haney Carr/CDC; 11.6a: © Lillian Mundt; 11.6b: © Marmaduke St. John/Alamy; 11.7a-b: © McGraw-Hill Education/Sandra Mesrine, photographer; 11.7c: © Terry Wild Studio; 11.9: © Total Care Programming, Inc.; 11.10, 11.11, Table 11.4(all), 11.12, 11.13: © Lillian Mundt; 11.14a: © Corbis RF; 11.14b: © SPL/Getty Images; 11.15: © Yoav Levy/Phototake; 11.16: © Lillian Mundt; 11.17: © Total Care Programming, Inc.; 11.18: © Marie Schmitt/BSIP/Corbis; p. 319: © Lillian Mundt.

Chapter 12

Opener: © mjjgm/Getty Images RF; 12.7: © Alamy RF.

Chapter 13

Opener: Adam Gault/Getty Images RF; 13.1, 13.2, 13.4, 13.5, 13.7: © Lillian Mundt; 13.8: © McGraw-Hill Education/Sandra Mesrine, photographer; 13.9: © Lillian Mundt; 13.10: Polymedco, Inc. Photo by Lillian Mundt; 13.11a: © Cliff Moore; 13.11b: Courtesy and © Becton, Dickinson and Company; 13.12: © Cliff Moore; 13.14: © McGraw-Hill Education/Sandra Mesrine, photographer; 13.15a: © Lisa Eastman/Alamy RF; 13.15b: © Leesa Whicker; 13.18: © Beckman Coulter; 13.20: © Total Care Programming, Inc.; 13.21a-b: © Terry Wild Studio; 13.22: © McGraw-Hill Education/Sandra Mesrine, photographer; 13.23, 13.24: © Terry Wild Studio; 13.25: © Quidel Corporation; 13.26: © Getty Images RF; 13.27: © Total Care Programming, Inc.; 13.28a-c: © Lillian Mundt; 13.29a-c: © McGraw-Hill Education/Take One Digital Media, photographer.

Chapter 14

Opener: © Digital Vision/PunchStock RF; 14.1: © Jon Feingersh/Getty Images RF; 14.2: © Tetra Images/Getty Images RF; 14.3: © Ingram Publishing RF; 14.5: © 68/Ocean/Corbis RF.

Appendix F

Figures F.1, F.2: © Interim LSU Hospital Pathology.

Index

Page numbers followed by *f* or *t* indicate material in figures or tables, respectively.

FSP; *see* Fibrin degradation/split products
Full-Scale Burnout Phase, 403
FUO; *see* Fever of unknown origin